Proprioception in Orthopaedics, Sports Medicine and Rehabilitation

Defne Kaya • Baran Yosmaoglu
Mahmut Nedim Doral
Editors

Proprioception in Orthopaedics, Sports Medicine and Rehabilitation

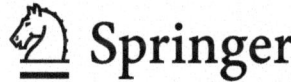 Springer

Editors
Defne Kaya
Department of Physiotherapy
and Rehabilitation
Uskudar University
Faculty of Health Sciences
Istanbul
Turkey

Baran Yosmaoglu
Department of Physiotherapy
and Rehabilitation
Baskent University
Faculty of Health Sciences
Baglıca/Ankara
Turkey

Mahmut Nedim Doral
Faculty of Medicine
Department of Orthopedics
and Traumatology
Ufuk University
Ankara
Turkey

ISBN 978-3-030-09776-9   ISBN 978-3-319-66640-2   (eBook)
https://doi.org/10.1007/978-3-319-66640-2

Printed on acid-free paper

This Springer imprint is published by the registered company Springer International Publishing
AG part of Springer Nature
The registered company address is: Gewerbestrasse 11, 6330 Cham, Switzerland

Preface

This book is dedicated to my father, Zekeriya Kaya, and to my mom, Ayse Kaya, with love. I have been extremely fortunate in my life to have parents who have shown me unconditional love and support.

A special word of thanks also goes to my dear professor, Mahmut Nedim Doral, for his contributions in my life and to be my icebreaker.

A special word of thanks also goes to my dear friend, Baran Yosmaoglu, for his contributions in the present book.

I am grateful for the love, encouragement, and tolerance of my love, Ceyhan Utlu, who has made all the difference in my life.

I am thankful for my sister, Duygu Kaya Yertutanol, the most precious gift in my life.

I wish to express a sincere thank you to all the authors who so graciously agreed to participate in the project.

I am also thankful for all who add value to my life.

Assoc Prof., İstanbul, Turkey, 2018   Defne Kaya

Acknowledgements

The editors would like to thank Mahmut Calik, P.T. and Research Assistant, of Uskudar University, for serving sincerely and for helping us in the process of publishing, especially editing.

Contents

About the Editors

Defne Kaya, Ph.D., M.Sc.   She was born on December 23, 1976, in Cide/ Kastamonu, Turkey. Dr. Kaya completed Master of Science program with her thesis entitled "Effectiveness of high voltage pulsed galvanic stimulation accompanying patellar taping on patellofemoral pain syndrome" in 2001. She worked in the Center for Rehabilitation Science of the University of Manchester for a postdoctoral project entitled "Optimizing physiotherapy in the treatment of patellofemoral pain syndrome" as a researcher for 6 months in 2007. In 2008, she completed her thesis entitled "Muscle strength, functional endurance, coordination, and proprioception in patellofemoral pain syndrome" and received her doctoral degree. Dr. Kaya worked on rehabilitation techniques for orthopedic problems and after orthopedic surgery when she worked as a research assistant from 1999 to 2008. She also worked on rehabilitation after medial patellofemoral ligament surgery in "Abteilung und Poliklinik für Sportorthopadie des Klinikum rechts der Isar der TUM" in September 2008. Dr. Kaya also worked as a researcher in Manchester University, Centre for Rehabilitation Science, Arthritis Research UK in November–December 2010 and September–November 2012.

In 2010, her and her colleagues' paper, which was published in the journal *Sports Health*, titled "The effect of an exercise program in conjunction with short-period patellar taping on pain, electromyogram activity, and muscle strength in patellofemoral pain syndrome," was selected as a suggestion paper by "Australian Sports Commission."

In 2010, at the 10th Turkish Society of Sports Traumatology Arthroscopy and Knee Surgery Congress, her and her colleagues' paper which was titled "Relation between the proprioception, muscle strength, and free-throw in professional basketball player" won the best presentation and young researcher award.

Defne Kaya worked as an associate professor in the Department of Sports Medicine, Faculty of Medicine, Hacettepe University. Now, Dr. Kaya is head of the Physiotherapy and Rehabilitation Department in the Faculty of Health Sciences in Uskudar University, Istanbul. She is also director of the NP Physiotherapy and Rehabilitation Clinic, İstanbul.

She currently studies on the techniques of rehabilitation after ankle injury/ surgery, knee injuries/surgery, shoulder injuries/surgery, rehabilitation after regenerative musculoskeletal surgery, and also patellofemoral pain syndrome.

She is an associate editor of the *Sports Injuries* published by Springer. She is also an editor of the book titled *Forgotten Sixth Sense: The Proprioception* published by OMICS Group.

She is on the editorial board of *Muscle Ligament Tendon Journal*.

Her Academic Members of the Scientific Institutes:

1. Turkish Physiotherapy Association
2. Turkish Sports Injuries, Arthroscopy and Knee Surgery Association
3. Research Center of Hacettepe University Sports Health and Performance.
4. Uskudar University Physical Therapy and Rehabilitation Research Center (USFIZYOTEM)

Hayri Baran Yosmaoglu, P.T., Ph.D. is an associate professor of physiotherapy at Baskent University, Ankara, Turkey. He received his Ph.D. degree from Hacettepe University Institute of Health Science in sports physiotherapy. He studied at Ghent University Motor Rehabilitation Department as an exchange Ph.D. student between 2005 and 2006. After his eight-year career as a research assistant at Hacettepe University, he worked as assistant professor at Baskent University between 2012 and 2013. His research is in the area of orthopedic rehabilitation, adolescent obesity, and sports injuries, particularly on rehabilitation after knee ligament injuries. He has published studies in various high impact journals. He acts as a member of editorial boards of international scientific journals, an executive committee member of Turkish Sport Physiotherapy Association, and a health committee member of Turkish Sports Federation of Disabled Athletes.

Mahmut Nedim Doral, M.D. is internationally recognized for his expertise in orthopedic sports medicine. He has authored over 150 scientific articles (more than 70 international and 100 national publications) in peer-reviewed journals and over 15 book chapters in internationally published books, and he acts as a referee in five international and four national journals. Recently, the book *Sports Injuries: Prevention, Diagnosis, Treatment and Rehabilitation* edited by Prof. Doral was published by Springer-Verlag. His major research interests are in sports injuries and rehabilitation, arthroscopic and endoscopic surgery, basic science research in tendon injuries, and knee arthroplasty since 1984. He was the Chairman of the Department of Orthopaedics and Traumatology at the Hacettepe University/Medical Faculty and the founder of the Department of Sports Medicine at the same University.

He has been the director of Hacettepe University Sports Medicine Center since 1995. He is the board member (2003–2009), program committee member and membership committee chairman (2007–2011), and archive committee member (2011–2019) of the International Society of Arthroscopy, Knee Surgery and Orthopaedic Sports Medicine (ISAKOS) and is on the scientific board of European Society of Sports Traumatology Knee Surgery and Arthroscopy (ESSKA). He also currently serves as Executive Council of Turkish National Olympic Committee.

Dr. Doral served as the President of Turkish Society of Orthopaedics and Traumatology (TOTBID) (2010–2011) and Turkish Arthroscopy, Knee Surgery and Sports Traumatology Society (2004–2006). He was the Past President of European Federation of Orthopaedic Sports Traumatology (EFOST) (2000–2003), Asia-Pacific Knee Society (APKS/Knee Section of APOA) (2004–2006), and Turkish Society of Sports Traumatology Arthroscopy and Knee Surgery (2002–2004); he is the elected president of APOA (Asia-Pacific Orthopaedic Society; 2018–2020). Prof. Doral is the Past Chief of Staff/Medical Committee Turkish Federation of National Basketball Team. He is the founder and current president of Turkish Society of Sports Traumatology. He was honored with distinguished visiting professor in the University of Pittsburgh School of Engineering in 2006 and Kentucky University in 2009.

Part I

Basics Knowledge of the Proprioception

Neurophysiology and Assessment of the Proprioception

Defne Kaya, Fatma Duygu Kaya Yertutanol, and Mahmut Calik

1.1 Introduction

Julius Caesar Scaliger was the first person who described the position-movement sensation as a "sense of locomotion" in 1557. After centuries in 1826, Charles Bell proposed that the information about the muscle's position were sent from muscles to brain which is in the opposite direction of motor comments. Bell's idea was noteworthy as explaining one of the first physiologic feedback mechanisms. In 1880, Henry Charlton Bastian suggested another term as "kinesthesia" instead of "muscle sense" to point out that afferent information was originating not only from muscles but also from joints, skin, and tendons. Alfred Goldscheider, a German neurologist, classified kinesthesia as muscle, tendon, and articular sensitivity in 1889. Finally in 1906, Charles Scott Sherrington introduced the terms "proprioception," "interoception,"

and "exteroception." "Exteroceptors" are sense organs such as eyes, ears, mouth, and skin that receive information from outside of the body, while "interoceptors" provide information about internal organs. On the other hand, "proprioception" is defined as awareness of movement and posture derived from muscle, tendon, and joint [1].

Movements of body parts are controlled by the functions of somatosensory and sensorimotor systems. Collective functioning of these systems is essential for an efficient proprioceptive sense. A *somatosensory system* consists of the sensory receptors, sensory neurons in the peripheral structures, and deeper neurons in the cortical structures. Receptors of somatosensory system are classified as thermoreceptors, photoreceptors, mechanoreceptors, and chemoreceptors. These receptors receive peripheral somesthetic (somatic) sense such as proprioceptive, tactile, thermal, and nociceptive information from skin and epithelia, skeletal muscles, bones and joints, internal organs, and cardiovascular system and transmit them to cortical structures. Meissner's corpuscles, Pacinian corpuscles, Merkel's disks, and Ruffini's corpuscles which encapsulated mechanoreceptors are specialized to provide information to the central nervous system about touch, pressure, vibration, and cutaneous tension [2]. *Sensorimotor system* functions in a highly ordered fashion, where association cortex executes general commands and lower levels as motor neurons and muscles are interested in the

D. Kaya, Ph.D., M.Sc., P.T. (✉) • M. Calik, P.T.
Department of Physiotherapy and Rehabilitation, Faculty of Health Sciences, Uskudar University, Istanbul, Turkey
e-mail: defne.kaya@uskudar.edu.tr; mahmut.calik@uskudar.edu.tr

F.D.K. Yertutanol, M.D., Ph.D.
Department of Psychology, Faculty of Humanities and Social Sciences, Uskudar University, Istanbul, Turkey
e-mail: fatmaduygu.kayayertutanol@uskudar.edu.tr

details. This hierarchical arrangement enables higher level structures to focus on complex functions. The role of the hierarchically organized sensorimotor system is to generate motor output that is guided by sensory input and to learn the changes of the nature and locus of sensorimotor control [3]. On the other hand, sensorimotor system is part of the peripheral nervous system associated with the voluntary control of body movements via skeletal muscles. This system consists of efferent nerves which stimulate muscle contraction, including all non-sensory neurons connected with skeletal muscles and skin [4]. Sensory information influences the way we execute motor responses.

Purpose of this chapter is to introduce neurophysiological pathway of the proprioceptive sense. Proprioception (metaphorically is also called the "sixth sense"), kinesthesia, and neuromuscular control are often used interchangeably.

Proprioceptive sense is more than just a feeling of movement, while proprioception represents the sense of awareness of joint position and kinesthesia describes the sensation of joint movement (see the summary of the proprioception in Fig. 1.1). Afferent signals from mechano- and cutaneous receptors are important to control joint movement (kinesthesia) and joint position (joint position sense). Massive proprioceptive input from specialized nerve endings originating from the muscles, fascia, tendons, ligaments, joints, and skin enters the dorsal horn of the spinal cord and is carried towards subcortical and cortical parts of the brain. Many neural pathways synapse at various levels of the nervous system, integrating all body position information to provide us with both a conscious and a nonconscious sense of where we are and how we are moving. We know where to place our extremities and how to move smoothly, accurately in different positions such as

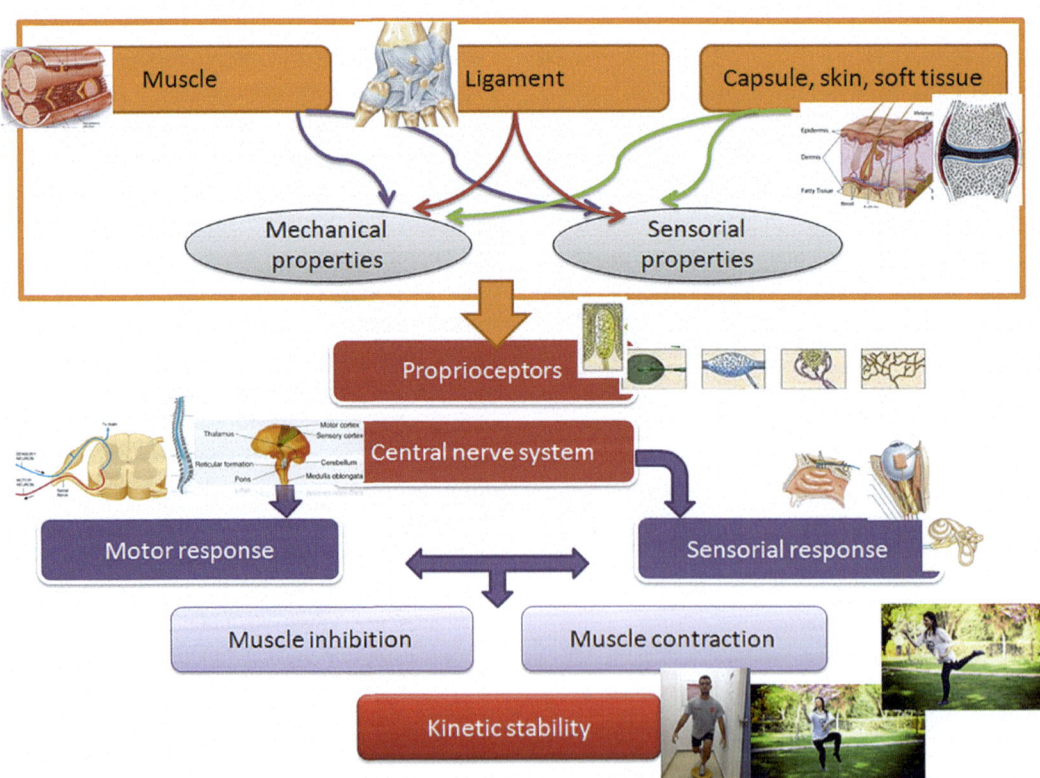

Fig. 1.1 Summary of the proprioception

standing, sliding, and turning with our eyes closed using proprioceptive or position-movement sense. In the case of an injury or a trauma, proprioceptors can be damaged. There is a discussion on whether proprioceptive deficits make individuals more vulnerable to injury or not [5]. Loss of this inner sense of timing and accuracy will lead to more severe injuries to occur and, of course, simple movements would take up an enormous amount of cognitive energy [5, 6].

1.2   Proprioceptive Receptors and Pathways

1.2.1   Peripheral Receptors and Pathway of Proprioception

Mechanoreceptors (proprioceptors) are also known as "receptors for self." Low-threshold mechanoreceptors such as muscle spindles, Golgi tendon organs, and joint mechanoreceptors receive sensory information and provide accurate complex body movements. Proprioceptors are also merged with the vestibular system to carry information about the position and motion of the head.

Muscle spindles are composed of approximately four to eight specialized intrafusal muscle fibers which are arranged in parallel with extrafusal fibers. The primary role of muscle spindles is to provide information about muscle length. Muscles that control fine movements contain more muscle spindles than do the muscles that control gross movements. Primary innervation is carried out by group I axons and the axon terminals are known as the primary sensory ending of the muscle spindle. Secondary innervation is provided by group II axons that innervate the nuclear chain fibers and give off a minor branch to the nuclear bag fibers. The intrafusal muscle fibers are innervated by γ motor neurons, which are derived from a pool of specialized neurons in the spinal cord. Unlike Golgi tendon organ, the muscle spindle doesn't relay signals through motor cortex; thus it isn't a feedback loop [7, 8].

Origin and insertion points of Golgi tendon organ (GTO), a sensory proprioceptor, are muscle fibers and tendons of skeletal muscles, respectively. Motor cortex inhibits muscle contraction in case of the excessive tension of the GTO. Muscle contractions which stimulate group Ib afferents lead the sensory terminals to compress by force. Group Ib sensory feedback generates spinal reflexes and supraspinal responses which control muscle contraction. Ib afferents synapse with interneurons that are within the spinal cord which also project to cerebellum and cerebral cortex. Golgi tendon organs are involved in cerebellar regulation of movement via dorsal and ventral spinocerebellar tracts [7, 8].

1.2.2   Ruffini Endings, Pacinian Corpuscles, and Golgi-Like Receptors Are Joint Mechanoreceptors

Ruffini endings, which are constantly reactive during joint motion, are slow-adapted and low-threshold receptors. Ruffini endings are very critical receptors in the regulation of stiffness and preparatory control of the muscles around the joint because they react to axial loading and tensile strain in the ligament [9]. *Pacinian corpuscles (deep pressure receptors)* (also known as lamellar corpuscles) are small, oval bodies that are found in deep layers of the skin and close to the GTOs. Pacinian corpuscles are rapidly adapted, high-threshold receptors and they are sensitive to mechanical disturbances such as joint acceleration/deceleration. They are also sensitive to quick movement and deep pressure [10]. Golgi-like ending, belonging to the same family as Ruffini ending, is silent during the rest and only active at the extremes of joint motion. Golgi-like receptors are important in monitoring tensile strain in the ligament during ultimate angles of joint motion [11].

Peripheral "ligamento-muscular reflexes" are also important for organizing peripheral proprioceptive reactions. These spinal reflexes are highly complex reactions that maintain adequate motor control of the joint [12]. Mono- and polysynaptic spinal reflexes between the ligaments in a joint and the muscles acting on that joint are well known and transmitted to the dorsal horn of the spinal cord [12, 13]. *Monosynaptic reflex* (such as a H-reflex), which is the fastest (within 20 ms after stimulation) and the simplest joint protective spinal reflex, can carry the peripheral information from skin, joints, ligaments, soft tissues, and tendons to the dorsal horn and directly stimulate the anterior horn for initial appropriate muscle contraction. As known, nerves carrying information from peripheral structures have the physiological properties necessary to compose initial joint protective reflexes. Delayed or earlier monosynaptic reflexes can cause uncontrolled joint motion and injury [14]. The efferent-muscular reaction can be caused by the *polysynaptic reflexes* with two or more interneurons [15]. The reflexes from cortical level are arranged by feed-forward inhibition, while reflexes from peripheral input are arranged by feed-back inhibition. Additionally, these inhibition systems are so critical to arrange the velocity, onset, and termination of motions. Spinal level reflexes can be controlled by muscle activity of the agonist and antagonist muscles which are influenced by feed-forward and feed-back inhibition systems [16].

1.3 Propriospinal Neurons and Pathway of Proprioception

Propriospinal system is a system that transmits motor inputs from supraspinal centers to motoneurons of spinal cord. Neurons of this system consist of spinal interneurons with their soma located in grey matter and their axons constitute white matter of spinal cord and terminate within it. These propriospinal neurons are settled rostral to motoneurons of spinal cord and can project to different locations like other spinal segments (intersegmental) or within that segment (intrasegmental). In contrary to the definition, it is important to note that some propriospinal neurons can also project to supraspinal areas [17].

Most of the studies related to propriospinal system come from studies on cats. Data coming from human studies are limited compared to animal studies. There are two basic kinds of propriospinal neurons: short axon propriospinal neurons and long axon propriospinal neurons [18]. Short axon propriospinal neurons project to within six spinal segments, whereas long axon propriospinal neurons reach beyond six spinal segments [18].

Short axon propriospinal projections may be classified as cervical and lumbosacral propriospinal projections, short thoracic propriospinal projections, and thoracic respiratory interneurons [18]. Cervical propriospinal projection which is also known as C3–C4 premotoneuronal system was defined in cats to mediate target-reaching movements [19]. The same system is thought to modulate corticospinal input to upper limb in humans [19]. On the other hand lumbosacral propriospinal projections transmit descending inputs to lower limb motoneurons. Short thoracic propriospinal projections were implicated for the control of axial muscles and thoracic respiratory interneurons were shown to receive respiratory drive to coordinate respiratory movements [18].

Long axon propriospinal projections are divided into long descending propriospinal tract projections, long ascending propriospinal tract projections, and upper cervical inspiratory interneurons [18]. Long descending propriospinal tract neurons are located in the cervical enlargement and project to the lumbosacral enlargement whereas long ascending propriospinal tract projections are located in the lumbosacral enlargement and project to the cervical enlargement. These neurons are thought to coordinate limb movements reciprocally during locomotion [17]. Upper cervical inspiratory interneurons project to intercostal and phrenic motoneurons and modulate inputs of brain stem to respiratory motoneurons [20].

In summary, the role of propriospinal system is to modulate descending and peripheral inputs for locomotion and autonomic and respiratory functions [18]. Thus, it functions as an integrating system for the inputs of cortical structures and the afferent feedback from limbs [19].

1.4 Cortical Receptors and Pathway of Proprioception

The excitatory and inhibitor synapses with afferent neurons help to carry peripheral proprioceptive information to higher cortical levels. Muscle, skin, ligament, and joint afferents and descending pathways are like a busy network of motorways. Somatosensorial information, which is sent from peripheral receptors via sensory nerves and tracts, is interpreted in the primary somatosensory area in the parietal lobe of cerebral cortex [2]. There are three neurons in somatosensory pathway. The first neuron is in dorsal root ganglion of spinal nerve. Ascending axons of the second neuron, which is in spinal cord, decussate to opposite side in the spinal cord. Axons of many of these neurons terminate in thalamus; others terminate in the reticular system or cerebellum. The third neuron is in thalamus and ends in postcentral gyrus of parietal lobe [21].

Corticospinal tract is the descending link between motor cortex and alfa and gamma motor neurons [22]. The kinesthetic information from muscle afferents of upper limbs is carried to cortex by *dorsal (posterior) columns*. The kinesthetic information from muscle afferents of lower limbs is carried to cortex by *Clarke's column* and *dorsal spinocerebellar tract*. The ascending pathways in spinal cord such as the *dorsal column medial lemniscal* and the *ventral spinothalamic pathways* carry information from body to brain and make a synapse in thalamus or reticular formation, before they reach cortex. The role of *ventral* and *dorsal spinocerebellar tracts*, which project to cerebellum, is to control posture and balance [21]. Cerebellum is responsible for coordinated motor movement. Cerebellum plans and modifies motor activities via *spinocerebellar tract*, which has a role in the regulation of gamma-MN drive to muscle spindles [23]. Spinocerebellar tract can carry peripheral information from skin, joint structures, and muscles to medulla, cerebellum, and dorsal column.

Kinesthesia and joint position sense (independent of vision) are provided by intact and appropriate cerebellar function, which is influenced by peripheral information from muscle spindles and skin-stretch receptors [24] (see the summary of supraspinal reactions of proprioception in Fig. 1.2).

1.5 Peripheral Assessment Techniques of Proprioception

Proprioceptive measurements are performed to assess the quality of the proprioceptive function. Measurements are usually based on testing the quality of perception for some of the above-mentioned deep sense by CNS in various ways. However a highly appreciated by all researchers in proprioception measurements, practical, easily repeatable testing method that provides complete measurement of perception or response is not developed yet. The most frequent proprioception measurement methods following orthopedic injury/surgery/rehabilitation are joint position reproduction (JPR)—also known as joint position matching—threshold to detection of passive motion (TTDPM), and active movement extent discrimination assessment (AMEDA) [25]. Joint position sense, kinesthesia, and tension (force) sense are considered as subtitles of conscious proprioceptive sense and evaluated by using various techniques. Proprioceptive sense is usually evaluated both with and without body weight on the extremity. While performing the test using weight on the extremity, functional position is used; therefore proprioceptive information received due to compression would be more [26]. Joint position sense is tested in such a way that the patient actively and passively repeats the tested degree. Joint position sense test measures the certainty of repeatability of a particular position and performed actively and passively both open and closed kinetic chain positions. Repeating joint degrees are measured with direct (goniometer, potentiometer, video) and indirect

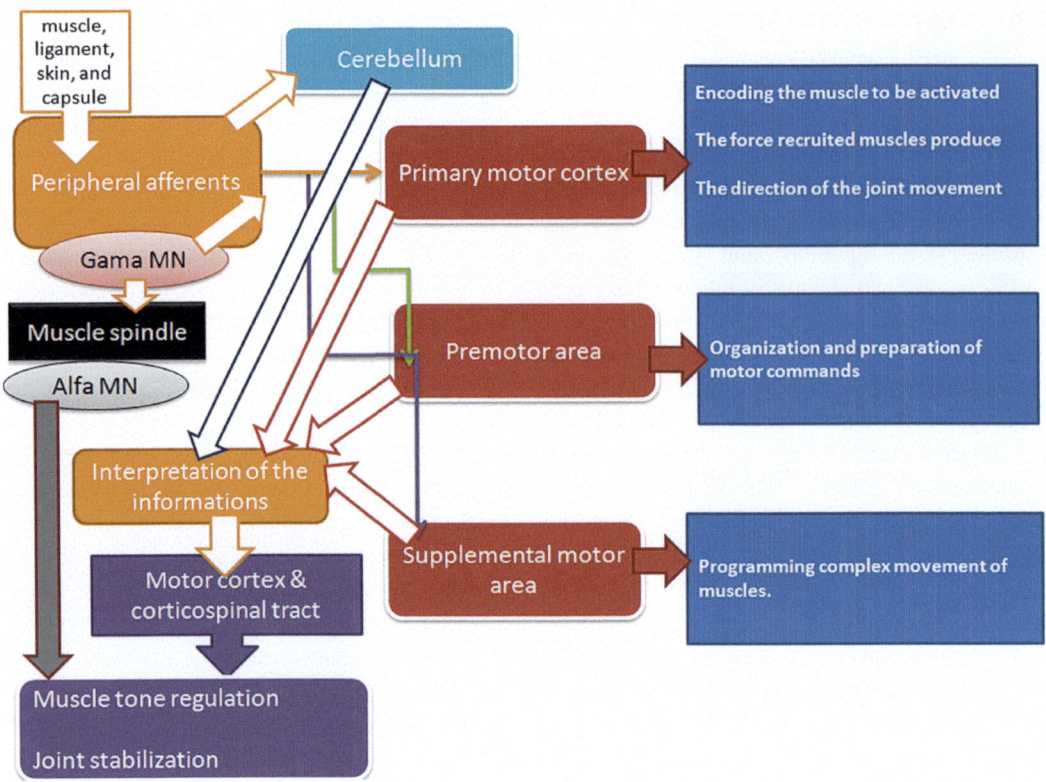

Fig. 1.2 Summary of the cortical pathways of the proprioception

(visual analog criterion) methods. Kinesthesia is evaluated by measuring threshold value for determining passive movement and more exclusively by finding out the threshold value of direction of movement. Accordingly not only the movement is defined but also the direction of the movement that generated. Tension (force) sense is measured by comparing the ability of people to repeat the magnitudes of torque that is produced under different circumstances by a group of muscles. To evaluate conscious proprioception, devices are built that follow various isokinetic dynamometers and electromagnetic trail. The objective of future studies is to verify conscious proprioceptive tension by measuring afferent pathway action potentials simultaneously (e.g., microneurography) and to compare the lack of sensorimotor control on dynamic joint stability and reduction in conscious proprioception [27]. Either rate of

perception or tension of movement is measured in proprioception tests. Vibration sense is as much important as other deep senses in perceiving a joint's position, movement, and forces effecting on that joint. Basic studies showed that low-frequency vibration is perceived with Meissner's corpuscles and high-frequency vibration is perceived with Pacini corpuscles and thus is participated in the proprioceptive process [28]. Gilman [29] stated that the neural paths of position and vibration senses are same; however, mechanoreceptors that perceive these senses are different, in some of the diseases, and receptors of one sense can be kept healthy while receptors of the other sense are damaged. Vibration is explained in such a way that it affects both kinesthesia and position sense and participates in proprioceptive process directly [30, 31].

Key Knowledge

Active joint degree repetition is objectively evaluated using isokinetic system. Before undergoing the test, normal warming process should be performed, person should be blindfolded through the test, and distal part of its extremity should be put into pressure splint. The degree to be evaluated must be shown to the person eyes-open and blindfolded three times before the test. Six times repetition of each degree is necessary and the result will be their averages.

Passive joint degree repetition is objectively evaluated using isokinetic system. Before undergoing the test, normal warming process should be performed, person should be blindfolded through the test, and distal part of its extremity should be put into pressure splint. Data collection begins with the joint placed in a starting position of 0°. The test begins with the tester passively moving the test limb into a position of target (reference) angle and maintaining that position for 10 s. After 10 s of static positioning, the joint is moved back passively from the target angle to the starting position. The subject is asked to passively reproduce the previously presented test angle as a target (reference) angle. Six trials are performed on each joint, with a mean value in degrees of passive movement calculated. Passive movement speed should be at 0.50° or less. Angular displacement is recorded as the error in degrees between the target angle and the repositioned angle. The mean of the six trials for each tested condition is calculated to determine an average error in scores.

1.6   Cortical Assessment Techniques of Proprioception

Joint mechanoreceptors are negatively affected after injury and/or surgery. A few studies showed decreased somatosensory evoked potentials

(SEPs) after anterior cruciate ligament injury and/or surgery [32, 33].

Electroencephalography (EEG) and functional magnetic resonance imaging (fMRI) techniques were used to determine decreased proprioceptive sense after injury and/or surgery at cortical level in very limited number of studies [34, 35]. Using EEG and fMRI techniques, the pattern of whole-brain activity during motion of isolated joints of lower limb, the somatotopic organization of lower limb joint representations in primary sensorimotor cortex and anterior lobe of the cerebellum, and the degree of overlap between these lower limb joint activations should be investigated [34, 36]. Large prospective longitudinal studies are needed to detect the influence of cortical and peripheral proprioceptive sense after injury and/or surgery.

Practical Key Points
Example 1: Ankle Joint Position Sense Measurement Technique:
Proprioception level after endoscopically guided percutaneous Achilles tendon [37].
Ankle proprioception was defined as the ability to match reference ankle joint angles (the "target angle") without visual feedback. Joint position sense was measured by active angle reproduction (AAR) using a Biodex system 3 dynamometer (Biodex Corp., Shirley, NY, USA). The dynamometer was calibrated according to the manufacturer's instructions prior to each testing session; data were read from the on-screen goniometer. Patients sat upright with knee flexed to approximately 20, the seat back tilted 100, and their barefoot in a neutral position. They were asked to close their eyes during testing to eliminate visual input. For each repetition, the patients moved their limb to the target angle of either 10 for dorsiflexion or 15 for plantar flexion actively. These midrange angles were selected in an attempt to maximize

sensory input from muscle proprioceptors. When patients felt they had reached the target angle, they activated the stop button and were not permitted to correct the angle. The angle was recorded from the on-screen goniometer; this process was repeated six times for each target angle. A total of six readings were taken, and the difference between the perceived angle and each of the target angles 10 for dorsiflexion or 15 for plantar flexion was noted as the absolute error and an average absolute error calculated for each trial.

Example 2: Knee Joint Position Sense Measurement Technique:

Is there a relationship between tracking ability, joint position sense, and functional level in patellofemoral pain syndrome? [38].

Joint position sense was measured by active reproduction test in the functional squat system. Functional squat system® is a valid tool assessing joint proprioception (2008, http://www.nhmi.net/validity_and_reliability_of_the_monitored_rehab.php) in clinical setting. Subjects were positioned in supine with the test knee flexed 90 while the opposite foot was resting on device. A load of 20% bodyweight as previously determined was applied during test performance. As they viewed the device monitor, subjects were instructed to keep the cursor on a defined pathway which provided them with continual knee position feedback. Following this, subjects were instructed to return to the start position of 90 knee flexion and attempt to replicate the reference knee position without visual feedback of the cursor. The difference in linear cursor position between the reference and reproduction trial was calculated by device software. This value represented error during active joint angle reproduction testing.

References

1. Smith R. "The sixth sense": towards a history of muscular sensation. Gesnerus. 2011;68(2):218–71.
2. Purves D. The somatic sensory system: touch and proprioception: primary somatic sensory cortex. In: Pulves D, Agustine GJ, Fitzpatrick D, et al., editors. Neuroscience. 5th ed. Sunderland, MA: Sinauer Associates; 2012. p. 202–3.
3. Weiss C, Tsakiris M, Haggard P, et al. Agency in the sensorimotor system and its relation to explicit action awareness. Neuropsychologia. 2014;52:82–92.
4. Riemann BL, Lephart SM. The sensorimotor system, part I: the physiologic basis of functional joint stability. J Athl Train. 2002;37(1):71–9.
5. Irrgang JJ, Whitney SL, Cox ED. Balance and proprioceptive training for rehabilitation of the lower extremity. J Sport Rehabil. 1994;3:68–83.
6. LaRiviere J, Osternig LR. The effect of ice immersion on joint sense position. J Sport Rehabil. 1994;3:58–67.
7. Taylor A, Durbaba R, Ellaway PH, et al. Static and dynamic gamma-motor output to ankle flexor muscles during locomotion in the decerebrate cat. J Physiol. 2006;571:711–23. https://doi.org/10.1113/jphysiol.2005.101634.
8. Prochazka A, Gorassini M. Ensemble firing of muscle afferents recorded during normal locomotion in cats. J Physiol. 1998;507:293–304.
9. Grigg P, Hoffman AH. Stretch-sensitive afferent neurons in cat knee joint capsule: sensitivity to axial and compression stresses and strains. J Neurophysiol. 1996;75:1871–7.
10. Collins DF, Refshauge KM, Todd G, et al. Cutaneous receptors contribute to kinesthesia at the index finger, elbow, and knee. J Neurophysiol. 2005;94:1699–706.
11. Johansson H, Sjolander P, Sojka P. A sensory role for the cruciate ligaments. Clin Orthop. 1991;268:161–78.
12. Hagert E, Persson JKE, Werner M, et al. Evidence of wrist proprioceptive reflexes elicited after stimulation of the scapholunate interosseous ligament. J Hand Surg Am. 2009;34:642–51.
13. Diederichsen LP, Norregaard J, Krogsgaard M, et al. Reflexes in the shoulder muscles elicited from the human coracoacromial ligament. J Orthop Res. 2004;22:976–83.
14. Solomonow M, Krogsgaard M. Sensorimotor control of knee stability. A review. Scand J Med Sci Sports. 2001;11:64–80.
15. Bawa P, Chalmers GR, Jones KE, et al. Control of the wrist joint in humans. Eur J Appl Physiol. 2000;83:116–27.
16. Alstermark B, Lundberg A, Sasaki S. Integration in descending motor pathways controlling the forelimb in the cat. 12. Interneurons which may mediate descending feed-forward inhibition and feed-back

inhibition from the forelimb to C3–C4 propriospinal neurones. Exp Brain Res. 1984;56:308–22.

17. Flynn JR, Graham BA, Galea MP, et al. The role of propriospinal interneurons in recovery from spinal cord injury. Neuropharmacology. 2011;60(5):809–22.

18. Conta A, Stelzner DJ. The propriospinal system. In: Watson C, Paxinos G, Kayalioglu G, editors. The spinal cord a Christopher and Dana Reeve foundation text and atlas. New York: Academic Press; 2009. p. 180–90.

19. Pierrot-Deseilligny E, Burke D. Propriospinal transmission of descending motor commands. In: Pierrot-Deseilligny E, Burke D, editors. The circuitry of the human spinal cord. 2nd ed. Cambridge: Cambridge University Press; 2012. p. 395–445.

20. Lipski J, Duffin J, Kruszewska B, et al. Upper cervical inspiratory neurons in the rat: an electrophysiological and morphological study. Exp Brain Res. 1993;95(3):477–87.

21. Augustine JR. Human neuroanatomy. San Diego: Academic Press; 2008.

22. Johansson H, Pedersen J, Bergenheim M, et al. Peripheral afferents of the knee: their effects on central mechanisms regulating muscle stiffness, joint stability and proprioception and coordination. In: Lephart SM, Fu FH, editors. Proprioception and neuromuscular control in joint stability. Champaign, IL: Human Kinetics; 2000. p. 5–22.

23. Dye SF. The functional anatomy of the cerebellum: an overview. In: Lephart SM, Fu FH, editors. Proprioception and neuromuscular control in: joint stability. Champaign, IL: Human Kinetic; 2000. p. 31–5.

24. Proske U, Gandevia SC. The kinaesthetic senses. J Physiol. 2009;587:4139–46.

25. Beynnon BD, Renström PA, Konradsen L, et al. Validation of techniques to measure knee proprioception. In: Lephart SM, Fu FH, editors. Proprioception and neuromuscular control in joint stability. Champaign, IL: Human Kinetics; 2000. p. 127–39.

26. Baker V, Bennell K, Stillman B, et al. Abnormal knee joint position sense in individuals with patellofemoral pain syndrome. J Orthop Res. 2002;20:208–14.

27. Riemann BL, Myers JB, Lephart SM. Sensorimotor system measurement techniques. J Athl Train. 2002;37:85–98.

28. Hall JE. Somatic sensations: I. General organization, the tactile and position senses. In: Guyton and hall textbook of medical physiology. 13th ed. Philadelphia, PA: Elsevier, Saunders; 2016. p. 607–21.

29. Gilman S. Joint position sense and vibration sense: anatomical organisation and assessment. J Neurol Neurosurg Psychiatry. 2002;73:473–7.

30. Collins DF, Refshauge KM, Gandevia SC. Sensory integration in the perception of movements at the human metacarpophalangeal joint. J Physiol. 2000;529:505–15.

31. Sorensen KL, Hollands MA, Patla E. The effects of human ankle muscle vibration on posture and balance during adaptive locomotion. Exp Brain Res. 2002;143:24–34.

32. Ochi M, Iwasa J, Uchio Y, et al. The regeneration of sensory neurones in the reconstruction of the anterior cruciate ligament. J Bone Jt Surg Br. 1999;81(5):902–6.

33. Valeriani M, Restuccia D, Di Lazzaro V, et al. Clinical and neurophysiological abnormalities before and after reconstruction of the anterior cruciate ligament of the knee. Acta Neurol Scand. 1999;99:303–7.

34. Kapreli E, Athanasopoulos S, Papathanasiou M, et al. Lower limb sensorimotor network: issues of somatotopy and overlap. Cortex. 2007;43(2):219–32.

35. Callaghan MJ, McKie S, Richardson P, et al. Magnetic resonance imaging knee joint proprioception tests using functional effects. Phys Ther. 2012;92:821–30.

36. Baumeister J, Reinecke K, Weiss M. Changed cortical activity after anterior cruciate ligament reconstruction in a joint position paradigm: an EEG study. Scand J Med Sci Sports. 2008;18:473–84.

37. Kaya D, Doral MN, Nyland J, et al. Proprioception level after endoscopically guided percutaneous Achilles tendon. Knee Surg Sports Traumatol Arthrosc. 2013;21(6):1238–44.

38. Yosmaoglu HB, Kaya D, Guney H, et al. Is there a relationship between tracking ability, joint position sense, and functional level in patellofemoral pain syndrome? Knee Surg Sports Traumatol Arthrosc. 2013;21(11):2564–71.

Posture, Kinesthesia, Foot Sensation, Balance, and Proprioception

2

John Nyland, Tiffany Franklin, Adam Short, Mahmut Calik, and Defne Kaya

2.1 Introduction

In their comparative model study, Freeman and Wyke [1] confirmed that activation of ankle joint mechanoreceptors in lightly anesthetized, neutrally intact cats leads to reciprocally coordinated leg muscle motor unit reflex activation changes. Destruction of articular mechanoreceptors or interruption of their afferent nerve fibers was found to abolish these reflexes during passive ankle joint movement [1]. Study findings supported the contention that articular mechanoreceptor reflexes functioned polysynaptically through the gamma motor neuron loop to control leg muscle tone and coordinate standing posture and movement [1].

Appreciation for the close synergism between capsuloligamentous and musculotendinous structures to maintain dynamic joint stability continues to grow [2–4]. The application of significant loads to ligament-embedded mechanoreceptors transmits neural signals via articular nerves directly to the central nervous system where synapses activate select muscles crossing the ankle joint to dynamically stiffen it, preserving dynamic joint stability. Restoration of dynamic joint stability is an essential component of functional rehabilitation programs.

J. Nyland, D.P.T., S.C.S., Ed.D., A.T.C. (✉)
T. Franklin, M.A., L.A.T., A.T.C.
Kosair Charities College of Health and Natural Sciences, Spalding University, Louisville, KY, USA
e-mail: jnyland@spalding.edu; tfranklin@spalding.edu

A. Short, M.D.
Department of Orthopaedic Surgery, University of Louisville, Louisville, KY, USA
e-mail: adamtylershort@gmail.com

M. Calik, P.T. • D. Kaya, Ph.D., M.Sc., P.T.
Department of Physiotherapy and Rehabilitation, Faculty of Health Sciences, Uskudar University, Istanbul, Turkey
e-mail: mahmut.calik@uskudar.edu.tr; defne.kaya@uskudar.edu.tr

2.2 Foot-Subtalar-Ankle Functional Anatomy

In the cat, a reflex arc exists from ankle deltoid ligament mechanoreceptors to the intrinsic muscles of the foot [4]. Pyar [5] first proposed the existence of a "ligamento-muscular protective reflex." In humans, as the deltoid ligament becomes stressed with eversion of the foot, intrinsic foot muscles such as the quadratus plantae, flexor digitorum brevis, abductor digiti minimi, and the halluces are activated to increase dynamic foot stability, control align-

© Springer International Publishing AG, part of Springer Nature 2018
D. Kaya et al. (eds.), *Proprioception in Orthopaedics, Sports Medicine and Rehabilitation*, https://doi.org/10.1007/978-3-319-66640-2_2

ment, regulate the rate of pronation, and maintain foot arch height, thereby relieving deltoid ligament stress [6]. Such a function provides a direct response to the instability created by the eversion and the biomechanical foundation that explains the reflex. The intrinsic foot muscles act as a single functional unit, are mostly active throughout the stance phase (from heel strike to toe off) and are highly active during toe off. Anatomically and biomechanically, these muscles, along with the lower leg muscles, stabilize the talonavicular, calcaneocuboid, and metatarsophalangeal joints. By stabilizing various foot joints, the arch is maintained during the weight-bearing portion of gait, thus preventing the load from flattening the foot, creating eversion stresses that increase mechanical instability [4, 7]. It is important to note that although the intrinsic foot muscles do not cross the ankle, they have a powerful effect on keeping the ankle, subtalar, and adjacent foot joints aligned and stable in the face of loads and forces that may cause eversion instability. This is in contrast to the ligamento-muscular reflex arcs that have been described at the knee and shoulder, which always make use of muscles that cross the joint to mitigate tibiofemoral or glenohumeral capsuloligamentous joint stresses, respectively.

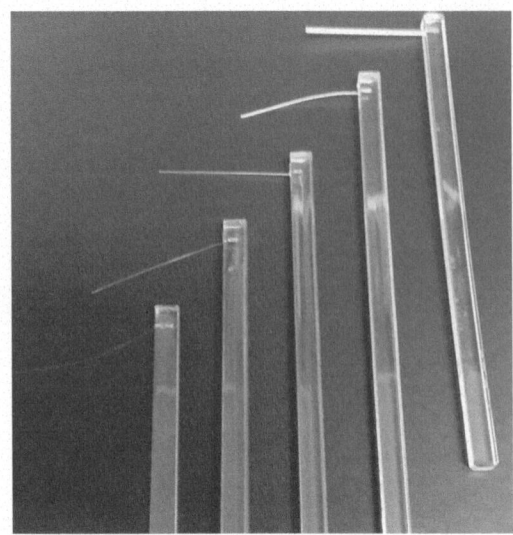

Fig. 2.1 Semmes-Weinstein monofilament sensory test instruments

2.3   Foot Mechanoreception

The detection of mechanical stimuli by the foot is vital to balance control during standing and walking in healthy subjects [8]. Clinically, sensory malfunction at the foot may cause substantial impairments and compensatory postures and movements, as in cases of patients with diabetes who suffer from neuropathic conditions. For standing balance control, especially under eyes-closed and unipedal stance conditions, foot-sole anesthesia increases the center of pressure length displacement and velocity and thus influences mediolateral as well as anteroposterior posture control [9].

Using Semmes-Weinstein monofilament test methods (Fig. 2.1), Hennig and Sterzing [10] reported that the least sensitive foot touch regions are the heel (P1), followed by the most proximal

site on the foot dorsum (D1), the medial and lateral malleoli (M1, L1), and the Achilles tendon (A1) (Fig. 2.2a, b). The medial longitudinal arch (P2) and the plantar (P8, P9, and P10) as well as the dorsal (D8, D9, D10) toe regions are the most sensitive touch regions. The most sensitive sites for vibration recognition are the heel and medial mid-foot area below the longitudinal arch (P1, P2, P3).

Fast-adapting mechanoreceptors which are particularly sensitive to sudden skin displacement changes are vital during initial foot strike [10]. Studies have reported [10, 12] a lower density of slowly adapting (Ruffini) mechanoreceptors compared to fast-adapting (Pacini) mechanoreceptors in the foot heel region. The vibration sensitivities of all plantar locations, except for the toes, had the lowest threshold values. These are structures that are essential to the recognition of foot placement throughout the contact phase of gait. Unevenness of the ground and unexpected slips can be detected by fast-adapting skin mechanoreceptors that serve as a feedback mechanism for balance maintenance and/or recovery. Kennedy and Inglis [12] reported that 70% of the mechanoreceptors under the foot represented the fast-adapting (Pacini) type. The recognition of sudden load and displacement changes under the foot is an important component of whole-body neuromo-

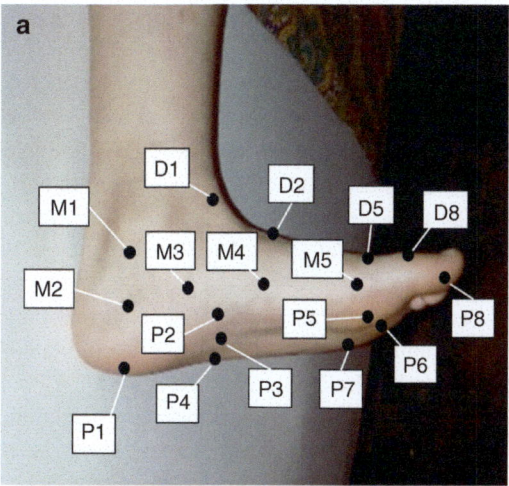

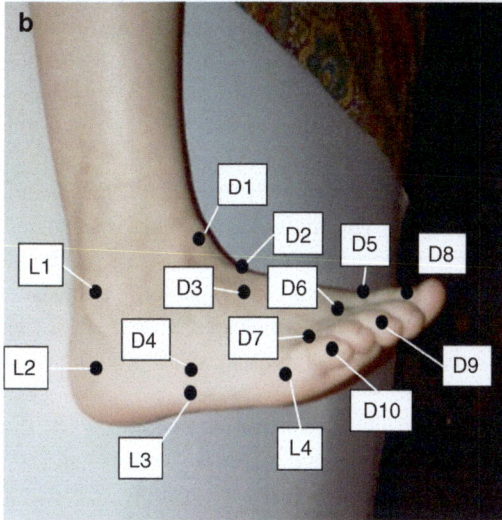

Fig. 2.2 (a) (medial view) and (b) (lateral view). Semmes-Weinstein filament test locations [11]. P1 = heel, P2 = medial arch, P3 = intermediate arch, P4 = lateral arch, P5 = first metatarsal head, P6 = third metatarsal head, P7 = fifth metatarsal head, P8 = center of hallux, P9 = distal phalanx 3 (not shown), P10 = distal phalanx 5 (not shown); D1 = articularis talocruralis, D2 = first metatarsal base, D3 = third metatarsal base, D4 = fifth metatarsal base, D5 = first metatarsal head, D6 = third metatarsal head, D7 = fifth metatarsal head, D8 = doral distal phalanx 1, D9 = dorsal distal phalanx 3, D10 = dorsal distal phalanx 5; M1 = medial malleolus, M2 = medial calcaneus, M3 = base of navicular, M4 = base of first metatarsal, M5 = head of first metatarsal; L1 = lateral malleolus, L2 = lateral calcaneus, L3 = base of fifth metatarsal, L4 = head of fifth metatarsal [11]

tor adjustments and learning [10]. Rehabilitation clinicians need to better consider these kinesiological relationships when designing therapeutic exercise programs for individuals who may have lower extremity neurosensory impairments.

Combined study findings [10, 12] suggest that vibration threshold sensitivity and therefore fast-adapting mechanoreceptor function are important in assisting balance control and movement adjustment during human locomotion. From the vibration sensitivity results, it appears that those structures which provide the least mechanoreceptor information about foot placement during ground contact show the lowest sensitivities. These are the medial and lateral malleolus (M1, L1), the dorsal area above the ankle (D1), and the Achilles tendon (A1). When wearing shoes, even the dorsal skin receptors provide useful information about foot position and behavior during ground contact. The least important sites for sensory feedback during ground contact D1, M1, L1, and A1 show the highest threshold values for touch as well as vibro-tactile stimuli. These anatomical locations have little functional importance for foot placement recognition. Based on this foot sensitivity map, a more systematic footwear, ankle-foot brace, or taping/support modification process may be considered to improve peripheral sensory feedback to the brain for better balance control during standing, locomotion, and athletic movement performance [10]. This foot sensitivity map helps improve our understanding of the vital role the foot serves as a sensory organ [10, 13] in addition to a source of load transfer, postural control, and movement generation.

2.4   Subtalar-Ankle Joint Region Mechanoreception

Using gold chloride technique, Michelson and Hutchins [14] observed mechanoreceptors in all the examined human ankle ligaments and in periligamentous connective tissue. Within the ligament, the mechanoreceptors tended to be located in connective tissue like septa which penetrated the ligaments. Using the classification system of Freeman and Wyke [1, 15], three of their four types of mechanoreceptors were detected in each ankle ligament (superficial and deep anterior talofibular, calcaneofibular, posterior talofibular, and deltoid).

Type I (Ruffini), thinly encapsulated globular mechanoreceptors were observed in all ligaments, but at a low frequency. Type II (Pacini), thickly encapsulated, more conical mechanoreceptors, thought to have a proprioceptive function, were the most common in all of the ankle ligaments. Type III (Golgi), thinly encapsulated fusiform mechanoreceptors were also observed in relatively high frequency in all ankle ligaments. There was no discernable segregation of mechanoreceptors within the ligaments, with several different types being observed in close proximity to one another [14]. Type I (Ruffini) mechanoreceptors were identified in small numbers throughout all five ankle ligaments with no frequency difference between ligaments. Type II (Pacini) and type III (Golgi) mechanoreceptors were observed with significantly greater frequencies than type I (Ruffini) in all ankle ligaments. The distribution of type II (Pacini) and type III (Golgi) mechanoreceptors was similar in all five ligaments; however the calcaneofibular ligament and the superficial deltoid ligament had the lowest density of these types. The difference between the superficial deltoid ligament and all other ligaments except the calcaneofibular ligament was significant. With respect to the calcaneofibular ligament, only the posterior talofibular ligament had significantly more type II (Pacini) or type III (Golgi) mechanoreceptors. Detailed examination of mechanoreceptor distribution within each ligament revealed no differences which could be related either to proximity to bone insertions or to depth within a ligament.

Using similar laboratory techniques, mechanoreceptors identified in the ankle ligaments of the feline [1] and humans [14] are mostly type II (Pacini) and type III (Golgi). In summary, these mechanoreceptor types were significantly more abundant than type I (Ruffini) mechanoreceptors in each individual ankle ligament, and in all ankle ligaments taken together. Since type I (Ruffini) mechanoreceptors probably mediate postural sense, it would appear that very few mechanoreceptors are required for the conveyance of static position at the ankle joint. In contrast, the abundance of type II (Pacini) mechanoreceptors in the ankle ligaments, which sense joint movement initiation, and type III (Golgi) mechanoreceptors which are more active at extremes of joint movement is consistent with the theory that they help alert the central nervous system to movement initiation and extremes of ankle joint movement, respectively. In a later study of human ankle ligaments using similar laboratory techniques, Wu et al. [16] reported that type II (Pacini) mechanoreceptors represented the predominant type in the ankle ligaments that they tested (anterior talofibular, posterior talofibular, and calcaneofibular).

In addition to movement initiation detection, type II (Pacini) mechanoreceptors have been associated with glomerular arteriovenous anastomoses [17–19]. When the vascular relationship between this mechanoreceptor type and an arteriovenous anastomosis is disturbed, a new mechanoreceptor is formed by retrograde growth on the same axon and the previous mechanoreceptor undergoes involution [17]. Type II (Pacini) mechanoreceptors can undergo morphologic changes in response to chemical, physical (trauma), and physiologic (vascular) stimuli. Neoplastic changes in type II (Pacini) mechanoreceptors can also be involved in sensory nerve compression syndromes.

Also using gold chloride laboratory methods and classification system, Moraes et al. [20] reported slightly different results. Although Michelson and Hutchins [14] did not identify type I (Ruffini) mechanoreceptors, this study identified their presence. Although they displayed less density than type II (Pacini) mechanoreceptors, in general they displayed a similar density as type III (Golgi) mechanoreceptors. Likewise, they did not identify any significant mechanoreceptor type density differences between the anterotalofibular, calcaneofibular, and posterotalofibular ligaments.

More recently, using enhanced laboratory methods, and the same classification system to evaluate human ankle ligament mechanoreceptor densities, Rein et al. [21, 22] reported a greater density of type IV (pain receptor/free nerve endings) in all ligaments compared to the other mechanoreceptor types, particularly in the lateral and medial ankle ligament complexes. Specifically, the inferior extensor retinaculum lateral root displayed significantly more type IV mechano-receptors and blood vessels than the canalis tarsi ligament (interosseous talocalcaneal ligament). The next more prevalent types in order of decreasing densities were type I (Ruffini), unclassifiable mechanoreceptors, type II (Pacini), and type III (Golgi) mechanoreceptors. Comparatively fewer type III (Golgi) mechanoreceptors were identified. Type I (Ruffini) mechanoreceptors were much more prevalent in the anterior tibiofibular ligament than in the medial complex and were more common than type II (Pacini) and type III (Golgi) mechanoreceptors in the lateral, medial, and sinus tarsi ligamentous complexes. There was also a significant negative correlation between type I (Ruffini) and unclassifiable mechanoreceptor densities and age.

As Golgi-like endings detect extreme joint movement ranges, they tend to appear more often in ligaments of big joints such as within the cruciate ligaments of the knee than in the ligaments of smaller joints [3]. In conclusion, sensory nerve endings were primarily located close to the ankle ligament bone insertion and the epiligamentous region. Several other studies at the ankle [20, 23] and other joints [24–26] have identified the highest mechanoreceptor densities near bony ligament insertions. Takabayashi et al. [23] reported

that 93% of the mechanoreceptors in cat lateral ankle ligaments were located near the fibular and calcaneus attachments. This polar distribution of mechanoreceptors allows them to act more sensitively as ligament tension monitors [23]. Based on studies such as these, it is clear that proprioceptive senses in terms of pain, joint position, movement, and detection of extreme injurious movements are each important at the ankle joint [27]. Clinicians are reminded to use care when attempting to interpret histological study findings based on differing study methods, or when attempting to extrapolate the findings of comparative animal studies to rehabilitation program planning.

2.5   Foot-Subtalar-Ankle Joint Contributions to Standing Balance and Neuromuscular Postural Control

Human upright postural stabilization is determined by central nervous system control strategies partially based on the visual, vestibular, and somatosensory afferent information that it receives [28–32]. The ensuing motor response attempts to match the ensemble cognitive appraisal of this sensory input (Fig. 2.3).

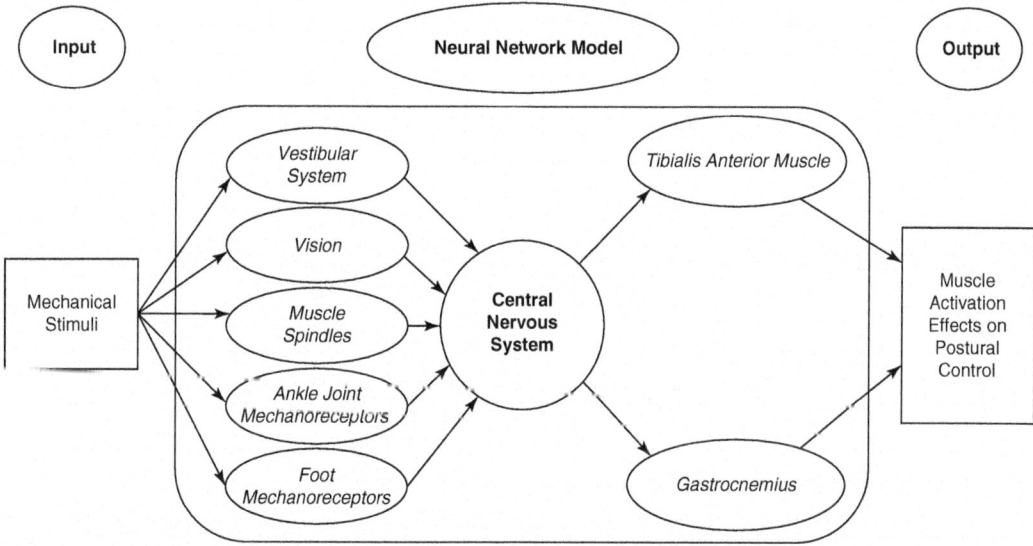

Fig. 2.3 Lower leg neuromuscular postural control model. Adapted from [4]

Ankle sprains are a common sports injury, with the vast majority of these injuries affecting the lateral ankle ligaments [33, 34]. Proprioception is a critical part of ankle and subtalar joint stability [7]. Since ligaments are more resistant to sprains close to their insertions, this better ensures that mechanoreceptor activation is triggered only by potentially noxious motions, remaining silent during ordinary joint activity [4]. Neurovascular elements near the bony ligament insertions may also be of importance to tissue healing following injury; therefore ligamentous insertion regions should be conserved during surgery [24, 35]. The elastic properties of lower leg tendons such as the Achilles tendon are well known, and their importance in running and jumping movements has been widely investigated and discussed [36, 37]. It is also well known that muscle spindle afferent responses may increase with increasing muscle or musculotendinous length or with a decrease in contractile force production [38–41]. However, the exact relationship between the joint capsuloligamentous mechanoreceptor activation and the precise manner in which muscle spindle responses contribute to composite lower extremity dynamic stability is less understood.

During weight bearing, unstable stance when leaning backward or forward involves activation of ventral muscles such as the tibialis anterior and quadriceps femoris or dorsal muscles such as the gluteus maximus and semitendinosus, respectively. Each of these events increases the demand for strong activation discharges from both primary and secondary muscle spindles due to co-activated gamma motor drive [42]. These neuromuscular responses, initiated by descending motor neuron activation, can be maintained by gradually increasing gamma motor neuron excitation and its influence on secondary muscle spindle activation levels [42, 43]. Secondary muscle spindle activation then links muscle groups acting at one joint to muscle groups operating at another adjacent joint (such as secondary muscle spindles from ankle plantar and dorsiflexors influencing both quadriceps and hamstring motor neurons at the knee) [43]. Selection of the appropriate heteronymous group II pathway for a given postural task, for example, quadriceps femoris activation but not hamstring activation while leaning backwards, might be ensured by the parallel activation of inhibitory pathways preventing the activation of muscles not required in this task [42, 43]. Several neural pathways may contribute to such a converging action: primary afferent depolarization interneurons and noradrenaline-releasing neurons activated from the brain stem, corticospinal activation of feedback inhibitory interneurons inhibiting lumbar propriospinal neurons [44], and selective control of heteronymous recurrent inhibition [45].

Because they are at the boundary between the body and the ground, the cutaneous mechanoreceptors of the soles play an important role in balance control [46]. Tactile messages from various foot areas contribute to balance control. Whole-body tilts occur when high-frequency vibration is applied to the skin covering the main foot supporting areas in a standing subject. Vibration-induced sensory messages from cutaneous and/or muscle proprioceptive receptors can provoke compensatory whole-body motor responses to regulate upright posture. This is functionally consistent with the fact that every inclination of the body in a given direction causes a lengthening of some specific muscles, which is coupled with a pressure increase in one or various particular sole areas [46].

As the lateral ankle ligaments are weaker than the medial ligaments and the invertor muscles are collectively stronger than the evertor muscles, the lateral ligaments are more likely to be injured, representing approximately 85% of total ankle sprain events [33]. However, both laboratory and clinical studies suggest that in many patients mechanical laxity may not correlate with functional or dynamic joint instability [47]. Although muscle spindles are well recognized for their role in detecting muscle stretch, they are considerably more complex, having a highly modifiable sensitivity to distinguish the immediate muscle length, changes in length, and velocity at which the muscle changes length [40].

During ankle anterior translation, Needle et al. [47] observed that nerve activity from muscle afferents increased at each level of force up to 90 N in healthy ankles. However, in mechanically unstable ankles, it did not increase until 60 N of anterior force was applied. Additionally, the amplitude of sensory traffic was less in the unstable ankles at 30 N of anterior force. These findings suggest that in patients with mechanical ankle instability, muscle spindles display a diminished response at lower levels of joint force compared to healthy ankles. This diminished response could potentially explain a mechanism by which patients with ankle mechanical instability are unable to properly detect force changes in the early stages of an impending rollover event. The signal from the muscle spindle afferent is directly influenced by sensory information from capsuloligamentous and musculotendinous mechanoreceptors. The researchers speculated that the decreased muscle spindle response in mechanically unstable ankles at lower tension force levels might be from decreased gamma motor neuron drive [47]. Preexisting capsuloligamentous mechanoreceptor injury could lead to decreased reflexive gamma motor drive and, therefore, less sensitive muscle spindle function when muscle length and tension changes occur, especially at low joint loads [47]. Following ankle sprain injury, injured mechanoreceptors may not repopulate the capsuloligamentous tissue in similar kind, quantity, and quality as before the injury [14, 23].

Repetitive capsuloligamentous ankle injury may also decrease ankle evertor musculotendinous Golgi tendon organ responses to low tension forces [23]. Prior to ankle injury, Golgi tendon organs can generally detect loads as low as 5 N and typically provide excitatory feedback to muscle spindles [48]. Additionally, the potential for plastic changes in the central nervous system at the spinal or supraspinal level after ligamentous injury could result in decreased gamma motor drive to muscle spindles, lowering their sensitivity to capsuloligamentous joint loading [3, 11, 49].

2.6 Therapeutic Interventions to Enhance Whole-Body Neuromuscular Postural Control Through the Foot

Through cutaneous mechanoreceptor activation, simple athletic tape application can help prevent sudden ankle inversion [50] and plantar flexion [34]. Ankle joint proprioception has a stronger relationship with sport performance and competitive level than shoulder or spinal proprioception [51]. Although athletic taping may improve proprioception through enhanced cutaneous mechanoreception, and both taping and bracing may help improve mechanical joint stability, active interventions, such as wobble or roller board training, are much more likely to improve dynamic, neuromuscularly controlled ankle joint stability [51]. Additionally, through a crossover effect, the benefits of dynamic or functional ankle joint stabilization training at the uninjured lower extremity can be transferred to the injured side through a central nervous system crossover training effect [51]. Since they have different effects on passive resistive torque and tendon stiffness, both static and dynamic musculotendinous stretching should be considered for training and rehabilitation purposes [52]. Subtalar joint position should be maintained in neutral alignment to focus the stretch on the muscular system that contributes to the Achilles tendon [53]. The need for bilateral lower extremity training following ankle injury cannot be emphasized enough.

To efficiently determine the influence of chronic ankle instability on functional movement patterns, Hertel et al. [54] determined that Star Excursion Balance Test performance moving the non-injured lower extremity as far as possible in anteromedial, medial, and posteromedial directions provided an accurate representation of performance deficits at the weight-bearing, injured ankle. Of all eight directions, moving the non-injured lower extremity as far as possible in the posteromedial direction was the single best functional performance capability indicator [54].

The return-to-play decision-making process following ankle injuries should include a variety of function tests. These include the dorsiflexion lunge test which confirms that sufficient ankle dorsiflexion during weight bearing exists to prevent adjacent lower extremity joint and neuromuscular compensations. If the foot cannot assume a position of at least 9–10 cm away from the wall at which the flexed knee is positioned, and if the tibial shaft angle is less than 35–38° anterior to the vertical axis, restricted ankle motion predictive of future ankle injury exists [55]. The agility T test is a standardized evaluation used to evaluate subject multidirectional agility while running through a prescribed course. High reliability has been demonstrated with the standardized test with average, non-injured test times ranging from 8.9 to 13.5 s [55]. The vertical jump test evaluates explosive power during single- or double-leg vertical jump performance. It also allows the rehabilitation clinician to verify the subject's willingness to perform a controlled single- or double-leg landing without evidence of maladaptive compensations such as favoring the injured

side or hesitance to attempt the task. In addition to physical performance readiness indicators, it is important that the rehabilitation clinician determine a subject's psychological readiness. Subjects should not display fear, or lack relevant task-specific confidence (Fig. 2.4a, b). Surveys such as the Trait Sport Confidence Inventory, the State Sport Confidence Inventory, and the Injury-Psychological Readiness to Return to Sport Scale are evidence-based tools that enable psychological readiness evaluation following lower extremity injury [55].

The foot core system described by McKeon et al. [6] parallels core development in the foot with core development in the axial-pelvic system. In this system, the "core" is made up of local plantar intrinsic muscles that both originate and insert within the foot. These muscles generally have small moment arms and small cross-sectional areas and serve primarily to stabilize foot arches. Foot core training focuses on activating these intrinsic plantar foot muscles to improve dynamic longitudinal foot arch control. Exercises progress from sitting to full weight-

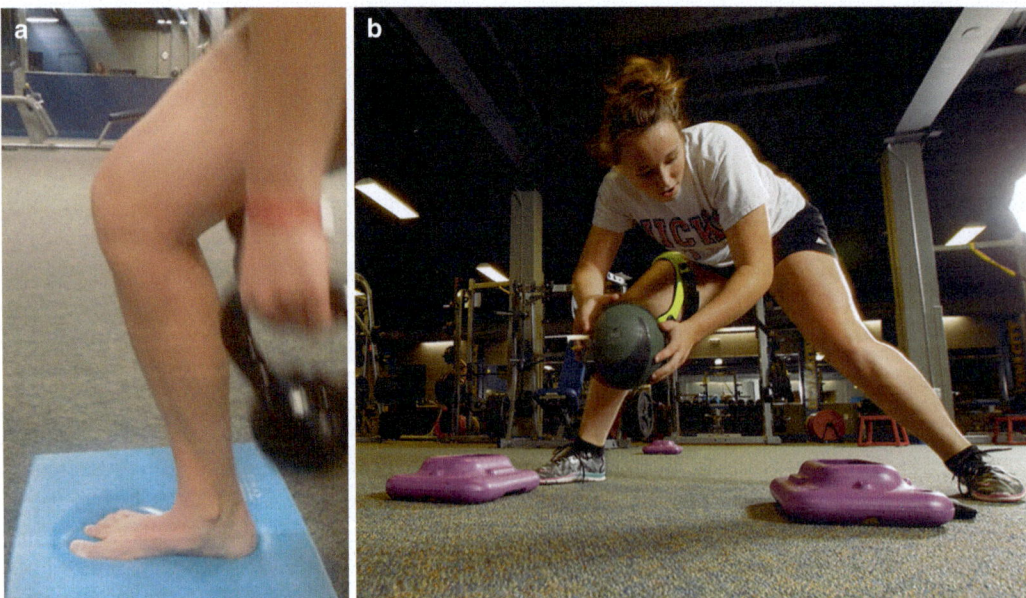

Fig. 2.4 (**a** and **b**) In addition to restoration of foot-ankle-subtalar joint segmental range of motion, strength, proprioception, and neuromuscular control (**a**), it is essen-

tial that the patient improves their task confidence, and minimizes fear of movement (**b**) bearing, standing positions. Impaired function of these stabilizers can adversely influence more proximal lower extremity and trunk function. With each footstep, the four layers of intrinsic muscles help control the magnitude and velocity of foot arch deformation. When they are not functioning properly, the foundation becomes unstable, and malaligned. When this occurs, the lower extremity mechanical loading axis changes position, and abnormal, potentially injurious movements ensue. This may manifest in foot-related problems. Plantar fasciitis is one of the most common overuse injuries of the foot. The importance of intrinsic foot muscles to control the foot arches and their significance to whole-body function are underappreciated. The description of "short foot" or "foot core" neuromuscular control exercises provides a framework for ankle-foot dynamic stability regulation that may improve both performance and lower extremity injury prevention. An advanced form of foot core training is barefoot running which may enhance whole-body postural stability when performed correctly.

Patients with mechanical ankle instability who participated in postural control [56], proprioception [57–59], or balance [60] focused exercises have demonstrated improved function based on Star Excursion Test, position sense, and associated postural control or sway measurements. Docherty et al. [61] reported that lateral hop test performance times among subjects with functional ankle instability were more valid return-to-play readiness indicators than single-leg hop or up-down hop tests.

2.7 Proprioception After Foot and Ankle Surgery

There is no consensus about proprioception level changes following foot-ankle surgical procedures such as internal fracture fixation, chondral repair of the talus, ligament repair, Achilles tendon repair, or arthroplasty. The majority of clinical studies following these interventions focus on neurosensory balance responses, not isolated joint proprioceptive sense.

2.8 Proprioception After Ligament Repair

Patients with unilateral chronic ankle instability are known to experience significant proprioceptive deficits compared to the contralateral side, or compared to a healthy control group [62]. The Hemi-Castaing ligamentoplasty technique uses a an approximately 8 cm, half-diameter peroneus brevis tendon graft with an intact distal insertion to reconstruct the lateral ankle ligament complex. Small ankle joint proprioceptive deficits have been reported at a minimum of six months post-surgery using this procedure [63]. Poor unilateral balance scores were correlated with the surgical side proprioception deficit. Balance and proprioceptive training exercises are essential for patients with chronic lateral ankle instability and for those who have undergone surgical lateral ankle ligament reconstruction.

2.9 Proprioception After Achilles Tendon Repair

Achilles tendon injury and surgery may lead to an ankle joint proprioception deficit. Kaya et al. [64] assessed patients at least one year following percutaneous Achilles tendon repair. They reported that ankle joint position sense at $10°$ dorsiflexion did not display significant side-to-side differences. However, ankle joint active angle replication position sense at $15°$ plantar flexion was impaired. Involved ankle joint position sense at $10°$ dorsiflexion and at $15°$ plantar flexion was the same as the healthy control group. Study findings suggest that proprioceptive exercises should be added to the early phases of post-Achilles tendon repair surgery [64]. Mezzarobba et al. [65] using podobarometric and optokinetic analysis methods reported decreased anterior foot pressure and increased anterior-posterior center of pressure oscillations compared to healthy control subjects at 24 month follow-up. Based on these findings they suggested that post-surgical tendon construct elongation increased the need to restore post-surgical propulsive gait strength and unilateral standing balance.

2.10 Proprioception After Osteochondral Surgery of the Talar Dome

The exact cause of atraumatic osteochondral talar dome defects remains unclear. Conceivably, these injuries may be associated with impaired joint proprioception and repetitive contact between the talus and the ankle mortise during foot pronation. In a group of subjects with a similar proportion of traumatic and atraumatic injury mechanisms, Nakasa et al. [66] identified significant involved ankle joint position sense impairments compared to the uninvolved side. To date, no study has investigated ankle joint proprioception following conservative or surgical management of patients with talar dome osteochondral injuries. Prospective, longitudinal studies are needed to evaluate the proprioception-enhancing efficacy of conservative, therapeutic interventions such as therapeutic exercises, use of functional bracing, and CAM walker use, compared to surgical approaches such as arthroscopic debridement, microfracture, and autologous or allograft osteochondral tissue transfer.

Conclusion

Whole-body postural control is directly dependent on the neuromuscular and capsuloligamentous proprioceptive structures of the foot-ankle and subtalar joints. Greater appreciation for the functional relationship between the afferent-efferent neural circuitry and the synergism that exists between intrinsic foot muscle activation and composite lower extremity dynamic joint stability and neuromuscular control during surgery and rehabilitation program planning will improve patient outcomes.

References

1. Freeman MAR, Wyke B. Articular reflexes at the ankle joint: an electro-myographic study of normal and abnormal influences of ankle-joint mechanoreceptors upon reflex activity in the leg muscles. Brit J Surg. 1967;54:990–1001.
2. Hogervorst T, Brand RA. Mechanoreceptors in joint function. J Bone Joint Surg Am. 1998;80:1365–78.
3. Johansson H, Sjolander P, Sojka P. A sensory role for the cruciate ligaments. Clin Orthop Relat Res. 1991;268:161–78.
4. Solomonow M, Lewis J. Reflex from the ankle ligaments of the feline. J Electromyogr Kinesiol. 2002;12:193–8.
5. Pyar E. Der heutige stand der gelenkchirugie. Arch Klin Chir. 1900;48:404–51.
6. McKeon P, Hertel J, Bramble D, et al. The foot core system: a new paradigm for understanding intrinsic foot muscle function. Br J Sports Med. 2015;49:290.
7. Stagni RA, Leardini A, O'Connor JJ, et al. Role of passive structures in the mobility and stability of the human subtalar joint: a literature review. Foot Ankle Int. 2003;24:402–209.
8. Perry SD, Mcllroy WE, Maki BE. The role of plantar cutaneous mechanoreceptors in the control of compensatory stepping reactions evoked by unpredictable, multi-directional perturbation. Brain Res. 2000;877:401–6.
9. Meyer PF, Oddsson LI, De Luca CJ. The role of plantar cutaneous sensation in unperturbed stance. Exp Brain Res. 2004;156:505–12.
10. Hennig EM, Sterzing T. Sensitivity mapping of the human foot: thresholds at 30 skin locations. Foot Ankle Int. 2009;30:986–91.
11. Hass CJ, Bishop MD, Doidge D, et al. Chronic ankle instability alters central organization of movement. Am J Sports Med. 2010;38:829–34.
12. Kennedy PM, Inglis JT. Distribution and behavior of glaborous cutaneous receptors in the human foot sole. J Physiol. 2002;538:995–1002.
13. Prochazka A, Trend P, Hulliger M, et al. Ensemble proprioceptive activity in the cat step cycle: towards a representative look-up chart. Prog Brain Res. 1989;80:61–74.
14. Michelson JD, Hutchins, C. Mechanoreceptors in human ankle ligaments. J Bone Joint Surg Br. 1995;77:219–24.
15. Wyke B. Articular neurology: a review. Physiotherapy. 1972;58:94–9.
16. Wu X, Song W, Zheng C, et al. Morphological study of mechanoreceptors in collateral ligaments of the ankle joint. J Orthop Surg Res. 2015;10:92.
17. Cauna N, Mannigan G. Developmental and post-natal changes of distal Pacinian corpuscles in three human hands. J Anat. 1959;93:271.
18. Cauna N, Mannigan G. The structure of human digital Pacinian corpuscle (corpuscular lamellosa) and its functional significance. J Anat. 1958;92:1–20.
19. Goldman F, Gardner R. Pacinian corpuscles as a cause for metatarsalgia. J Am Podiatry Assoc. 1980;70:561–7.
20. Moraes MRB, Cavalcante LC, Leite JAD, et al. Histomorphometric evaluation of mechanoreceptors and free nerve endings in human lateral ankle ligaments. Foot Ankle Int. 2008;29:87–90.
21. Rein S, Hagert E, Hanisch U, et al. Immunohistochemical analysis of sensory nerve endings in ankle ligaments: a cadaver study. Cells Tissues Organs. 2013;197:64–76.

22. Rein S, Hanisch U, Zwipp H, et al. Comparative analysis of inter- and intraligamentous distribution of sensory nerve endings in ankle ligament: a cadaver study. Foot Ankle Int. 2013;34:1017–24.
23. Takebayashi T, Yamashita T, Minaki Y, et al. Mechanosensitive afferent units in the lateral ligaments of the ankle. J Bone Joint Surg Br. 1997;79:490–3.
24. Del Valle ME, Harwin SF, Maestro A, et al. Immunohistochemical analysis of mechanreceptors in the human posterior cruciate ligament: a demonstration of its proprioceptive role and clinical relevance. J Arthroplast. 1998;13:916–22.
25. Morisawa Y. Morphological study of mechanoreceptors on the coracoacromial ligament. J Orthop Sci. 1988;3:102–10.
26. Tomita K, Berger EJ, Berger RA, et al. Distribution of nerve endings in the human dorsal radiocarpal ligament. J Hand Surg Am. 2007;32:466–73.
27. Konradsen L. Sensori-motor control of the uninjured and injured human ankle. J Electromyogr Kinesiol. 2002;12:199–203.
28. Bessou P, Bessou M, Dupui PH, et al. Le pied organe de l'equilibre et posture. Parie: Frison-Roches; 1996. p. 21–32.
29. Burcal CJ, Wikstrom EA. Plantar cutaneous sensitivity with and without cognitive loading in people with chronic ankle instability, copers, and uninjured controls. J Orthop Sports Phys Ther. 2016;46:270–6.
30. Ribot-Ciscar E, Hospod V, Roll JP, et al. Fusimotor drive may adjust spindle feedback to task requirements in humans. J Neurophysiol. 2009;101:633–40.
31. Wu G, Chiang JH. The significance of somatosensory stimulations to the human foot in the control of postural reflexes. Exp Brain Res. 1997;114:163–9.
32. Wu G, Haugh L, Sarnow M, et al. A neural network approach to motor-sensory relations during postural disturbance. Brain Res Bull. 2006;69:365–74.
33. Ferran NA, Maffuli N. Epidemiology of sprains of the lateral ankle ligament complex. Foot Ankle Clin. 2006;11:659–62.
34. Simoneau GG, Degner RM, Kramper CA, et al. Changes in ankle joint proprioception resulting from strips of athletic tape applied over the skin. J Athl Train. 1997;32:141–7.
35. Halasi T, Kynsburg A, Ta'lley A, et al. Changes in joint position sense after surgically treated chronic lateral ankle instability. Br J Sports Med. 2005;39:818–24.
36. Alexander RMN, Vernon A. The dimensions of knee and ankle muscles and the forces they exert. J Hum Mov Stud. 1975;1:115–23.
37. Rack PMH, Ross HF, Thilmann AF, et al. Reflex responses at the human ankle: the importance of tendon compliance. J Physiol. 1983;344:503–24.
38. Banks RW. An allometric analysis of the number of muscle spindles in mammalian skeletal muscles. J Anat. 2006;208:753–68.
39. Banks RW, Hulliger M, Saed HH, et al. A comparative analysis of the encapsulated end-organs of mammalian skeletal muscles and of their sensory nerve endings. J Anat. 2009;214:859–87.
40. Bergenheim M, Johansson H, Pedersen J. The role of the gamma-system for improving information transmission in populations of Ia afferents. Neurosci Res. 1995;23:207–15.
41. Matthews BHC. Nerve endings in mammalian muscle. J Physiol. 1933;78:1–53.
42. Marchand-Pauvert V, Nicolas G, Marque P, et al. Increase in group II excitation from ankle muscles to thigh motoneurones during human standing. J Physiol. 2005;566:257–71.
43. Simonetta-Moreau M, Marque P, Marchand-Pauvert V, et al. The pattern of excitation of human lower limb motoneurons by probable group II muscle afferents. J Physiol. 1999;517:287–300.
44. Marchand-Pauvert V, Simonetta-Moreau M, Pierrot-Deseilligny E. Cortical control of spinal pathways mediating group II excitation to human thigh motoneurons. J Physiol. 1999;517:301–13.
45. Barbeau H, Marchand-Pauvert V, Meunier S, et al. Posture-related changes in heteronymous recurrent inhibition from quadriceps to ankle muscles in humans. Exp Brain Res. 2000;130:345–61.
46. Kavounoudias A, Roll R, Roll JP. The plantar sole is a 'dynamometric map' for human balance control. Neuroreport. 1998;9:3247–52.
47. Needle AR, Swanik CB, Farquhar WB, et al. Muscle spindle traffic in functionally unstable ankles during ligamentous stress. J Athl Train. 2013;48:192–202.
48. Grigg P. Peripheral neural mechanisms in proprioception. J Sport Rehabil. 1994;3:2–17.
49. Courtney C, Rine RM, Kroll P. Central somatosensory changes and altered muscle synergies with anterior cruciate ligament deficiency. Gait Posture. 2005;22:69–74.
50. Karlsson J, Andreasson GO. The effect of external ankle support in chronic lateral ankle joint instability. An electromyographic study. Am J Sports Med. 1992;20(3):257–61.
51. Han J, Anson J, Waddington G, et al. The role of ankle proprioception for balance control in relation to sports performance and injury. Biomed Res Int. 2015;2015:842804. https://doi.org/10.1155/2015/842804.
52. Mahieu NN, McNair P, De Muynck M, et al. Effect of static and ballistic stretching on the muscle-tendon tissue properties. Med Sci Sports Exerc. 2007;39:494–501.
53. Edama M, Kubo M, Onishi H, et al. Differences in the degree of stretching applied to Achilles tendon fibers when the calcaneus is pronated or supinated. Foot Ankle Online J. 2016;9(3):5.
54. Hertel J, Braham R, Hale S, et al. Simplifying the star excursion balance test: analyses of subjects with and without chronic ankle instability. J Orthop Sports Phy Ther. 2006;36(3):131–7.
55. Clanton T, Matheny I., Jarvis H, et al. Return to play in athletes following ankle injuries. Sports Health. 2012;4(6):471–4.
56. Hale S, Hertel J, Olmsted-Kramer L. The effect of a 4-week comprehensive rehabilitation program on postural control and lower extremity function in individuals with chronic ankle instability. J Orthop Sports Phys Ther. 2007;37(6):303–11.

57. Goble DJ, Coxon JP, Van Impe A, et al. Brain activity during ankle proprioceptive stimulation predicts balance performance in young and older adults. J Neurosci. 2011;31:16344–52.

58. Lephart S, Pincivero D, Giraldo J, et al. The role of proprioception in the management and rehabilitation of athletic injuries. Am J Sports Med. 1997;25(1):130–7.

59. Matsusaka N, Yokoyama S, Tsurusaka T, et al. Effects of ankle disk training combined with tactile stimulation to the leg and foot on functional instability of the ankle. Am J Sports Med. 2001;29(1):25–30.

60. Bernier J, Perrin D. Effect of coordination training on proprioception of the functionally unstable ankle. J Orthop Sports Phys Ther. 1998;27(4):264–75.

61. Docherty C, Arnold B, Gansneder B, et al. Functional-performance deficits in volunteers with functional ankle instability. J Athl Train. 2005;40(1):30–4.

62. Nakasa T, Fukuhara K, Adachi N, et al. The deficit of joint position sense in the chronic unstable ankle as measured by inversion angle replication error. Arch Orthop Trauma Surg. 2008;128(5):445–9.

63. Baray AL, Philippot R, Farizon F, et al. Assessment of joint position sense deficit, muscular impairment and postural disorder following hemi-Castaing ankle ligamentoplasty. Orthop Traumatol Surg Res. 2014;100:271–4. https://doi.org/10.1016/j.otsr.2014.02.014.

64. Kaya D, Doral MN, Nyland J, et al. Proprioception level after endoscopically guided percutaneous Achilles tendon. Knee Surg Sports Traumatol Arthrosc. 2013;21(6):1238–44. https://doi.org/10.1007/s00167-012-2007-5.

65. Mezzarobba S, Bortolato S, Giacomazzi A, et al. Percutaneous repair of Achilles tendon ruptures with Tenolig: quantitative analysis of postural control and gait pattern. Foot (Edinb). 2012;22(4):303–9. https://doi.org/10.1016/j.foot.2012.09.001.

66. Nakasa T, Adachi N, Shibuya H, et al. Evaluation of joint position sense measured by inversion angle replication error in patients with an osteochondral lesion of the talus. J Foot Ankle Surg. 2013;52(3):331–4. https://doi.org/10.1053/j.jfas.2013.01.009.

Treatment of the Proprioception and Technology

3

Zeynep Bahadir Ağce, Adnan Kara, and Baris Gulenc

Proprioception is defined as detecting and processing the stimulus and initiating a reactive output (kinesthesia) through the neuromuscular system [1, 2]. The proprioceptive information in varying degrees depending on the environment and condition is provided by skin, joint, and muscle mechanoreceptors and transmitted to the central nervous system [1, 3, 4].

Proprioception is vital to creating voluntary control, smoothing, and coordination on movements, motor learning, and error correction during movements and providing postural stabilization and balance control [3, 5–7]. It is difficult to maintain the static posture due to postural oscillation increase in the proprioceptive disorders that occur in the lower extremity [5, 7].

Proprioceptive sensory impairment can develop with neurological disorders such as multiple sclerosis and parkinson or various damage caused by orthopaedic causes such as direct swelling, ACL deficiency, knee osteoarthritis, idiopathic neck pain, and inflammation [1, 4–6, 8–13]. It also leads to loss of proprioception in chronic diseases which affects soft tissue such as rheumatoid arthritis and complex regional pain syndrome or causes neuropathic problems such as diabetes [14, 15]. There are significant decreases in the proprioception due to changes in the central and peripheral nervous system along with progressive aging [3, 15, 16]. Proprioception is related to functional movements of the upper extremity, rate of the physical activity, and perceived level of social isolation [17]. Particularly in the proprioceptive losses of neurological origin, motor problems also contribute to the decrease in the quality of life and the participation of the individual in daily-life activity [2, 18].

For improving the proprioceptive sensory training, vibrotactile feedback, biofeedback, goal-directed movements, robotic device applications, and virtual reality applications are made [18–22]. Repetitive and active exercises have a positive effect on enhancing proprioception; therefore, goal-oriented, frequent rehabilitation practices with technological applications support proprioceptive development [23]. It is accepted that proprioceptive sensory training can improve motor performance and proprioception has a fundamental role in motor control [19, 23]. Technological advances are being used in rehabilitation applications for a variety of reasons, such as assistive device technologies, complex haptic perception, and proprioception [24]. Technology is essential

Z. Bahadir Ağce, P.T., M.Sc. (✉)
Department of Occupational Therapy, Faculty of Health Sciences, Uskudar University, İstanbul, Turkey
e-mail: zeynep.bahadiragce@uskudar.edu.tr

A. Kara, M.D. • B. Gulenc, M.D.
Department of Orthopedics and Traumatology, Faculty of Medicine, Istanbul Medipol University, Istanbul, Turkey
e-mail: adnan.kara@medipol.com.tr; barisgulenc@yahoo.com

because it can help to optimize motor learning in a safe environment and help improve the functional activities of everyday life by replicating real-life scenarios [25].

Also technology-based rehabilitation can increase individual participation to intervention with encouraging personalized, motivating, amusing, and engaging [26]. The tools used in technology rehabilitation are basically classified as endpoint robots and exoskeletons [24, 27]. Exoskeletons are used to assist the movement of the user through actuators placed outside the extremity, to increase the power and rehabilitation performance [28]. Endpoint robots are linked to the body's only limb, such as the trunk, arm, or leg, and the device creates structural force fields that provide perturbation, resistance, or motion assistance in the virtual environment [24, 27].

3.1   Enhancement of Proprioception with Robot Training, Virtual Reality, and iProprio

Robotic technology is used to determine the degree of rehabilitation disorder, create goal for intervention, make the desired movement repetitive, and create progressive goals [27]. The robotic devices are supported to control the patient's own movement via proprioceptive, visual, and tactile inputs [29]. Virtual reality with robotics is used in the rehabilitation of lots of impairments such as hands and fingers, wrist, gait, position sense, motion dynamics, proprioception, and upper and lower extremity motor control [21]. Robotic devices and virtual reality, together with such as VR-based treadmill locomotor system, have the ability to train individuals in different environments safely [30].

The virtual reality [VR] technique contributes to rehabilitation applications by providing interaction between motion and virtual objects in different virtual environments [31]. It is mentioned that VR application reduces the pain threshold and increases the daily physical activity levels of the patients [32]. Recent studies have shown that motor function, everyday life, and quality of life increase after virtual reality applications, especially at the upper extremities [33]. VR technology aims to stimulate movement with computer-based games such as Nintendo Wii, Xbox Kinect, and PlayStation [26, 33]. VR technique uses the interaction between virtual objects and motion, in rehabilitation, by providing various visual environments and using motion tracking [34]. In this way VR practices will create an environment that encourages and motivates the patient who is not observing the exercise treatment due to lack of motivation [27, 32]. The game consoles and interactive computer games have been shown to increase motivation and fun during exercise [27].

VR's clinical practice aims to encourage motor learning using visual, auditory, and haptic inputs [33, 35]. VR can also support to compared with environmental feedback, internal proprioceptive senses, and performance information obtained [33]. Many studies use both visual feedback and tactile feedback to enhance realism in virtual environment [36]. And virtual reality applications are recommended for upper and lower extremity proprioceptive rehabilitation in patients after neurological or orthopaedic disease [31, 33, 37]. Moreover, it is emphasized that the use of proprioceptive feedback in rehabilitation programs to improve motor control is more effective than visual feedback in addition to its low cost being an advantage in using them [31, 38].

The Nintendo Wii [NW] is designed as a popular video game with a Wii Balance Board [WBB] [Nintendo, Kyoto, Japan], and it is used with a game console and associated software [39]. It is a simple and affordable virtual therapy application that can be used at home and in stroke rehabilitation units around the world [40–42]. In NW, proprioceptive stimulation is provided with visual biofeedback to allow the individual to self-correct [41]. However, caution should be exercised when using NW at home, as injuries such as ischemic stroke and vertebral, shoulder, and knee fracture are reported [40].

The Xbox Kinect uses microphone, cameras, and depth infrared sensors to translate body movement on the play; there is no need for a balance pad or handheld instruments [38, 43]. When compared to Wii and Xbox Kinect, it is advantageous as it offers capability for bespoke software that can be designed appropriately; it has the disadvantage as to there is less research about it [43]. With evidence in Xbox Kinect, it is stated that Wii rehabilitation programs are particularly reliable and valid to predict the risk of falling [37, 44].

The PlayStation EyeToy that can be displayed on a standard TV monitor includes USB interface, color digital camera, DualShock with pressure sensitivity, and Analog Controller [45]. The PlayStation EyeToy brings in higher motion intensities than the Nintendo Wii [27]. The literature does not have enough study on the PlayStation games, and need to investigate in more target-based action have been studied for dynamic balance and motor planning with stroke or hemiparetic children [35, 45].

The smartphones that we use commonly in our daily lives have started to be used for rehabilitation and home exercise programs. "iProprio" system is used to improve and evaluate the proprioceptive system. This system uses the internal motion unit sensors that are found on the smartphones, and it gives adjustable vibrotactile biofeedback for users; therefore it can be an alternative for improving proprioception at home exercise. With the multimodal interface, the user can use different sensory modalities as feedback by using visual, auditory, or vibration options. It is a new application but can be appropriate for use in home exercise [46].

3.1.1 New Technological Materials for Proprioception

Simply defined as perceiving the spatial location of any body part, proprioception is a subject on which orthopaedic surgeons and physical therapy specialists spend long working hours. In the last two decades, the number of studies on this subject has steadily increased. The importance of proprioception has been appreciated after noticing the differences among athletes' return to sport and reinjury rates [47].

Proprioception is usually assessed with sensation of joint position and kinesthesia. Loss of proprioception may cause prolonged rehabilitation, inadequate treatment response, and prolonged hospital stay, leading to increased cost of care and recurrent injuries. It also adversely affects postural stability and motor functional recovery [48].

Proprioceptive afferent nerves are principal elements for movement control. Impaired grip strength and coordination have been shown even in patients who had sensory nerve injury but not motor nerve injury. While visual stimuli are the primary factor for wrist proprioception, proprioceptive impairment has also been reported in disorders where motor neurons are also involved, such as parkinson's disease, dystonia, and stroke. Apart from these, it has been reported that robotic rehabilitation devices providing continuous passive movement can be effectively used for loss of proprioception after traumatic injuries and orthopaedic operations [49–51].

Preservation or regain of the sensation of position in patients with stroke has been reported among some important indicators of a high likelihood of motor recovery. In patients with stroke who have a diminished or lost proprioceptive afferent conduction, the response to sensorial stimuli originating from the contralateral side of the cortex is reduced or lost altogether. The ultimate result of all these effects combined is a worsened functional performance and difficulties in performing daily tasks during rehabilitative process [34, 52, 53].

Today, with technological advances, the use of robots in medicine has become increasingly widespread. Robots devised for rehabilitative purposes are widely utilized for regulating wrist proprioception in disorders including stroke which may involve upper extremity. Even though it is expensive than the classical methods, the measurement of the sensation of joint position with rehabilitation robots has been reported to be more sensitive than measurements done by clinical measurement tools and techniques. These devices not only take measurements, but also make patients exercise, thus making an important contribution to neuromotor rehabilitation [54, 55].

3.2 Assessment of Proprioception with Robotic Devices

Proprioception involves two main components, namely kinesthesia [joint motion] and sensation of joint position. Their variability is determined by their measurement. Both parameters are formed via afferent data generated by mechano-receptors found within and around joints [56].

Two separate systems have been widely used for the measurement and use of robotic proprioception. Endpoint-based systems such as MIT-MANUS, MIME, and GENTLE/S, and Exoskeleton robots such as ARMin, T-WREX, Pneu-WREX, L-Exos, and Selford Rehabilitation Exoskeleton, have been designed to support patients during performance of upper extremity exercises [57, 58].

Several studies have examined the change in proprioception in association with the use of wrist and the ability of grip force following robotic rehabilitation in patients with stroke. In a study by Piovesan, the ability of patients with stroke to use plegic arms at the beginning of and after rehabilitation measured by a robotic manipulandum was compared with that of the control group. The researchers demonstrated that the muscle strength necessary to perform a certain task was markedly reduced at the latest sessions. Voluntary control, motor recovery, and motion planning were improved by continuous passive motion with robotic rehabilitation of patients with stroke [56].

Caimmi et al. assessed cortical activation level using EEG during active voluntary motion in patients with stroke. The authors required the control and chronic stroke groups to make active motion followed by the robot-assisted "hand-to-mouth" exercise using an end effector-based robot [Pa10–7, Mitsubishi, Japan]. They found that there were no significant differences between the unaffected hand and healthy subjects with regard to EEG patterns and movement speed; they also demonstrated that no significant difference occurred in cortical activation during robot-assisted movements in healthy subjects whereas a significant level of EEG-recorded cortical activation occurred in patients with chronic stroke; the

authors also noted that the patient obtained huge benefit and achieved functional recovery [59].

Casadio et al. sought to find an answer to the question to what degree patients with stroke needed robotic support. They designed a mechanism to provide patients with assistance to perform a certain task (with the help of a planar manipulandum [Braccio di Ferro]), and they asked patients to perform a certain movement with and without taking visual assistance. At the subsequent sessions, the level of strength applied by patients to perform that task was reduced and their movement speed increased; they also performed the task more properly. It was observed that two patients who were least affected by the disease became able to perform the assigned task without any external assistance at the end of the study; and the authors stated that the proprioception developing robot-assisted therapy performed without a visual assistance may be more beneficial for stroke patients than the classical visual assisted trainings [23].

In a study by Ozkul et al., where elbow proprioception was assessed in two different healthcare professions, healthy volunteer physiotherapists and engineers were assigned tasks in which they would flex their elbows at certain angles with the help of an exoskeleton robot (RehabRoby), with their eyes open versus shut. Then, the values by which they were capable of doing that task and their mistake rates were recorded. All groups' biceps brachii strengths were recorded prior to the start of the experiment. The results of the study indicated that the physiotherapy students made fewer mistakes in assigned tasks with eyes both open and shut; the results also suggested that biceps brachii muscle strength at $20°$ flexion movement played an active role on the sensation of proprioception [60].

Two-sided exoskeleton robots (KINARM [BKIN Technologies Ltd., Kingston, Ontario]) are also commonly used for proprioception studies and rehabilitation therapy. They were designed particularly for poststroke proprioception measurement. They may provide movement on horizontal plane, monitor elbow and shoulder movements, and provide mechanical loading on the same joints. KINARM can measure the sensation of position more sensitively in patients with stroke [61, 62].

MIT-Manus is an end effector-based system that has been used for rehabilitation for the last 30 years. The system allows patients to perform two-dimensional movements with their hands and can record these movements. Having the ability to control patients' hand movements, this system facilitates movement as necessary and strengthens weakened extremity sensation [57, 63].

GENTLE/s is another end effector-based robot that determines the elbow's position in space and allows patients to perform three-dimensional arm movements. Having visual and tactile manipulators, this device aids patients to make movements towards the goal and can finish the movement [64].

Mechatronic system for Motor recovery after Stroke [MEMOS] is a robot that provides and hastens motor recovery in patients with hemiplegia. MEMOS records velocity and directional data and aids in observation of treatment efficacy during rehabilitation process [65].

ARMin is an exoskeleton robot used for arm rehabilitation that possesses strength sensors. It allows elbow flexion-extension and shoulder movements. ARMin II is a new version with passive movement, game therapy, and task-based training modes and is effectively used for treatment of patients with stroke [66].

References

1. Clark VM, Burden AM. A 4-week wobble board exercise programme improved muscle onset latency and perceived stability in individuals with a functionally unstable ankle. Phys Ther Sport. 2005;6:181–7.
2. Semrau JA, Herter TM, Scott SH, Dukelow SP. Robotic identification of kinesthetic deficits after stroke. Stroke. 2013;44:3414–21.
3. Hughes CML, Tommasino P, Budhota A, Campolo D. Upper extremity proprioception in healthy aging and stroke populations, and the effects of therapist and robot-based rehabilitation therapies on proprioceptive function. Front Hum Neurosci. 2015;9:120.
4. Cappello L, Elangovan N, Contu S, Khosravani S, Konczak J, Masia L. Robot-aided assessment of wrist proprioception. Front Hum Neurosci. 2015;9:198.
5. Fling BW, Dutta GG, Schlueter H, Cameron MH, Horak FB. Associations between proprioceptive neu-
ral pathway structural connectivity and balance in people with multiple sclerosis. Front Hum Neurosci. 2014;8:814.
6. Mahmoudian A, van Dieen JH, Baert IA, Jonkers I, Bruijn SM, Luyten FP, et al. Changes in proprioceptive weighting during quiet standing in women with early and established knee osteoarthritis compared to healthy controls. Gait Posture. 2016;44:184–8.
7. Ingemanson ML, Rowe JB, Chan V, Wolbrecht ET, Cramer SC, Reinkensmeyer DJ. Use of a robotic device to measure age-related decline in finger proprioception. Exp Brain Res. 2016;234:83–93.
8. Chen L, Lo WLA, Mao YR, Ding MH, Lin Q, Li H, et al. Effect of virtual reality on postural and balance control in patients with stroke: a systematic literature review. Biomed Res Int. 2016;2016:7309272.
9. Haas CT, Buhlmann A, Turbanski S, Schmidtbleicher D. Proprioceptive and sensorimotor performance in Parkinson's disease. Res Sports Med. 2006;14:273–87.
10. Teasdale H, Preston E, Waddington G. Proprioception of the ankle is impaired in people with Parkinson's disease. Mov Disord Clin Pract. 2017;4(4):524–8.
11. Cooper R, Taylor N, Feller J. A randomised controlled trial of proprioceptive and balance training after surgical reconstruction of the anterior cruciate ligament. Res Sports Med. 2005;13:217–30.
12. Stanton T, Leake H, Bowering K, Moseley G. Evidence of impaired proprioception in chronic idiopathic neck pain: a systematic review and meta-analysis. Physiotherapy. 2015;101:1432–3.
13. Lefaivre SC, Almeida QJ. Can sensory attention focused exercise facilitate the utilization of proprioception for improved balance control in PD? Gait Posture. 2015;41:630–3.
14. Harem Sadaqat SA, Malik AN. Kinesthetic and proprioceptive impairments in diabetic patients. J Riphah Coll Rehabil Sci. 2013;1:12–6.
15. Packer M, Williams M, Samuel D, Adams J. Hand impairment and functional ability: a matched case comparison study between people with rheumatoid arthritis and healthy controls. Hand Therapy. 2016;21:115–22.
16. Bank PJ, Peper CLE, Marinus J, Beek PJ, van Hilten JJ. Motor dysfunction of complex regional pain syndrome is related to impaired central processing of proprioceptive information. J Pain. 2013;14:1460–74.
17. Meyer S, Karttunen AH, Thijs V, Feys H, Verheyden G. How do somatosensory deficits in the arm and hand relate to upper limb impairment, activity, and participation problems after stroke? A systematic review. Phys Ther. 2014;94:1220.
18. Lee Y, Chen K, Ren Y, Son J, Cohen BA, Sliwa JA, et al. Robot-guided ankle sensorimotor rehabilitation of patients with multiple sclerosis. Mult Scler Relat Disord. 2017;11:65–70.
19. Cuppone A, Squeri V, Semprini M, Konczak J. Robot-assisted training to improve proprioception does benefit from added vibro-tactile feedback. Engineering in Medicine and Biology Society [EMBC], 37th Annual International Conference of the IEEE; 2015.

20. Jones SA, Fiehler K, Henriques DY. A task-dependent effect of memory and hand-target on proprioceptive localization. Neuropsychologia. 2012;50(7):1462–70.
21. Wade E, Winstein CJ. Virtual reality and robotics for stroke rehabilitation: where do we go from here? Top Stroke Rehabil. 2011;18:685–700.
22. Senanayake SA. Negative biofeedback for enhancing proprioception training on wobble boards. In: Soft computing in industrial applications. Berlin, Heidelberg: Springer-Verlag; 2011. p. 163–72.
23. Casadio M, Morasso P, Sanguineti V, Giannoni P. Minimally assistive robot training for proprioception enhancement. Exp Brain Res. 2009;194:219–31.
24. Masia L, editor. Novel trends in rehabilitation of proprioception and actuation for assistive technology. Ubiquitous Robots and Ambient Intelligence [URAI], 2014 11th International Conference on; 2014.
25. Kim S, Hwang J, Xuan J, Jung YH, Cha H-S, Kim KH. Global metabolite profiling of synovial fluid for the specific diagnosis of rheumatoid arthritis from other inflammatory arthritis. PLoS One. 2014;9:e97501.
26. Dockx K, Bekkers EM, Van den Bergh V, Ginis P, Rochester L, Hausdorff JM, et al. Virtual reality for rehabilitation in Parkinson's disease. Cochrane Database Syst Rev. 2016;12:CD010760.
27. Laut J, Porfiri M, Raghavan P. The present and future of robotic technology in rehabilitation. Curr Phys Med Rehabil Rep. 2016;4:312–9.
28. Pazzaglia M, Molinari M. The embodiment of assistive devices—from wheelchair to exoskeleton. Phys Life Rev. 2016;16:163–75.
29. Mokienko O, Lyukmanov RK, Chernikova L, Suponeva N, Piradov M, Frolov A. Brain–computer interface: the first experience of clinical use in Russia. Hum Physiol. 2016;42:24–31.
30. Fung J, Richards CL, Malouin F, McFadyen BJ, Lamontagne A. A treadmill and motion coupled virtual reality system for gait training post-stroke. Cyberpsychol Behav. 2006;9:157–62.
31. Kim SI, Song I-H, Cho S, Kim IY, Ku J, Kang YJ, et al. Proprioception rehabilitation training system for stroke patients using virtual reality technology. Engineering in Medicine and Biology Society [EMBC], 2013 35th Annual International Conference of the IEEE; 2013.
32. Camargo C, Cardoso A, Lamounier E Jr, Camargo V, Cavalheiro G, Adriano O. Protocols of virtual rehabilitation for women in post-operative breast cancer stage, São Paulo, SP, Brazil: XII SBGames; 2013 October 16–18, pp. 61–64.
33. Abbruzzese G, Trompetto C, Mori L, Pelosin E. Proprioceptive rehabilitation of upper limb dysfunction in movement disorders: a clinical perspective. Front Hum Neurosci. 2014;8:961.
34. Cho S, Ku J, Cho YK, Kim IY, Kang YJ, Jang DP, et al. Development of virtual reality proprioceptive rehabilitation system for stroke patients. Comput Methods Prog Biomed. 2014;113:258–65.
35. Rand D, Kizony R, Weiss PTL. The Sony PlayStation II EyeToy: low-cost virtual reality for use in rehabilitation. J Neurol Phys Ther. 2008;32:155–63.
36. Wu C-M, Hsu C-W, Lee T-K, Smith S. A virtual reality keyboard with realistic haptic feedback in a fully immersive virtual environment. Virtual Reality. 2017;21:19–29.
37. Ruff J, Wang TL, Quatman-Yates CC, Phieffer LS, Quatman CE. Commercially available gaming systems as clinical assessment tools to improve value in the orthopaedic setting: a systematic review. Injury. 2015;46:178–83.
38. Levinger P, Zeina D, Teshome AK, Skinner E, Begg R, Abbott JH. A real time biofeedback using Kinect and Wii to improve gait for post-total knee replacement rehabilitation: a case study report. Disabil Rehabil Assist Technol. 2016;11:251–62.
39. Baltaci G, Harput G, Haksever B, Ulusoy B, Ozer H. Comparison between Nintendo Wii Fit and conventional rehabilitation on functional performance outcomes after hamstring anterior cruciate ligament reconstruction: prospective, randomized, controlled, double-blind clinical trial. Knee Surg Sports Traumatol Arthrosc. 2013;21:880–7.
40. da Silva Ribeiro NM, Ferraz DD, Pedreira É, Pinheiro Í, da Silva Pinto AC, Neto MG, et al. Virtual rehabilitation via Nintendo Wii® and conventional physical therapy effectively treat post-stroke hemiparetic patients. Top Stroke Rehabil. 2015;22:299–305.
41. Dos Santos LRA, Carregosa AA, Masruha MR, Dos Santos PA, Coêlho MLDS, Ferraz DD, et al. The use of Nintendo Wii in the rehabilitation of poststroke patients: a systematic review. J Stroke Cerebrovasc Dis. 2015;24:2298–305.
42. Bonnechère B, Jansen B, Omelina L, Van Sint J. The use of commercial video games in rehabilitation: a systematic review. Int J Rehabil Res. 2016;39:277–90.
43. Taylor MJ, Griffin M. The use of gaming technology for rehabilitation in people with multiple sclerosis. Mult Scler J. 2015;21:355–71.
44. Barry G, van Schaik P, MacSween A, Dixon J, Martin D. Exergaming [XBOX Kinect™] versus traditional gym-based exercise for postural control, flow and technology acceptance in healthy adults: a randomised controlled trial. BMC Sports Sci Med Rehabil. 2016;8:25.
45. Flynn S, Palma P, Bender A. Feasibility of using the Sony PlayStation 2 gaming platform for an individual poststroke: a case report. J Neurol Phys Ther. 2007;31:180–9.
46. Mourcou Q, Fleury A, Diot B, Vuillerme N, editors. iProprio: a Smartphone-based system to measure and improve proprioceptive function. Engineering in Medicine and Biology Society, 2016 IEEE 38th Annual International Conference of the; 2016.
47. Nowak DA, Glasauer S, Hermsdörfer J. How predictive is grip force control in the complete absence of somatosensory feedback? Brain. 2004;127:182–92.
48. Hermsdörfer J, Elias Z, Cole J, Quaney B, Nowak D. Preserved and impaired aspects of feed-forward

grip force control after chronic somatosensory deafferentation. Neurorehabil Neural Repair. 2008;22:374–84.

49. Rickards C, Cody F. Proprioceptive control of wrist movements in Parkinson's disease. Reduced muscle vibration-induced errors. Brain. 1997;120:977–90.

50. Putzki N, Stude P, Konczak J, Graf K, Diener HC, Maschke M. Kinesthesia is impaired in focal dystonia. Mov Disord. 2006;21:754–60.

51. Carey LM, Matyas TA, Oke LE. Sensory loss in stroke patients: effective training of tactile and proprioceptive discrimination. Arch Phys Med Rehabil. 1993;74:602–11.

52. Kusoffsky A, Wadell I, Nilsson B. The relationship between sensory impairment and motor recovery in patients with hemiplegia. Scand J Rehabil Med. 1981;14:27–32.

53. Tyson SF, Hanley M, Chillala J, Selley AB, Tallis RC. Sensory loss in hospital-admitted people with stroke: characteristics, associated factors, and relationship with function. Neurorehabil Neural Repair. 2008;22:166–72.

54. Smith DL, Akhtar AJ, Garraway WM. Proprioception and spatial neglect after stroke. Age Ageing. 1983;12:63–9.

55. Taub E, Berman A. Avoidance conditioning in the absence of relevant proprioceptive and exteroceptive feedback. J Comp Physiol Psychol. 1963;56:1012.

56. Piovesan D. A computational index to describe slacking during robot therapy. In: Progress in Motor Control. Cham: Springer; 2016. p. 351–65.

57. Krebs HI, Ferraro M, Buerger SP, Newbery MJ, Makiyama A, Sandmann M, et al. Rehabilitation robotics: pilot trial of a spatial extension for MIT-Manus. J Neuroeng Rehabil. 2004;1:5.

58. Housman SJ, Le V, Rahman T, Sanchez RJ, Reinkensmeyer DJ, editors. Arm-training with T-WREX after chronic stroke: preliminary results of a randomized controlled trial. Rehabilitation

Robotics, 2007 ICORR 2007 IEEE 10th International Conference on; 2007.

59. Caimmi M, Visani E, Digiacomo F, Scano A, Chiavenna A, Gramigna C, et al. Predicting functional recovery in chronic stroke rehabilitation using event-related desynchronization-synchronization during robot-assisted movement. Biomed Res Int. 2016;2016:7051340.

60. Özkul F, Erol BD, Badıllı DŞ, Inal S. Evaluation of elbow joint proprioception with RehabRoby: a pilot study. Acta Orthop Traumatol Turc. 2011;46:332–8.

61. Huang VS, Krakauer JW. Robotic neurorehabilitation: a computational motor learning perspective. J Neuroeng Rehabil. 2009;6:5.

62. Wilson JL, Slieker FJ, Legrand V, Murray G, Stocchetti N, Maas AI. Observer variation in the assessment of outcome in traumatic brain injury: experience from a multicenter, international randomized clinical trial. Neurosurgery. 2007;61:123–9.

63. Krebs HI, Volpe BT, Williams D, Celestino J, Charles SK, Lynch D, et al. Robot-aided neurorehabilitation: a robot for wrist rehabilitation. IEEE Trans Neural Syst Rehabil Eng. 2007;15:327–35.

64. Loureiro R, Amirabdollahian F, Topping M, Driessen B, Harwin W. Upper limb robot mediated stroke therapy—GENTLE/s approach. Auton Robot. 2003;15:35–51.

65. Micera S, Sergi PN, Zaccone F, Cappiello G, Carrozza M, Dario P, et al., editors. A low-cost biomechatronic system for the restoration and assessment of upper limb motor function in hemiparetic subjects. Biomedical Robotics and Biomechatronics, 2006 BioRob 2006 The First IEEE/RAS-EMBS International Conference on; 2006.

66. Nef T, Mihelj M, Kiefer G, Perndl C, Muller R, Riener R, editors. ARMin-Exoskeleton for arm therapy in stroke patients. Rehabilitation Robotics, 2007 ICORR 2007 IEEE 10th International Conference on; 2007.

Part II

Clinical Knowledge of the Proprioception

Proprioception After Shoulder Injury, Surgery, and Rehabilitation

4

Irem Duzgun and Egemen Turhan

4.1 Proprioceptive Sense in Glenohumeral Joint

Neuromuscular control aims to prepare dynamic stabilizers for joint motion and overload with subconscious activation, its response, and continuity of joint stability [1]. This neuromuscular control mechanism is provided by the coordination of muscle activation during the functional movements with coactivation of shoulder muscles (strength pairs), muscular reflex, regulation of muscular tone, and induration [1, 2]. Thus, shoulder muscles allow mobility at high levels by providing the centralization of humerus head in glenoid cavity. In addition, the joint position sense is an important participant in maintaining muscle induration and coordination and it reduces the risk of injury by creating steady motion for optimal performance [3, 4]. This is particularly important for enabling stabilization in broad joint motion in shoulder functions [5, 6].

I. Duzgun, Ph.D., M.Sc., P.T. (✉)
Faculty of Health Sciences, Department of Physiotherapy and Rehabilitation, Hacettepe University, Ankara, Turkey
e-mail: iremduzgun@yahoo.com

E. Turhan, M.D. (✉)
Faculty of Medicine, Department of Orthopaedics and Traumatology, Hacettepe University, Ankara, Turkey
e-mail: dregementurhan@yahoo.com

Receptors have an important function for maintaining neuromuscular control. Our body consists of Meissner and Ruffini (type I), Pacini and Krause (type II), Golgi tendon organ (type III), and free nerve ending (type IV) receptors [7]. In the shoulder, Pacinian corpuscles, Ruffini endings, Golgi tendon organ, and muscle spindle mechanoreceptors have been identified [8, 9]. In the histological studies conducted on humans, Vangness et al. [8] have suggested that there are slowly adapting Pacinian corpuscles and Ruffini endings on the glenohumeral ligament complex. They have also discovered that labrum and subacromial bursa include free nerve endings but do not include mechanoreceptors. It has been shown that there are type IV mechanoreceptors on supraspinatus muscle and tendon of the rabbits. These receptors are responsible for nociceptive stimulus and closely related to afferent pain stimulation. Besides, it has been suggested that supraspinatus muscle has more of these receptors than infraspinatus does [10].

The muscle spindle is one of the primary providers of joint position sense in the midranges of joint motion. Capsuloligamentous mechanoreceptors (e.g., Ruffini endings, Pacinian corpuscles, and Golgi endings) are inactive at these angles [11] and stimulated by the deformation on the tissues they are located [12]. Many authors have stated that these receptors are stimulated at the end range of the joint motion in which the tissue is stretched the most rather than the midrange of the motion [8, 13].

This mechanism is also true for the glenohumeral joint. Janwantanakul et al. reported that, like other authors, receptors are more stimulated at the end range of the shoulder external rotation [5].

The reason why the joint position sense is related to the scapular muscle activation in the midrange of the motion can be that more muscle spindles are related to joint position sense. It has been thought that a scapular muscle disorder causes a deterioration of the joint position sense in these angles. However, in the end range of the motion, the activation of mechanoreceptors in the capsuloligamentous structures can compensate the wrong information [14].

Blaiser et al. have stated that shoulder external rotation is more sensitive than internal rotation and this is related to the mechanism that proprioceptive signals go to the central nervous system more as a result of the stretching of the capsule [12]. In addition, it has been suggested that joint position sense gets better with the increase of joint torque and elevation angles [15] and external overload [16] and this can be associated with the increase in the muscle activation level and muscle spindle signals. Another study, which examines the effect of isometric contraction intensity, has suggested that there is more deviation in the high contraction intensity [17, 18].

There is a consensus among the researchers about that with the increase of shoulder elevation angle the soft-tissue strain increases and this results in the increase of proprioceptive sense [5, 16]. This mechanism has a great importance in limiting the joint translation forces that occur at the end range of the joint motion border. Effective motor response is necessary for optimal suitability in active position repetition sense [19].

4.2   Effect of Injury on Proprioceptive Sense

Mechanic instability occurs as a result of the injury of traumatic or nontraumatic mechanisms and stabilizer structures of the glenohumeral joint [2]. This causes mechanic deficit and sensorimotor change and functional stability deficit

[2]. It has been previously stated that glenohumeral joint capsule, glenohumeral ligaments, and glenoid labrum include mechanoreceptors which provide proprioceptive information for the sensorimotor system that generates glenohumeral joint stability and neuromuscular control. Accordingly, joint injury affects not only the mechanic limiters, but also sensorimotor contribution and dynamic stability. Many studies have shown that shoulder instability and proprioceptive sense are affected negatively [18, 20]. For the patients with glenohumeral joint instability, both joint position sense and kinesthesia are affected [18, 20]. It has been thought that this is because mechanoreceptor stimulation decreases with the injury of capsuloligamentous tissues [20].

Warner et al. have stated that increase of the translation on the joints in glenohumeral instabilities causes changes in the motions of glenohumeral and scapulothoracic joints. Proprioceptive sense disorder that is seen in this pathology can be related to unsynchronized scapulothoracic motions, neuromuscular tasks, or both [21].

Acuity of capsuloligamentous mechanoreceptors decreases based on their physical laxity and differentiation. Previous studies have shown the differentiation in the proprioceptive sense on normal and pathological shoulders, normal and surgical repair, and normal and highly trained groups [2, 18, 20]. There have been contradictory results in rotator cuff pathologies. A study has shown that proprioceptive sense decreases during the shoulder elevation in chronic cuff pathologies. It has been found out that the maximum disorder is in the scapular plan at 100° elevation; the place aches the most in impingement syndrome. This is the opposite case of the asymptomatic adults. It has been known that with the increase in the elevation of capsuloligamentous and muscular tension, proprioceptive stimulation and related sense increase in the asymptomatic individuals [5, 16]. Machner et al. have shown that kinesthesia decreases in the patients with phase 2 subacromial impingement syndrome and stated that the deficit in subacromial bursa is related to the sense of motion [22]. Besides, it has been stated that loss occurs both in the proprioceptive sense and the strength in the athletes with isolated infraspinatus muscle atrophy, and it is necessary to give proprioceptive training in the rehabilitation of these patients [23]. However, Maenhout et al. have shown with the strength sense test conducted with anisokinetic tool that there is no difference between the patients with rotator cuff tendinopathy and the asymptomatic individuals [24]. Rotator cuff pathologies include different pathologies from tendinopathy to full-thickness tear. It has been thought that the studies conducted with the homogenous groups would provide more precise results.

The proprioceptive deficit has been shown in the patients with osteoarthritis [25]. Cuomo et al. have related this deficit to the decrease of the activation level of the shoulder muscles [25]. The increase of the afferent stimulations coming from the pain receptors has been also thought to decrease proprioceptive afferents by suppressing them. It has been shown that with the increase of nociceptive activity, the proprioception decreases in the baseball players with shoulder ache [26].

Joint position sense differs in frozen shoulder problem. A relation has been found especially between joint position sense in the midrange of the joint motion and the scapular muscle activation. It has been shown that the deterioration in joint position sense is related to the functional level of the individuals [14].

Shoulder dynamic stability is significant for overhead athletes. However, these athletes often face mobility deteriorations, changes in shoulder muscle strength, and proprioceptive deficit [27]. But the existence of proprioceptive deficit is controversial. While some writers state that repetitive motions improve proprioceptive sense, other writers state that capsular laxity and extreme joint motion decrease proprioceptive sense [28]. Exercise programs provide improvements in joint position sense as a result of increased central and neural adaptation [27]. In addition, overhead throwing activity includes plyometric motions and this is thought to provide functional stability by improving central and peripheral adaptation. With the long-term training, Golgi tendon organ becomes desensitized and muscle spindle sensitivity increases. During the throwing motion, repetitive stimulation of articular mechanoreceptors which are at the end range of the motion can enable peripheral adaptation. Thus, it has been thought that proprioception increases with the modification of muscle spindle and articular mechanoreceptors [1, 29].

4.3 Evaluation of the Proprioceptive Sense

It is quite difficult to evaluate proprioception on the glenohumeral joint because it is the most mobile joint in our body. Different techniques have been developed for evaluation [19, 30, 31].

Passive and active position repetition test (joint position sense), kinesthesia, and strength repetition tests are used for evaluation [1, 32, 33].

Isokinetic systems and robotic systems are used in passive position repetition test [34]. The joint is passively moved at 2°/s or 0.5°/s speed. After waiting at the previously mentioned angles for a while, it is moved to the previous position again. Then, while the system joint is passively moving at the same speed, the person is asked to stop the system at the previous position. The angular deviation at this point gives us information about the proprioceptive sense. As the motion is passively done, it has been thought that the capsuloligamentous mechanoreceptors are more responsible for this sense.

In the active position repetition test, individual's ability to actively repeat the reference position is evaluated. This test has shown that capsuloligamentous and musculotendinous mechanoreceptors are maximal sensitive [19, 30, 35]. In the evaluation of this sense, isokinetic systems, robotic systems, three-dimensional analysis methods, propriometer, and laser pointer-assisted angle repetition tests which can be easily used in clinics are used [34, 36–38].

Kinesthesia sense is investigated during the passive motion. Isokinetic systems are often used in the evaluation of this sense. While the joint is passively moved with the 0.1°/s speed, the person is asked to state at which point he/she feels the motion. This point gives information about the kinesthesia sense of the person.

Isokinetic systems and dynamometers (myometers) are used in strength repetition test. The person is often asked to perform isometric contraction. This value is recorded; 50% of this recorded maximum isometric contraction or another particular value is repeated. The patient is asked to comprehend and repeat this contraction. Deviations at the created force are recorded. Dover et al. have shown that isokinetic system is highly reliable and repeatable for measuring the force sense of the shoulder external and internal rotators [39].

It is highly important to provide standardization while applying the proprioceptive tests. It has to be taken into account that the body orientation during the test can affect the test results. Janwantanakul et al. have suggested that there has not been a difference between sitting and supine position in passive joint position repetition test but the results of the test in sitting position with three repetitions are more coherent [5]. Martijn et al. have stated that body position shows no difference in active and passive joint position repetition test results. However, they have found that the deviation in active joint position repetition test is higher than passive joint position test [33].

Apart from that, the proprioceptive sense can be affected from tiredness. Especially extreme activation of the receptors in the musculotendinous structure is thought to cause a decrease in the transmission of the proprioceptive information after a while. The studies conducted show that the muscle tiredness affects the result negatively for both active and passive position sense evaluation [30, 40, 41].

In the evaluations that were conducted by taking this factor into account, it has been shown that joint position sense changes between 3° and 9° in unrestricted protocols [15, 16, 42, 43]. Failure in shoulder joint position sense varies from 2° to 7° [5, 42, 44].

In the active angle repetition test conducted with the laser pointer, it has been suggested that the worst angle repetition capacity was seen while the shoulder is at 55° elevation (both stable and unstable shoulders), and the best results were gathered at 90° [36].

4.4 Restoration of Proprioceptive Sense

It has been known that proprioception has a great importance in providing shoulder joint stability, protecting it from injuries and preventing the repetition of the injury. The aim of the surgical and conservative practices applied after the injury is to provide the right biomechanics. Thus, it is aimed to both increase the functional activity level and eliminate the possible symptoms that can occur because of wrong biomechanics.

Right biomechanics will provide the right motion pattern. This shall form the appropriate sense input from the receptors present at the capsuloligamentous and musculotendinous structures.

Shoulder complex consists of four joints. The steady motion occurs as a result of the coordinated motion of these joints. The studies have suggested that the proprioceptors mostly appear in the joint capsule, glenohumeral ligaments, rotator cuff, and shoulder muscles. The receptors on this structure shall create the appropriate motor activities by providing the related sense input. It has been accepted that it is necessary to provide steady motion on the scapulothoracic joint for the individual with a shoulder problem in rehabilitation. Thus, it is aimed to decrease the possible symptoms (pain, inflammation, joint motion restriction, etc.) and provide the right biomechanics. Besides, we shouldn't forget that the proprioceptive sense is related to scapular muscle activation in the midrange of the motion. The dominant idea is that the injury or the risk of repetition of it can be eliminated with the appropriate sensorimotor system.

Physiotherapy and rehabilitation and surgical practices are preferred for providing the right biomechanics in the restoration of the proprioceptive sense.

4.4.1 Role of Surgery on Shoulder Proprioception

Shoulder proprioception can be differently affected from the underlying pathology. The common surgical interventions for shoulder are based on instability, rotator cuff problems, subacromial pathologies, and biceps tendon diseases. Unfortunately literature is lack of evaluation of proprioception alterations before and after surgical procedures for shoulder when compered with knee joint. Aydin et al. [45] investigate proprioception of the shoulder in groups of individuals with healthy and surgically repaired shoulders in instability cases. They reported that there is no difference between the operated and nonoperated shoulders. Surgery might restore proprioception indeed but to evaluate this parameter may differ from the chosen method.

Neuromuscular dysfunction is expressed in the different muscle recruitment patterns during elevation and external rotation, shown in patients with subacromial impingement. Common findings include decreased activity in the rotator cuff muscles and serratus anterior and increased activity in the middle deltoid and the upper trapezius. The rotator cuff plays an important role in opposing the superior translation force of the deltoid. A lack of good control of muscle force could compromise dynamic stability of the shoulder joint resulting in altered glenohumeral kinematics. Anterosuperior translation of the humerus has already been demonstrated in patients with rotator cuff tendinopathy. This affects the proprioception indeed but again literature is not satisfactory to evaluate the impact of surgery on neural control of shoulder. According to our experience after rotator cuff surgery shoulder joint proprioception recovery is rapid. The history of the patients and chronicity of the tear affect proprioception.

Performing shoulder arthroplasty did negatively affect one component of shoulder proprioception that was measured by the active angle reproduction test. This might be related to the surgical approach that includes division of the subscapularis muscle and the glenohumeral ligaments. In order to be able to diminish negative influences on postoperative proprioception further prospective studies will have to evaluate pre- and intraoperative variables to improve proprioception after shoulder replacement. Although proprioception does not improve many after implantation of shoulder arthroplasty, a pain-free increase of range of motion in activities of daily living is the main improvement for the patient after surgery [46, 47].

4.4.2 Physiotherapy and Rehabilitation

The primal purpose of the rehabilitation is to suppress pain and inflammation. Some studies have researched the effect of applying cold for this purpose on the joint position sense. However, there is no consensus about it. Three studies have found that the cold has no effect on joint position sense while four studies have stated that it decreases the sense [48]. A study conducted in 2016 suggested that applying ice to the shoulder for 15 min negatively affected the muscle strength and impaired joint position sense [49]. This is thought to relate to the decreased speed of neural transmission.

The second purpose of rehabilitation after suppressing the pain and inflammation is to increase the peripheral muscle activation and to use the right biomechanics. All these applications provide the restoration of proprioceptive sense. Proprioceptive training regenerates the system between mechanoreceptors and central nervous system and tries to compensate the proprioceptive deficit resulted from injury [1]. Effective shoulder exercises provide the restoration of the sensorimotor mechanism.

It has been known that open and closed kinetic chain exercises improve the joint position sense [50]. Closed kinetic chain exercises facilitate the coactivation of the shoulder muscles on upper extremities and increase functional joint stability. This is thought to result from the stimulation of the articular mechanoreceptors during closed kinetic chain exercises [51]. However, a study showed that after a 4-week-long closed and open kinetic exercise conducted on the rotator cuff and scapular muscles of the healthy individuals, the muscular force was increased but the joint position sense showed no difference [52]. When thinking that this study was conducted with healthy individuals (with no proprioceptive sense influence), it is not surprising that the sense did

Fig. 4.1 Closed kinetic chain exercises

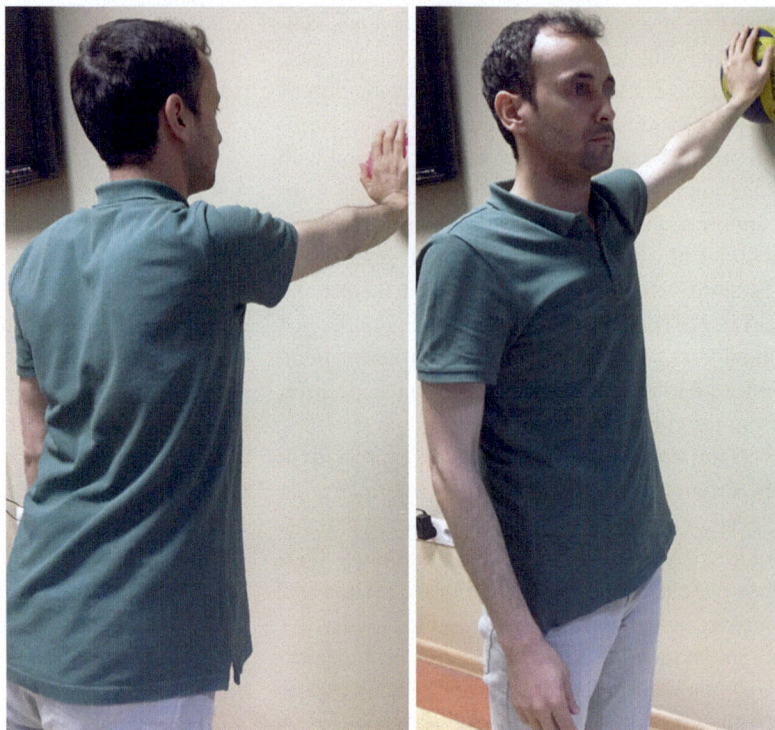

not show any differences after the training. The general idea is that the exercise training on pathological shoulders is effective on proprioceptive sense.

Various exercises are used in the clinics to increase the proprioceptive sense. The active motion used in the first step is thought to provide proprioceptive input. It has been thought that based on the compression stress applied to the joint capsule in the closed kinetic chain exercises, which are preferred in the primary steps of rehabilitation, the stimulation of the receptors can be provided (Fig. 4.1). In the later steps of proprioceptive training, the exercises conducted on different surfaces both increase the somatosensorial sense input and help the improvement of the reflexive responses that can be formed against the fulminant stresses (Fig. 4.2). However, a study has suggested that there are minimal changes in EMG activity with the exercises conducted on unstable surfaces [53] while another study has shown that compensatory muscle activity decreases after the vibration application to the Achilles tendon [54]. More studies are needed on this subject.

Strengthening exercises are frequently used in rehabilitation. The purpose is to increase the neuromuscular control besides muscular strength. Particularly these exercises are thought to increase the sensitivity of Golgi tendon organ and muscle spindle. Various exercise equipment can be used for this purpose (exercise band, free weights, etc.). A study assessed the effect of external overload on the joint position sense and suggested that the joint position sense only increased in the direction of the overload. There was no difference in the joint position sense on other surfaces [16]. It has been suggested to exercise on multiplanes to generally increase the joint proprioception. In this respect, rhythmic stabilization, one of the proprioceptive neuromuscular facilitation techniques, can be preferred because it allows sense input on different directions (Fig. 4.3).

Physical activity causes overload on both musculotendinous and capsuloligamentous tissues. As a result of this overload, the increase in the sensitivity of the receptors in these tissues improves the proprioceptive sense. Pochini et al.

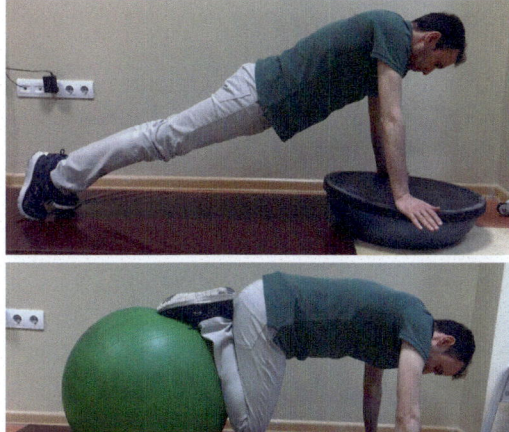

Fig. 4.2 Closed kinetic chain exercises on the different surfaces

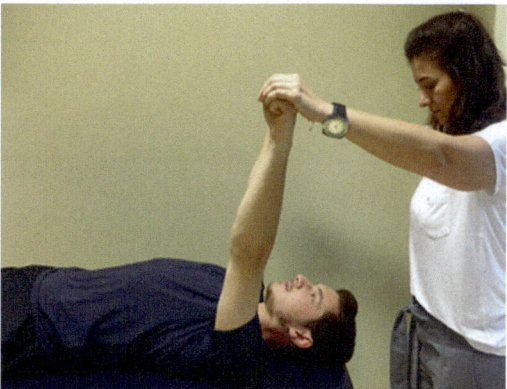

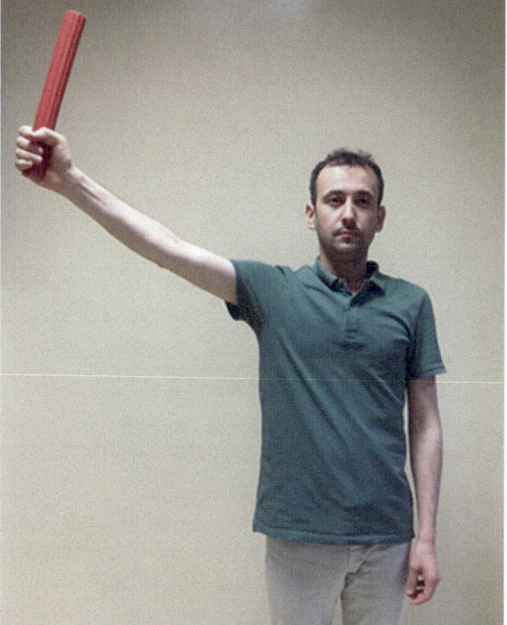

Fig. 4.3 Rhythmic stabilization

have shown that extreme physical activity increased the number of the proprioceptors in the supraspinatus tendon in the mice [55]. Proprioceptive training also includes the increase of the physical activity level of the individuals.

Upper extremity rehabilitation programs often include plyometric exercises to provide neuromuscular control and functional joint stability (Fig. 4.4). It has been shown that the plyometric activities increase the lower extremity muscle performance characteristics [29, 56]. Besides, they increase proprioception and kinesthesia and help stability. The data regarding the effect of plyometric exercises on neuromuscular adaptation in upper extremities is limited [29]. These exercises focus on dynamic restriction and muscle performance. By enabling reflexive muscular recruitment pattern, elastic energy storage and force-creating capacity are aimed to improve. Thus, the relation between the force pairs necessary for the dynamic limitation is enabled [29, 53–56].

Plyometric activities consist of three parts: eccentric loading, amortization, and concentric contraction phase. Theoretically, it is thought to provide peripheral and chronic neural adaptation. Dynamic restriction increases 10–15% by voluntary muscle contraction with the reflexive activity of muscle spindle during eccentric load-

ing [29]. With the chronic adaptation of plyometric training, the joint proprioception and kinesthesia increase; thus, restoration of functional stability is provided. It has been thought that chronic exercise desensitizes Golgi tendon organ, neutralizes the effect of inhibition, and increases the sensitivity of muscle spindle. The modification in the sensitivity of muscle spindle can increase proprioceptive and kinesthetic awareness [29]. Swanik et al. have shown that both proprioception and kinesthesia improve after 6-week-long plyometric training. This difference has shown that joint position sense and joint motion perception improve as a result of

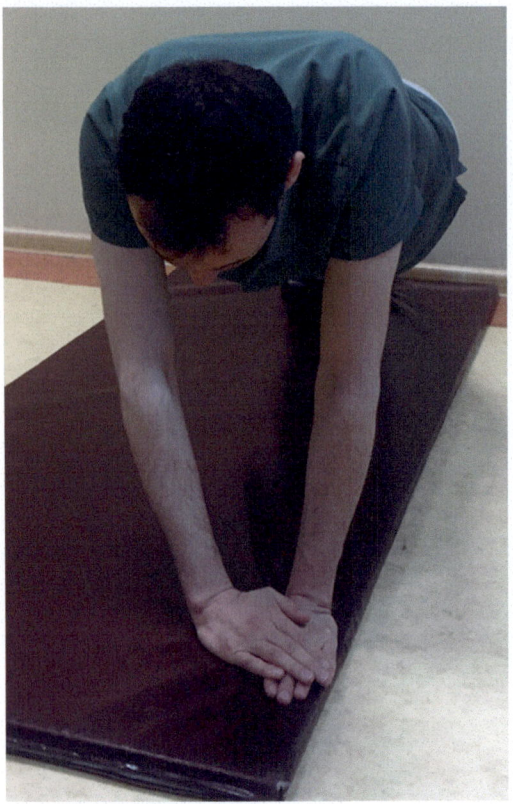

Fig. 4.4 Plyometric exercises

peripheral and central neural adaptation with plyometric training [29]. However, Heiderscheit et al. gave plyometric training to the internal rotators for 8 weeks in the study they conducted with sedentary individuals. They stated that they there was no difference in joint position sense before and after the training [57]. Besides, it has been shown that shoulder plyometric exercises increase proprioception in the swimmers. It has been though that it is related to the increase in the proprioceptive awareness resulted from length/tension changes of shoulder stabilizers with repetitive eccentric overload [29]. In the literature, there have been various studies that stated that training and rehabilitation increase the joint position sense [29, 58].

Peripheral adaptation is thought to result from the repetitive stimulation of the articular mechanoreceptors with plyometric training [56]. It has been shown that articular mechanoreceptors are stimulated maximum at the end range of shoulder

rotation [19, 34]. Besides, fast length/tension changes in the tenomuscular structures can facilitate the adaptation of muscle spindle and Golgi tendon organ [29].

One of the practices frequently used in the rehabilitation of the injuries is banding. It has been thought that the sense input increases due to the stimulation of the receptors especially on the skin with banding. In addition, one of the aims of banding is to enable right mechanics. This is thought to provide steady motion input and increase neuromuscular control. We have previously stated the importance of the steadiness in scapular motions of the shoulder complex. Lin et al. have found out that scapular banding increases the scapular muscle activation and proprioceptive feedback in their study. They explained this situation as scapular banding enables neuromuscular control [59].

The harmony between the activation of force pairs on shoulder joint is important. The studies have shown that upper trapezius activation increases in the individuals with a shoulder problem, while middle and lower trapezius activation decreases. The deterioration in the activation rate affects the steadiness of scapular motion. Morin et al. have shown that scapular banding decreases the upper trapezius activity and increases middle trapezius activity. This shall restore the scapular motions and provide somatosensorial input [60]. Lin et al. have shown that banding increases serratus anterior activity while lower trapezius activity does not change and upper trapezius activity decreases [57]. In consideration of these results, it has been thought that banding is effective in creating appropriate motor activity and increasing proprioceptive sense by providing the right somatosensorial input.

Kinesio tape application has been highly popular in recent years. However, a consensus couldn't be reached in the studies conducted. While a study stated that joint position sense error decreased in shoulder flexion and external rotation [61], another study suggested that it was not effective [62]. More studies are needed on this subject. Tiredness is accepted to affect proprioceptive sense negatively [63, 64]. Kinesio tape is claimed to decrease muscle tiredness. But it has been shown that kinesio tape applied to deltoid muscle does not compensate the decrease in joint position sense resulted from tiredness [65]. A study conducted in 2017 also showed that tiredness resulted from eccentric or concentric exercise does not affect proprioceptive sense [66].

With these practices, the increase in the proprioceptive sense can be explained by various factors. Probable mechanisms based on the increase of the sensitivity of local receptors have been tried to be explained above. In addition to these, we should not forget that personal learning has a great role in increasing the performance. Individuals proceed learning from cognitive to associative and to the automatic learning phase after months or perhaps years of repetition. The most critical part is to learn in the right motion pattern. After the activity proceeds to the automatic phase, it will be harder to reverse it.

Consequently, glenohumeral joint is a complex joint with a broad range of motion. Because the static stabilization cannot be provided sufficiently, dynamic stabilization and neuromuscular control are highly significant. Appropriate proprioceptive input is necessary to provide neuromuscular control. It should be kept in mind that first anatomical uniformity and then right motion patterns should be provided to enable right proprioceptive input.

References

1. Myers JB, Lephart SM. The role of the sensorimotor system in the athletic shoulder. J Athl Train. 2000;35(3):351–63.
2. Myers JB, Lephart SM. Sensorimotor deficits contributing to glenohumeral instability. Clin Orthop Relat Res. 2002;400:98–104.
3. Madhavan S, Shields RK. Influence of age on dynamic position sense: evidence using a sequential movement task. Exp Brain Res. 2005;164:18–28.
4. Sainburg RL, Poizner H, Ghez C. Loss of proprioception produces deficits in interjoint coordination. J Neurophysiol. 1993;70:2136–47.
5. Janwantanakul P, Magarey ME, Jones MA, Dansie BR. Variation in shoulder position sense at mid and extreme range of motion. Arch Phys Med Rehabil. 2001;82:840–4.
6. Suprak DN. Shoulder joint position sense is not enhanced at end range in an unconstrained task. Hum Mov Sci. 2011;30:424–35.
7. Freeman MAR, Wyke B. The innervation of the knee joint: an anatomical and histological study in cat. J Anat. 1967;101:505–32.
8. Vangness CT Jr, Ennis M, Taylor JG, Atkinson R. Neural anatomy of the glenohumeral ligaments, labrum, and subacromial bursa. Arthroscopy. 1995;11(2):180–4.
9. Ide K, Shirai Y, Ito H, Ito H. Sensory nerve supply in the human subacromial bursa. J Shoulder Elb Surg. 1996;5:371–82.
10. Windhorst U. Muscle proprioceptive feedback and spinal networks. Brain Res Bull. 2007;73:155–202.
11. Shields RK, Madhavan S, Cole K. Sustained muscle activity minimally influences dynamic position sense of the ankle. J Orthop Sports Phys Ther. 2005;35:443–51.
12. Blaiser RB, Carpenter JE, Huston LJ. Shoulder proprioception. Effect of joint laxity, joint position, and direction of motion. Orthop Rev. 1994;23(1):45–50.
13. Steinbeck J, Brüntrup J, Greshake O, Pötzl W, Filler T, et al. Neurohistological examination of the inferior glenohumeral ligament of the shoulder. J Orthop Res. 2003;21(2):250–5.
14. Yang JI, Jan MH, Hung CJ, Yang PL, Lin JJ. Reduced scapular muscle control and impaired shoulder joint position sense in subjects with chronic shoulder stiffness. J Electromyogr Kinesiol. 2010;29:206–11.
15. Suprak DN, Ostering LR, Donkelaar PV, Karduna AR. Shoulder joint position sense improves with elevation angle in a novel, unconstrained task. J Orthop Res. 2006;24:559–68.
16. Suprak DN, Ostering LR, Donkelaar PV, Karduna AR. Shoulder joint position sense improves with external load. J Mot Behav. 2007;39(6):517–25.
17. Walsh LD, Smith JL, Gandevia SC, Taylor JL. The combined effect of muscle contraction history and motor commands on human position sense. Exp Brain Res. 2009;195:603–10.
18. Zuckerman JD, Gallagher MA, Cuomo F, Rokito A. The effect of instability and subsequent anterior shoulder repair on proprioceptive ability. J Shoulder Elb Surg. 2003;12(2):105–9.
19. Anderson VB, Wee E. Impaired joint proprioception at higher shoulder elevations in chronic rotator cuff pathology. Arch Phys Med Rehabil. 2011;92:1146–51.
20. Barden JM, Balyk R, Raso VJ, Moreau M, Bagnall K. Dynamic upper limb proprioception in multidirectional shoulder instability. Clin Orthop Relat Res. 2004;420:181–9.
21. Warner JJ, Micheli LJ, Arslanian LE, Kennedy J, Kennedy R. Patterns of flexibility, laxity, and strength in normal shoulders and shoulders with instability and impingement. Am J Sports Med. 1990,18(4).366–75.
22. Machner A, Merk H, Becker R, Rohkohl K, Wissel H, et al. Kinesthetic sense of the shoulder in patients with impingement syndrome. Acta Orthop Scand. 2003;74(1):85–8.
23. Contemori S, Biscarini A, Botti FM, Busti D, Panichi R, Pettorossi VE. Sensorimotor control of the shoulder in professional volleyball players with

isolated infraspinatus muscle atrophy. J Sport Rehabil. 2017;12:1–29.

24. Maenhout AG, Palmans T, De Muynck M, De Wilde LF, Cools A. The impact of rotator cuff tendinopathy on proprioception, measuring force sensation. J Shoulder Elb Surg. 2012;21:1080–6.

25. Cuomo F, Birdzell MG, Zuckerman JD. The effect of degenerative arthritis and prosthetic arthroplasty on shoulder proprioception. J Shoulder Elb Surg. 2005;14(4):345–8.

26. Safran MR, Borsa PA, Lephart SM, Fu FH, Warner JJ. Shoulder proprioception in baseball pitchers. J Shoulder Elb Surg. 2001;10(5):438–44.

27. Wilk KE, Meister K, Andrews JR. Current concepts in the rehabilitation of the overhead throwing athlete. Am J Sports Med. 2002;30(1):136–51.

28. Moghadam AN, Khaki N, Kharazmi A, Eskandri Z. A comparative study on shoulder rotational strength, range of motion and proprioception between the throwing athletes and non-athletic persons. Asian J Sports Med. 2013;4:34–40.

29. Swanik KA, Lephart SM, Swanik B, Lephart SP, Stone DA, et al. The effects of shoulder plyometric training on proprioception and selected muscle performance characteristics. J Shoulder Elb Surg. 2002;11:579–86.

30. Voight ML, Hardin JA, Blackburn TA, Tippett S, Canner GC. The effects of muscle fatigue on and the relationship of arm dominance to shoulder proprioception. J Orthop Sports Phys Ther. 1996;23(6):348–52.

31. Ramsay JR, Riddoch MJ. Position-matching in the upper limb: professional ballet dancers perform with outstanding accuracy. Clin Rehabil. 2001;15:324–30.

32. Lephart SM, Myers JB, Bradley JP, Fu FH. Shoulder proprioception and function following thermal capsulorraphy. Arthroscopy. 2002;18:770–8.

33. Niessen MH, Veeger DHE, Janssen TWJ. Effect of body orientation on proprioception during active and passive motions. Am J Phys Med Rehabil. 2009;88:979–85.

34. Erickson RIC, Karduna AR. Three-dimensional repositioning tasks show differences in joint position sense between active and passive shoulder motion. J Orthop Res. 2012;30:787–92.

35. Alvemalm A, Furness A, Wellington L. Measurement of shoulder joint kinesthesia. Man Ther. 1996;1:140–5.

36. Balke M, Liem D, Dedy N, Thorwesten L, Balke M, et al. The laser-pointer assisted angle reproduction test for evaluation of proprioceptive shoulder function in patients with instability. Arch Orthop Trauma Surg. 2011;131:1077–84.

37. Duzgun I, Simsek IE, Yakut Y, Baltaci G, Uygur F. Assessing shoulder position sense using angle reproduction test in healthy individuals: a pilot study. Fizyoterapive Rehabilitasyon. 2011;22(3):240–4.

38. Lubiatowski P, Ogrodowicz P, Wojtaszek M, Kaniewski R, Stefaniak J, et al. Measurement of active shoulder proprioception: dedicated system and device. Eur J Orthop Surg Traumatol. 2013;23:177–83.

39. Dover G, Powers ME. Reliability of joint position sense and force-reproduction measures during internal and external rotation of the shoulder. J Athl Train. 2003;38(4):304–10.

40. Allen TJ, Ansems GE, Proske U. Effects of muscle conditioning on position sense at the human forearm during loading or fatigue of elbow flexors and role of the sense of effort. J Physiol. 2007;15:423–34.

41. Lee HM, Liau JJ, Cheng CK, Tan CM, Shih JT. Evaluation of shoulder proprioception following muscle fatigue. Clin Biomech. 2003;18(9):843–7.

42. Tripp BL, Boswell L, Gansneder BM, Shultz SJ. Functional fatigue decreases 3-dimensional multijoint position reproduction acuity in the overhead-throwing athlete. J Athl Train. 2004;39(4):316–20.

43. Yang JL, Chen S, Jan MH, Lin YF, Lin JJ. Proprioception assessment in subjects with idiopathic loss shoulder range of motion: joint position sense and a novel proprioceptive feedback index. J Orthop Res. 2008;26(9):1218–24.

44. Tripp BL, Yochem EM, Uhl TL. Functional fatigue and upper extremity sensorimotor system acuity in baseball athletes. J Athl Train. 2007;42(1):90–8.

45. Aydin T, Yildiz Y, Yanmiş I, Yildiz C, Kalyon TA. Shoulder proprioception: a comparison between shoulder joint in healthy and surgically repaired shoulders. Arch Orthop Trauma Surg. 2001;121(7):422–5.

46. Maier MW, Niklasch M, Dreher T, Wolf SI, Zeifang F, Loew M, Kasten P. Proprioception 3 years after shoulder arthroplasty in 3D motion analysis: a prospective study. Arch Orthop Trauma Surg. 2012;132(7):1003–10.

47. Kasten P, Maier M, Retting O, Raiss P, Wolf S, Loew M. Proprioception in total, hemi- and reverse shoulder arthroplasty in 3D motion analyses: a prospective study. Int Orthop. 2009;33(6):1641–7.

48. Costello JT, Donnelly AE. Cryotherapy and joint position sense in healthy participants: a systematic review. J Athl Train. 2010;45(3):306–16.

49. Torres R, Silva F, Pedrosa V, Ferreira J, Lopes A. The acute effects of cryotherapy on muscle strength and shoulder proprioception. J Sport Rehabil. 2016;11:1–24.

50. Rogol IM, Ernst G, Perrin DH. Open and closed kinetic chain exercises improve shoulder joint reposition sense equally in healthy subjects. J Athl Train. 1998;33(4):315–8.

51. Myers JB, Wassinger CA, Lephart SM. Sensorimotor contribution to shoulder stability: effect of injury and rehabilitation. Man Ther. 2006;11:197–201.

52. Lin YL, Karduna A. Exercise focusing on rotator cuff and scapular muscles do not improve shoulder joint position sense in healthy subjects. Hum Mov Sci. 2016;49:248–57.

53. Uribe BP, Coburn JW, Brown LE, Judelson DA, Khamoui AV, et al. Muscle activation when performing the chest press and shoulder press on a stable bench vs. a Swiss ball. J Strength Cond Res. 2010;24(4):1028–33.

54. Mohapatra S, Krishnan V, Aruin AS. Postural control in response to an external perturbation: effect of altered proprioceptive information. Exp Brain Res. 2012;217:197–208.

55. Pochini AC, Ejnisman B, Alves MTS, Uyeda LF, Nouailhetas VLA, et al. Overuse of training increases mechanoreceptors in supraspinatus tendon of rats SHR. J Orthop Res. 2011;29:1771–4.

56. Wilk KE, Voight ML, Keirns MA, Gambette V, Andrews JR, et al. Stretch-shortening drills for the upper extremities: theory and clinical application. J Orthop Sports Phys Ther. 1993;17(5):225–39.

57. Heiderscheit BC, McLean KP, Davies GJ. The effects of isokinetic vs plyometric training on the shoulder internal rotators. J Orthop Sports Phys Ther. 1996;23(2):125–33.

58. Wilk KE, Arrigo CA, Andrews JR. Current concepts: the stabilizing structures of the glenohumeral joint. J Orthop Sports Phys Ther. 1997;25(6):364–79.

59. Lin JJ, Hung CJ, Yang PL. The effects of scapular taping on electromyographic muscle activity and proprioception feedback in healthy shoulders. J Orthop Res. 2011;29:53–7.

60. Morin GE, Tiberio D, Austin G. The effect of upper trapezius taping on electromyographic activity in the upper and middle trapezius region. J Sport Rehabil. 1997;6:309–19.

61. Burfeind SM, Chimera N. Randomized control trial investigating the effects of kinesiology tape on shoulder proprioception. J Sport Rehabil. 2015;24(4):405–12.

62. Keenan KA, Akins JS, Vrnell M, Abt J, Lovalekar M, Lephart S, Sell TC. Kinesiology taping does not alter shoulder proprioception, or scapular kinematics in healthy, physically active subjects and subjects with Subacromial Impingment syndrome. Phys Ther Sport. 2017;24:60–6.

63. Ju YY, Wang CW, Cheng HY. Effects of active fatiguing movement versus passive repetitive movement on knee proprioception. Clin Biomech. 2010;25(7):708–12.

64. Ribeiro F, Venancio J, Quintas P, Oliveira J. The effect of fatigue on knee position sense is not dependent upon the muscle group fatigued. Muscle Nerve. 2011;44(2):217–20.

65. Zanca GG, Mattiello SM, Karduna AR. Kinesio taping of the deltoid does not reduce fatigue induced deficits in shoulder joint position sense. Clin Biomech. 2015;30(9):903–7.

66. Spargoli G. The acute effects of concentric versus eccentric muscle fatigue on shoulder active repositioning sense. Int J Sports Phys Ther. 2017;12(2):219–26.

Proprioception After Elbow Injury, Surgery, and Rehabilitation

5

Tüzün Firat and Özgün Uysal

5.1 Proprioception After Elbow Injury/Surgery and Rehabilitation

Elbow joint acts as an intermediate joint between shoulder and hand. It is mainly responsible for positioning of the hand in space [1]. Proprioceptive ability of elbow does not depend on its structures solely; it is nourished by hand and shoulder elements. Thereby the assumption that elbow joint complex has an independent proprioceptive function is not a valid view. Many studies suggest that injury of shoulder and wrist complex can affect elbow function [2, 3]. In addition to elbow pathologies, pathologies of the hand and shoulder should be analysed before assessment and treatment. Moreover, some injury models do not only contain elbow joint itself although injury mainly affects elbow structures. For example radial head fractures associated with medial collateral ligament injury generally occur with falling, and wrist structures including radioscaphoid ligament can be affected.

When falling pattern is examined it can be seen that it is an expected result of protective

extension reaction [4, 5]. This reaction is also connected with contralateral activations of the primary sensory and motor cortex, and of the supplementary motor area in addition to the midbrain structures. These kinds of injuries may be the result of disturbance of whole proprioceptive system [6, 7]. Accordingly, assessment and treatment of elbow proprioception should be planned in a complementary approach and should not be focused only on elbow joint.

5.2 Elbow Structures Containing Proprioceptive Afferents

The elbow complex is a modified hinge joint and consists of three bones and two joints. The articular capsule is reinforced anteriorly by oblique bands of fibrous tissue and strengthened by collateral ligaments which augment structural stability [1]. Medial collateral ligaments consist of anterior, posterior and transverse bundles; anterior bundle is the strongest and stiffest of all and resists valgus loading. Anterior bundles provide articular stability throughout the entire range of motion. Posterior bundles are resisting valgus forces and become taut in extreme flexion ranges. Because they start and end in the same bone, they do not provide structural stability to articulation [8–10].

Lateral collateral ligament is made of two bundles originating from lateral epicondyle. One

T. Firat, Ph.D., M.Sc., P.T. (✉) • Ö. Uysal, P.T.
Faculty of Health Sciences, Department of
Physiotherapy and Rehabilitation, Hacettepe
University, Ankara, Turkey
e-mail: tuzun75@gmail.com; uysalozgun@gmail.com

© Springer International Publishing AG, part of Springer Nature 2018
D. Kaya et al. (eds.), *Proprioception in Orthopaedics, Sports Medicine and Rehabilitation*,
https://doi.org/10.1007/978-3-319-66640-2_5

Table 5.1 Mechanoreceptors, types, and their stimulation [21]

Mechanoreceptors	Type	Stimulation
Muscle-tendon unit	Muscle spindle Golgi tendon organ	Muscle length Velocity of change of muscle length Active muscle tension
Joint	Ruffini ending Pacinian ending Mazzoni ending Golgi ending	Low and high load tension Compression loads throughout the entire ROM
Fascia	Ruffini ending Pacinian ending	Low and high tension loads During joint movement
Skin	Hair follicle receptor Ruffini ending Pacinian ending Merkel ending Meissner ending	Superficial tissue deformation/stretch or compression during joint movement

is known as "radial collateral ligament" and blends with annular ligament. The other is named as "lateral collateral ligament (LCL)" which attaches to ulna. These fibres become stretched in full flexion. Both LCL and lateral side of capsule resist varus-producing forces [8, 11].

Within capsule, radial head is held against proximal ulna by a fibro-osseous ring that is formed by 75% annular ligament and 25% radial notch of ulna.

These structures give elbow joint passive stability and muscles give dynamic stability. In order to achieve stability, these structures are being loaded and tensed with movements. Amount of load and tension stimulates proprioceptors and plays an important role in the extremity positioning and joint stability.

Proprioception can be defined as brain's ability to interpret sensory signals from muscles, joints and skin receptors to determine body segments positions and movements in space [12–17].

Proprioception is the product of sensory information supplied by specialized nerve endings termed mechanoreceptors, i.e. transducers converting mechanical stimuli to action potentials for transmission to the central nervous system (CNS) [18, 19]. Mechanoreceptors specifically contributing to proprioception are termed proprioceptors and are found in muscle, tendon, joint and fascia; receptors in the skin can also contribute to proprioception, which is shown in Table 5.1 [18, 20].

The muscle spindles, located in all skeletal muscles in parallel with the extrafusal muscle fibres [22–24], are considered the most important source of proprioception [25, 26]. They are highly sensitive and their density varies throughout the body, reflecting different functional demands. Importantly the sensitivity of the muscle spindles can be adjusted via innervation of the polar ends of the intrafusal muscle fibres by gamma motor neurons [25]. Other sources of proprioception are the ligaments surrounding elbow endowed with mechanoreceptors consisting of Golgi organs, Ruffini terminals, Pacinian corpuscles and free nerve endings. These receptors supply important information to CNS to augment proprioception and detect safe limits of passive tension in structures around the elbow [27]. They have been considered "limit detectors", stimulated at the extremes of joint range of motion (ROM) [28]. However it is now known that joint proprioceptors provide input throughout a joint's entire ROM under both low- and high-load conditions stimulating strong discharges from the muscle spindle and are thus vital for joint stability [29–31].

5.3 Injury Models of Elbow

5.3.1 Trauma

Elbow injuries are common in many sports, recreational activities and repetitive motions. Elbow fractures can involve any bone within the elbow joint. These fractures usually result from a fall on an outstretched arm. Involvement of each bone depends on the nature, magnitude, location and direction of force. Also age of patient is important. Generally soft-tissue injuries accompany the fracture and augment the level of disability.

Passive stabilizers of elbow usually injured by high-velocity trauma, mostly by falling. The medial collateral ligament (MCL) is usually injured by violently forcing fully extended elbow into excessive valgus (often falling on to outstretched arm). There can be an accompanying fracture in humeroradial joint or radius head. If the joint is excessively hyperextended, anterior capsule can be injured too. MCL can be injured by repetitive trauma/stress, which is commonly seen in sportspeople (especially in baseball pitchers) [32–34]. Lateral collateral ligament (LCL) often ruptures in a sports trauma and as a result increased valgus and posterior-lateral rotary instability occur. This instability results with excessive rotation of forearm followed by subluxation of the joints [35, 36].

5.3.2 Idiopathic

Lateral epicondylitis (LE) presents as lateral elbow pain arising from extensor carpi radialis brevis and longus tendons at the lateral epicondyle. Primary pathology is collagen disorganization in the origin of extensor carpi radialis brevis and extensor digitorum communis. It's a degenerative process than inflammatory process. With continued loading partial tears may occur. LE can also be characterized as an enthesopathy. Entheses are close to many sensory nerve endings that affect proprioceptive input. It can occur

with striking sports as well as occupations involving repetitive motions of wrist and elbow during pinching and grasping [37–39].

5.3.3 Elbow's Response to Injury, Trauma, and Rehabilitation

Frequently after trauma, musculoskeletal tissues and innervating mechanoreceptors are damaged [40, 41]. Therefore after resolving trauma, persistent pain and swelling, the loss of musculoskeletal tissue and its mechanoreceptors causes impairment in proprioception [42–44]. In surgically treated dislocations, cortical deafferentation causes alterations in the motor scheme due to anaesthesia and immobilization period [45]. Soon after surgery, giving perceptive rehabilitation including mental imagery techniques for recovering the perception of movement should be planned for recovering fast reflex responses after external stimulations [46].

5.3.4 Surgery or Conservative Treatment? Which Is Better for Proprioception?

Treatments aim functional recovery as early as possible either surgical or conservative. Sometimes surgery may seem harmful in regard of damaging the mechanoreceptors as a consequence of incision, oedema, pain and immobilization. Also, anaesthesia procedures may affect cortical representation in surgical exposure area. Nonetheless, surgery generally accelerates the duration of functional recovery. For example in the case of persistent LE problem surgery may improve the quality of life and function more early than conservative follow-up. Some elbow surgeries such as total elbow arthroplasty are quite traumatic. Medial and lateral skin flaps are raised, triceps is reflected, both flexors and extensors are released, collateral ligaments are released and the capsule is excised. This means that a huge damage to the main sources of proprioceptive afferent system can be expected. This kind of extensive surgery affects the proprioception of elbow. Besides, anaesthetic method also affects joint position sense. Also, anaesthetics may lead deafferentation in cortex and diminish joint position sense [47].

For these reasons, main factors to consider for proprioception when deciding surgery are preservation of afferents, promotion of regeneration of mechanoreceptors and modification of protective reflex arcs as possible.

- **Preservation of afferents**: While operating around elbow joint, mechanoreceptors and afferent nerves of joint structures must be preserved as much as possible. For this purpose, arthroscopy may offer better results than open surgery.
- **Promotion of regeneration of mechanoreceptors**: After surgery, density of afferents may decline. To prevent this loss, preserving original tissue tensions during repairing structures is crucial.
- **Modification of protective reflex arcs**: In the inadequacy of ligamentous stabilization, muscles undertake the function as dynamic stabilizer of the joint, i.e. hamstring function as in anterior cruciate ligament rupture [48].

Although it is well known that surgery deteriorates proprioception, it is not possible to make a comparison with conservative management of selected pathologies. Firstly, surgical decision-making is quite easy in pathologies such as multiple fractures, advanced degenerative diseases, dislocations with multiple ligamentous injury, instabilities and tumours. Secondly, painful pathologies including overuse injuries, nerve compression syndromes and rheumatic conditions are generally followed with conservative approach. However this rough distinction is not always correct. In the light of this discussion, a paradigm can be developed: Whole upper extremity should be evaluated and treated in all localized pathologies with conservative approaches. Because surgery targets only affected part, where

the symptoms arising from other parts of extremity can be underestimated.

5.4 Assessing Proprioception in Elbow

Specific tests of proprioception assess an individual's status with regard to joint position sense (**JPS**), kinaesthesia or force sense [26, 49]. Tests can be performed under passive (biasing joint mechanoreceptors) or active conditions (stimulating joint and muscle-tendon mechanoreceptors) [49, 50]. The joint position error (**JPE**) test is considered the primary measure of upper limb proprioception and has been widely used as an outcome indicator especially for patients with cervical spinal cord injury. JPE tests assess precision or accuracy in repositioning a joint at a predetermined target angle [51, 52]. A decrease in JPE indicates increased ability to reposition the joint after active movement.

Kinaesthesia tests assess the ability to perceive joint movement measured using threshold to detection of passive motion (**TTDPM**) [51, 52], movement discrimination tests [53, 54] or acuity of a tracking task [55]. Force sense tests assess the ability to perceive and produce a previously generated and predetermined sub-maximal quantity of force [52, 56, 57].

Threshold testing and joint position matching methods examine different physiological aspects of proprioceptive function. Because threshold testing is based on passive motion, it most closely reflects afferent sensory feedback processing (i.e. proprioception). Matching methods require active motion and are consequently influenced by additional sensorimotor processes. Factors such as working memory and transmission between brain hemispheres also influence joint matching task outcomes.

Several variables are commonly calculated in JPS, TTDPM and force sense tests. Variables include constant error (CE), variable error (VE) and absolute error (AE) [58]. These variables are intended to describe different aspects of JPS and force sense. Acuity at a pursuit or tracking task is commonly presented as deviation from target, or time on target [58]. Researchers have used three to five test trials to generate reliable mean values at the extremity joints [52, 56, 59]. A limitation of these proprioception tests is that they involve cognitive components and provide an indirect measure of proprioception. Other factors can also affect results. The size and speed of the movement should be standardized, or specific to a functional task [60, 61]. Larger errors can be expected when assessing children and the elderly compared to younger adults [62]. Muscle thixotropy, which is history-dependent passive stiffness of the muscle [63], can also affect the results and thus isometric contraction of the muscle at the test position before assessment, especially in passive tests, i.e. prior to the passive movement, is recommended [26].

5.5 Rehabilitation Approaches After Elbow Injury

Regardless of injury model (due to surgery, trauma and idiopathic), connective tissues undergo inflammatory, fibroblastic and remodelling phases [5]. During the inflammatory phase treatment should be focused on protecting the healing structures, maintaining stability, controlling pain, minimizing oedema and moving the elbow through a stable arc of motion by performing active assisted ROM exercises.

In the fibroblastic phase, the tensile strength of the healing tissue is minimal and progressively increases with time. Increased collagen density contributes to contracture formation [64]. Gentle passive ROM exercises together with active ROM exercises are added to this program to influence the collagen remodelling in a way that allows motion of the joints. As the patient advances through the fibroblastic phase, light activities of daily living are encouraged. Patients are cautioned with respect to the intensity of exercise to prevent a new inflammatory response. Static progressive splinting to gain ROM is considered, depending on the pathology.

During the remodelling phase passive, active and progressive strengthening exercises enhance collagen orientation and plastic elongation of

musculotendinous and capsular tissues. Low-grade joint mobilization techniques should be started initially [65, 66]; progressing to high grades is also effective in increasing joint mobility and ROM. Static progressive splinting together with progressive resistive muscle strengthening increases mobility and strength. Endurance training and work hardening then are added to the program.

Rehabilitation approaches should be designed as painless as possible for preventing adverse affect of pain on proprioception. Almost all rehabilitation regimes focus on motor performance-based functional improvement. However a sensorial input-based proprioceptive function should be the first step in elbow injuries. Especially after surgery, mental imagery can be initiated during the immobilization period and it can be maintained during whole rehabilitation to preserve communication between cortical and peripheral structures. Although mirror therapy is a preferred method for providing sensorial input after injury [5, 67], however it may be difficult to prepare a mirror box for elbow.

After trauma, basic principles of rehabilitation are containing drawbacks of immobilization, avoiding stress of the healing tissue over a certain limit, fulfilling defined criteria before moving to next stage and keeping programme patient based and up to date [68]. Rehabilitation principles can be chronologically grouped into four stages: stage of early mobilization, intermediate stage of recovery, stage of advanced strengthening and return to working/sports activity [45].

In a rehabilitation programme, proprioceptive retraining is used to improve dynamic stability of the joints. Dynamic stability is proprioception's duty in regulation of joint function. Normally, in excessive joint movements, ligament tension increases which causes proprioceptive stimuli followed by response of muscle contraction to stabilize and protect the joint [5]. In this situation, any disruption on ligaments may disrupt this function.

Reducing causes of "inhibition" of proprioception should be aimed; pain, effusion and fatigue are known inhibitors of proprioception. So any intervention on these inhibitors would improve proprioception [21].

Mobilization of the humeroradial, proximal radioulnar and humeroulnar joints in rehabilitation of elbow trauma has a role in reducing pain, decreasing muscle spasm and gaining motion if followed immediately by active or passive motion. Initially oscillatory motions of the elbow are effective in stimulating tendon and proprioceptive end organs, which inhibits muscle spasm and muscle co-contraction [65, 66, 69].

After resolving causes for inhibition of proprioception, improving awareness of joint position and joint motion or kinaesthesia should be the new focus of rehabilitation programme. Mimicking a specific position angle of healthy side with affected elbow and remembering the previosly shown elbow angle with or without vision can be preferred as basic proprioceptive exercises. Mirror therapy can be used to enhance this process. Creating illusion of motion of the involved side would influence cortical areas of sensorimotor control which will increase motor performance [5]. If possible, rhythmic stabilization, exercises for the shoulder, wrist and elbow can be started in the early-stage to provide correct neuromuscular control of the whole upper limb [45].

Closed kinetic chain exercises with minimal loading should be started as early possible. Pain-free loading and ROM are important to avoid afferent suppression due to pain.

When the elbow reaches a painless and stable function regardless of ROM, proprioceptive rehabilitation can also be started in order to obtain fast reflex responses to external stresses. Closed kinetic chain exercises with loading should be initiated [45].

The next stage involves focusing on the muscles that aids/protects ligaments and joint in order to support and increase joint stabilization and improve proprioception. Open kinetic chain exercises with resistive tools should be started.

The concept of total arm strengthening is encouraged using proximal stability and enabling distal mobility, to ensure adequate muscular performance and dynamic joint stability. In addition, neuromuscular control exercises are performed to enhance dynamic stability and proprioceptive skill. These exercise protocols include proprioceptive neuromuscular facilitation exercises such as rhythmic stabilizations and slow reversal holds, which can progress as tolerated to rapid diagonal movements [69, 70].

Neuromuscular joint facilitation (NJF) is a new therapeutic exercise based on kinesiology that integrates the facilitation element of proprioceptive neuromuscular facilitation (PNF) and joint composition movement, aiming to improve the movement of the joint through passive, active and resistance exercises. NJF is used to increase strength, flexibility and ROM, and improve elbow function. NJF uses the same motion pattern as PNF, but the location of resistance of NJF is different, i.e. proximal resistance is applied to the biceps or to the brachialis muscle tendon attachment point in elbow patterns [71–73].

5.5.1 Effects of Taping/Orthotics on Elbow Proprioception

Application of an elastic bandage improved elbow position sense in the study of Khabie. Although it does not provide mechanical support, it's believed that it stimulates skin receptors and enhances proprioceptive function during application. However its effect ends with removing the bandage [74]. Similarly, effect of taping on proprioception has been investigated in many studies involving different joints. Bae showed that spiral kinesio taping was effective on functional ankle instability within 30 min after application [75]. It affects sensory modulation and may organize synaptic organization through afferent stimulation in short-term duration in pathological conditions. However, Long et al. stated that kinesio taping may impair proprioception in healthy people via input overload [76]. It can be concluded that kinesio taping provides significant sensory stimulus on afferent system and its usage in pathological conditions is recommended.

Augmentation of somatosensory information via passive techniques such as manual therapy, soft tissue techniques and taping or braces can be valuable as they stimulate the mechanoreceptors in joints, soft tissues and skin to send a barrage of sensory information to the CNS [77].

The peripheral somatosensory receptors located in the superficial skin layers and their relationship to pain, proprioception and motor control have been investigated, and recent studies support the reported physical effects of kinesio taping on skin, lymphatics, and muscle and joint functions [5].

Skin envelops the body with sensory receptors that signal to the CNS changes in the environment, which then elicits a response. These responses can range from simple reflexes, such as shivering to control heat loss, to reflexes as complicated as intricate muscle control to walk a tightrope blindfolded. Each of these responses requires a different degree of cortical control but functions on the same neurologic pathways. Cutaneous sensory receptors include mechanoreceptors, thermoreceptors and nociceptors. CNS responses are determined by the type and extent of stimulation to these receptors. The elastic properties of Kinesio Tex Tape provide increased low-threshold excitement to these somatosensory receptors during movement and at rest, thereby increasing somatosensory input to the CNS [5].

The application of an elastic bandage is shown to improve elbow proprioception [74]. Similar findings have been reported in studies investigating proprioception in other joints. A study of proprioception of osteoarthritic knees [78] demonstrated an improvement in joint awareness when an elastic bandage was applied. They concluded that wearing an elastic bandage improves joint position sense in knees.

Taping affects the inflammatory responses. Pain and oedema which are inhibitors of proprioception can be decreased by taping. The anterolateral system transmits information from the skin on crude touch and pressure, contributing to touch and limb proprioception. This pathway also transmits thermal and nociception information to higher brain centres, much like the medial lemniscal system. The gate theory for pain control views the neurologic system as a simple three-axon chain system. This theory supports the idea that superficial stimulation of first-order afferent receptors in the skin can inhibit the transmission of pain at the spinal cord level. Theoretically, kinesio taping may stimu-

late the somatosensory system to reduce pain. When properly applied to stretched skin, the elastic recoil of the tape may accomplish the following:

- Increases sensory stimuli to mechanoreceptors, thereby activating the endogenous analgesic system
- Possibly activates the spinal inhibitory system through stimulation of touch receptors
- Possibly activates the descending inhibitory system
- Decreases pain by reducing inflammation, thereby decreasing pressure on nociceptors [5]

References

1. Neumann DA. Kinesiology of the musculoskeletal system-E-book: foundations for rehabilitation. London: Elsevier Health Sciences; 2013.
2. Werner FW, An KN. Biomechanics of the elbow and forearm. Hand Clin. 1994;10(3):357–73.
3. Cooper JE, Shwedyk E, Quanbury AO, Miller J, Hildebrand D. Elbow joint restriction: effect on functional upper limb motion during performance of three feeding activities. Arch Phys Med Rehabil. 1993;74(8):805–9. https://doi.org/10.1016/0003-9993(93)90005-U.
4. Brukner P. Brukner & Khan's clinical sports medicine. North Ryde: McGraw-Hill; 2012.
5. Skirven TM, Osterman AL, Fedorczyk J, Amadio PC. Rehabilitation of the hand and upper extremity, 2-volume set E-book: expert consult. London: Elsevier Health Sciences; 2011.
6. Shumway-Cook A, Woollacott MH. Motor control: theory and practical applications. Philadelphia: Lippincott Williams & Wilkins; 2001.
7. Ghez C, Krakauer J. Voluntary movement. Princ Neural Sci. 1991;3:609–25.
8. Regan WD, Korinek SL, Morrey BF, An KN. Biomechanical study of ligaments around the elbow joint. Clin Orthop Relat Res. 1991;271:170–9.
9. Dugas JR, Ostrander RV, Cain EL, Kingsley D, Andrews JR. Anatomy of the anterior bundle of the ulnar collateral ligament. J Shoulder Elb Surg. 2007;16(5):657–60. https://doi.org/10.1016/j.jse.2006.11.009
10. Callaway GH, Field LD, Deng XH, Torzilli PA, O'Brien SJ, Altchek DW, et al. Biomechanical evaluation of the medial collateral ligament of the elbow. J Bone Joint Surg Am. 1997;79(8):1223–31.
11. Olsen BS, Søjbjerg JO, Dalstra M, Sneppen O. Kinematics of the lateral ligamentous constraints of

the elbow joint. J Shoulder Elb Surg. 1996;5(5):333–41. https://doi.org/10.1016/S1058-2746(96)80063-2.

12. Goodwin GM, McCloskey DI, Matthews PB. Proprioceptive illusions induced by muscle vibration: contribution by muscle spindles to perception? Science (New York, NY). 1972;175(4028):1382–4.

13. Burke D, Hagbarth KE, Lofstedt L, Wallin BG. The responses of human muscle spindle endings to vibration of non-contracting muscles. J Physiol. 1976;261(3):673–93.

14. Roll JP, Vedel JP. Kinaesthetic role of muscle afferents in man, studied by tendon vibration and microneurography. Exp Brain Res. 1982;47(2):177–90.

15. Ferrell WR, Gandevia SC, McCloskey DI. The role of joint receptors in human kinaesthesia when intramuscular receptors cannot contribute. J Physiol. 1987;386:63–71.

16. Edin BB. Cutaneous afferents provide information about knee joint movements in humans. J Physiol. 2001;531(Pt1):289–97.https://doi.org/10.1111/j.1469-7793.2001.0289j.x.

17. Edin BB, Abbs JH. Finger movement responses of cutaneous mechanoreceptors in the dorsal skin of the human hand. J Neurophysiol. 1991;65(3):657–70.

18. Martin JH, Jessell TM. Modality coding in the somatic sensory system. Princ Neural Sci. 1991;3:341–52.

19. Yahia LH, Rhalmi S, Newman N, Isler M. Sensory innervation of human thoracolumbar fascia. Acta Orthop Scand. 1992;63(2):195–7. https://doi.org/10.3109/17453679209154822.

20. Rothwell JC. Control of human voluntary movement. Netherlands: Springer Science & Business Media; 2012.

21. Röijezon U, Clark NC, Treleaven J. Proprioception in musculoskeletal rehabilitation. Part 1: basic science and principles of assessment and clinical interventions. Man Ther. 2015;20(3):368–77.

22. Peck D, Buxton DF, Nitz A. A comparison of spindle concentrations in large and small muscles acting in parallel combinations. J Morphol. 1984;180(3):243–52. https://doi.org/10.1002/jmor.1051800307.

23. Kulkarni V, Chandy M, Babu K. Quantitative study of muscle spindles in suboccipital muscles of human foetuses. Neurol India. 2001;49(4):355.

24. Banks RW. An allometric analysis of the number of muscle spindles in mammalian skeletal muscles. J Anat. 2006;208(6):753–68. https://doi.org/10.1111/j.1469-7580.2006.00558.x.

25. Gordon J, Ghez C. Muscle receptors and spinal reflexes: the stretch reflex. Princ Neural Sci. 1991;3:565–80.

26. Proske U, Gandevia SC. The proprioceptive senses: their roles in signaling body shape, body position and movement, and muscle force. Physiol Rev. 2012;92(4):1651–97. https://doi.org/10.1152/physrev.00048.2011.

27. Petrie S, Collins JG, Solomonow M, Wink C, Chuinard R, D'Ambrosia R. Mechanoreceptors in the human elbow ligaments. J Hand Surg Am. 1998;23(3):512–8. https://doi.org/10.1016/s0363-5023(05)80470-8.

28. Burgess PR, Clark FJ. Characteristics of knee joint receptors in the cat. J Physiol. 1969;203(2):317–35. https://doi.org/10.1113/jphysiol.1969.sp008866.

29. Sojka P, Johansson H, Sjölander P, Lorentzon R, Djupsjöbacka M. Fusimotor neurones can be reflexy influenced by activity in receptor afferents from the posterior cruciate ligament. Brain Res. 1989;483(1):177–83.https://doi.org/10.1016/0006-8993(89)90051-6.

30. Johansson H. The anterior cruciate ligament: a sensor action on the γ-muscle-spindle systems muscles around the knee joints. Neuro-Orthopedics. 1990;9:1–23.

31. Needle AR, Swanik CB, Farquhar WB, Thomas SJ, Rose WC, Kaminski TW. Muscle spindle traffic in functionally unstable ankles during ligamentous stress. J Athl Train. 2013;48(2):192–202. https://doi.org/10.4085/1062-6050-48.1.09.

32. Cohen MS, Bruno RJ. The collateral ligaments of the elbow: anatomy and clinical correlation. Clin Orthop Relat Res. 2001;383:123–30.

33. Sabick MB, Torry MR, Lawton RL, Hawkins RJ. Valgus torque in youth baseball pitchers: a biomechanical study. J Shoulder Elb Surg. 2004;13(3):349–55. https://doi.org/10.1016/s1058274604000308.

34. Williams RJ 3rd, Urquhart ER, Altchek DW. Medial collateral ligament tears in the throwing athlete. Instr Course Lect. 2004;53:579–86.

35. Dunning CE, Zarzour ZD, Patterson SD, Johnson JA, King GJ. Ligamentous stabilizers against posterolateral rotatory instability of the elbow. J Bone Joint Surg Am. 2001;83-a(12):1823–8.

36. O'Driscoll SW, Jupiter JB, King GJW, Hotchkiss RN, Morrey BF. The unstable elbow. JBJS. 2000;82(5):724.

37. Freivalds A. Biomechanics of the upper limbs: mechanics, modeling and musculoskeletal injuries. London: CRC press; 2011.

38. Snijders CJ, Volkers A, Mechelse K, Vleeming A. Provocation of epicondylalgia lateralis (tennis elbow) by power grip or pinching. Med Sci Sports Exerc. 1987;19(5):518–23.

39. Hong Y, Bartlett R. Routledge handbook of biomechanics and human movement science. Londres: Routledge; 2008.

40. Dhillon MS, Bali K, Vasistha RK. Immunohistological evaluation of proprioceptive potential of the residual stump of injured anterior cruciate ligaments (ACL). Int Orthop. 2010;34(5):737–41. https://doi.org/10.1007/s00264-009-0948-1.

41. Bali K, Dhillon MS, Vasistha RK, Kakkar N, Chana R, Prabhakar S. Efficacy of immunohistological methods in detecting functionally viable mechanoreceptors in the remnant stumps of injured anterior cruciate ligaments and its clinical importance. Knee Surg Sports Traumatol Arthrosc. 2012;20(1):75–80. https://doi.org/10.1007/s00167-011-1526-9.

42. Smith RL, Brunolli J. Shoulder kinesthesia after anterior glenohumeral joint dislocation. Phys

Ther. 1989;69(2):106–12. https://doi.org/10.1093/ptj/69.2.106.

43. Borsa PA, Lephart SM, Irrgang JJ, Safran MR, Fu FH. The effects of joint position and direction of joint motion on proprioceptive sensibility in anterior cruciate ligament-deficient athletes. Am J Sports Med. 1997;25(3):336–40. https://doi.org/10.1177/036354659702500311.

44. Willems T, Witvrouw E, Verstuyft J, Vaes P, De Clercq D. Proprioception and muscle strength in subjects with a history of ankle sprains and chronic instability. J Athl Train. 2002;37(4):487–93.

45. Fusaro I, Orsini S, Kantar SS, Sforza T, Benedetti M, Bettelli G, et al. Elbow rehabilitation in traumatic pathology. Musculoskelet Surg. 2014;98(1):95–102.

46. James RY, Throckmorton TW, Bauer RM, Watson JT, Weikert DR. Management of acute complex instability of the elbow with hinged external fixation. J Shoulder Elb Surg. 2007;16(1):60–7.

47. Ettinger LR, Shapiro M, Karduna A. Subacromial Anesthetics increase proprioceptive deficit in the shoulder and elbow in patients with subacromial impingement syndrome. Clin Med Insights Arthritis Musculoskelet Disord. 2017;10:1179544117713196.

48. Safran MR, Caldwell GL Jr, Fu FH. Proprioception considerations in surgery. J Sport Rehabil. 1994;3(1):105–15.

49. Riemann BL, Myers JB, Lephart SM. Sensorimotor system measurement techniques. J Athl Train. 2002;37(1):85–98.

50. Clark NC, Röijezon U, Treleaven J. Proprioception in musculoskeletal rehabilitation. Part 2: clinical assessment and intervention. Man Ther. 2015;20(3):378–87. https://doi.org/10.1016/j.math.2015.01.009.

51. Lephart SM, Warner JJP, Borsa PA, Fu FH. Proprioception of the shoulder joint in healthy, unstable, and surgically repaired shoulders. J Shoulder Elb Surg. 1994;3(6):371–80. https://doi.org/10.1016/S1058-2746(09)80022-0.

52. Benjaminse A, Sell TC, Abt JP, House AJ, Lephart SM. Reliability and precision of hip proprioception methods in healthy individuals. Clin J Sport Med. 2009;19(6):457–63. https://doi.org/10.1097/JSM.0b013e3181bcb155.

53. Waddington G, Adams R, Jones A. Wobble board (ankle disc) training effects on the discrimination of inversion movements. Aust J Physiother. 1999;45(2):95–101. https://doi.org/10.1016/S0004-9514(14)60341-X.

54. Waddington G, Seward H, Wrigley T, Lacey N, Adams R. Comparing wobble board and jump-landing training effects on knee and ankle movement discrimination. J Sci Med Sport. 2000;3(4):449–59. https://doi.org/10.1016/S1440-2440(00)80010-9.

55. Kristjansson E, Oddsdottir GL. "The fly": a new clinical assessment and treatment method for deficits of movement control in the cervical spine: reliability and validity. Spine. 2010;35(23):E1298–E305. https://doi.org/10.1097/BRS.0b013e3181e7fc0a.

56. Dover G, Powers ME. Reliability of joint position sense and force-reproduction measures during inter-nal and external rotation of the shoulder. J Athl Train. 2003;38(4):304–10.

57. O'Leary SP, Vicenzino BT, Jull GA. A new method of isometric dynamometry for the craniocervical flexor muscles. Phys Ther. 2005;85(6):556–64.

58. Schmidt RA, Lee TD. Motor control and learning: a behavioral emphasis. Champaign, IL: Human Kinetics; 2005.

59. Nagai T, Sell TC, Abt JP, Lephart SM. Reliability, precision, and gender differences in knee internal/external rotation proprioception measurements. Phys Ther Sport. 2012;13(4):233–7. https://doi.org/10.1016/j.ptsp.2011.11.004.

60. Preuss R, Grenier S, McGill S. The effect of test position on lumbar spine position sense. J Orthop Sports Phys Ther. 2003;33(2):73–8. https://doi.org/10.2519/jospt.2003.33.2.73.

61. Suprak DN, Osternig LR, van Donkelaar P, Karduna AR. Shoulder joint position sense improves with external load. J Mot Behav. 2007;39(6):517–25. https://doi.org/10.3200/JMBR.39.6.517-525.

62. Goble DJ. Proprioceptive acuity assessment via joint position matching: from basic science to general practice. Phys Ther. 2010;90(8):1176–84. https://doi.org/10.2522/ptj.20090399.

63. Lakie M, Walsh EG, Wright GW. Resonance at the wrist demonstrated by the use of a torque motor: an instrumental analysis of muscle tone in man. J Physiol. 1984;353(1):265–85. https://doi.org/10.1113/jphysiol.1984.sp015335.

64. Boyer MI. Green's operative hand surgery. J Hand Surg. 1999;24(3):649.

65. Kaltenborn FM, Evjenth O. Manual mobilisation of the extremity joints: basic examination and treatment techniques. Oslo Norway: O.N. Bokenhandel; 1989.

66. Chinchalkar SJ, Szekeres M. Rehabilitation of elbow trauma. Hand Clin. 2004;20(4):363–74. https://doi.org/10.1016/j.hcl.2004.06.004.

67. Ramachandran VS, Altschuler EL. The use of visual feedback, in particular mirror visual feedback, in restoring brain function. Brain. 2009;132(7):1693–710.

68. Wilk KE, Arrigo C, Andrews JR. Rehabilitation of the elbow in the throwing athlete. J Orthop Sports Phys Ther. 1993;17(6):305–17.

69. Wilk KE, Arrigo CA, Andrews JR, Azar FM. Rehabilitation following elbow surgery in the throwing athlete. Oper Tech Sports Med. 1996;4(2):114–32.

70. Wilk KE, Voight ML, Keirns MA, Gambetta V, Andrews JR, Dillman CJ. Stretch-shortening drills for the upper extremities: theory and clinical application. J Orthop Sports Phys Ther. 1993;17(5):225–39. https://doi.org/10.2519/jospt.1993.17.5.225.

71. Huang Q, Li D, Yokotsuka N, Zhang Y, Ubukata H, Huo M, et al. The intervention effects of different treatment for chronic low back pain as assessed by the cross-sectional area of the multifidus muscle. J Phys Ther Sci. 2013;25(7):811–3.

72. Huo M, Maruyama H, Kaneko T, Naito D, Koiso Y. The immediate effect of lumbar spine pat-

terns of neuromuscular joint facilitation in young amateur baseball players. J Phys Ther Sci. 2013;25(12):1523–4.

73. Huang Q, Wang K-Y, Yu L, Zhou Y, Gu R, Cui Y, et al. Evaluation of the effects of different treatments for the elbow joint using joint proprioception and surface electromyography. J Phys Ther Sci. 2015;27(12):3907–9.

74. Khabie V, Schwartz MC, Rokito AS, Gallagher MA, Cuomo F, Zuckerman JD. The effect of intraarticular anesthesia and elastic bandage on elbow proprioception. J Shoulder Elb Surg. 1998;7 (5):501–4.

75. Bae Y-S. Effects of spiral taping on proprioception in subjects with unilateral functional ankle instabil-

ity. J Phys Ther Sci. 2017;29(1):106–8. https://doi. org/10.1589/jpts.29.106.

76. Long Z, Wang R, Han J, Waddington G, Adams R, Anson J. Optimizing ankle performance when taped: effects of kinesiology and athletic taping on proprioception in full weight-bearing stance. J Sci Med Sport. 2017;20(3):236–40.

77. Haavik H, Murphy B. The role of spinal manipulation in addressing disordered sensorimotor integration and altered motor control. J Electromyogr Kinesiol. 2012;22(5):768–76. https://doi.org/10.1016/j. jelekin.2012.02.012.

78. Barrett D, Cobb A, Bentley G. Joint proprioception in normal, osteoarthritic and replaced knees. J Bone Joint Surg Br. 1991;73(1):53–6.

Proprioception After Hand and Wrist Injury, Surgery, and Rehabilitation

6

Cigdem Oksuz, Deran Oskay, and Gazi Huri

6.1 Assessment of Proprioception in the Hand

Three main testing techniques in the literature have been reported for assessing proprioception of proximal joints and hand/wrist. These techniques are threshold detection of passive motion, joint position reproduction also known as joint position matching, and active movement extent discrimination assessment [1, 2]. However, standardization of these tests is poor and it is really hard to detect small changes which is an important issue in hand within these tests [3, 4].

Threshold to detection of passive movement direction discrimination test is assessed as the body segment is passively moved in a predetermined direction. Participants are instructed to press a stop button as soon as they perceive the movement and direction. This can be named as the evaluation of kinesthesia as well. The assessment of kinesthesia is the smallest change in joint angle needed to elicit conscious awareness of joint motion, as related to time (Δ/s) [5]. So by evaluating the threshold to detection of passive motion you are assessing the ability of detecting the slow motion. However hand joints could not be aware of slow motions like the knee joints did. It is shown that hand isometric flexion/extension contractions caused 6–7° of perceived hand displacement. So in clinical practice it is advised to use a professional device like the Upper limb exerciser (Biometrics Ltd., Ladysmith, VA) or a Biodex Dynamometer (Biodex Medical Systems Inc., Shirley, NY) to be able to detect the minimal change and speed of motion or kinesthesia [6].

Joint position reproduction testing technique could be conducted either passively or actively which may involve either ipsilateral limb movements called "ipsilateral remembered matching test" or contralateral limb movements called "contralateral remembered matching test." This technique measures subject's ability to detect passive movement or the ability to reposition a joint to a predetermined position [7]. This method requires some basic cognitive capacities so it may not be a suitable method for neurological problems [8, 9].

Active movement extent discrimination assessment is conducted using active movements. Participants are asked to make a judgement as to the position number of each test movement [1].

C. Oksuz, Ph.D., M.Sc., P.T. (✉)
Department of Occupational Therapy, Faculty of Health Science, Hacettepe University, Ankara, Turkey
e-mail: cigdemoksuz@yahoo.com

D. Oskay, Ph.D., M.Sc., P.T.
Department of Physiotherapy and Rehabilitation, Faculty of Health Sciences, Gazi University, Ankara, Turkey
e-mail: deranoskay@yahoo.com

G. Huri, M.D.
Department of Orthopaedics and Traumatology, Faculty of Medicine, Hacettepe University, Ankara, Turkey
e-mail: gazihuri@gmail.com

© Springer International Publishing AG, part of Springer Nature 2018
D. Kaya et al. (eds.), *Proprioception in Orthopaedics, Sports Medicine and Rehabilitation*,
https://doi.org/10.1007/978-3-319-66640-2_6

Studies on assessing proprioception in the upper extremity have mainly concentrated on the proximal joints like elbow and shoulder. There is still a lack of consensus in the literature about simple, clinically suitable, and reliable method to assess proprioception of hand or wrist. Although its reliability and validity are still criticized, using a goniometer to easily assess joint position sense of the hand and wrist seems to be the simple and reliable method. Reproducibility of wrist motion with a simple goniometer was reported for intra-observer as 5–8° and for interobserver as 6–10° [10]. To assess active joint position sense with a simple goniometer the patient is asked to actively move his wrist till the predetermined target position. For passive assessment, the therapist moves the wrist and the patient signals when it has reached the target position [11]. Some studies in the literature describe the measurement technique of joint position sense of wrist joint. Gay in his study described wrist joint position measurement device by avoiding cutaneous and visual inputs which may affect joint position sense. According to his study "this system allows the researcher to decrease extraneous influences that may affect joint position sense awareness and therefore improve the knowledge of the mechanisms underlying kinesthesia and proprioception" [12]. Figure 6.1: Magnetic motion tracking system for the measurement of proprioception following stroke is also described by Leibowitz [13].

In a clinical setting, static and dynamic "up or down test" at the distal interphalangeal joint is the only widely acknowledged clinical test of finger proprioception. This is a simple test but it is able to recognize proprioceptive loss only from gross sensory deficit. In this test therapist holds the patient's finger and gently flexes and extends and asks the end position of the finger [4]. Since speed and displacement cannot be precisely measured within this test, it is not a reliable and valid test for the measurement of hand proprioception. Some clinicians use the thumb localizing test. Other studies use paradigms like pointing, reaching, matching, or other judgement tasks to analyze proprioception in healthy subjects or neurological deficit patients. Despite their advantage of being simple and quick these methods all have very poor inter-rater reliability and sensitivity and lack of sensitivity to change and value criteria [4, 14].

Recent studies focused on assessing position sense displacing joints below the sensory threshold, at an angular velocity of <2/min. Other authors emphasize that examining dynamic motion better simulates joint activity during functional tasks [15].

Portable novel devices are also introduced in the literature to assess proprioception of the hand and wrist. The device called "proprioceptor meter" is reported in the literature as a new portable device with a high intra-rater and inter-rater reproducibility for measuring proprioception in the hand. It requires the subject to observe a target angle and actively match the position with a hidden index finger [16]. See Fig. 6.1: Han described a novel device for measuring functional proprioception at the fingertips. This device was constructed for measuring pinch movement discrimination between index finger and thumb (Fig. 6.1) [17].

In recent years robotic systems are used to evaluate and also train the proprioception of the upper extremity [18]. They are launched as quantitative and sensitive and can detect motor and sensory compared with the conventional assessment methods. Different systems have been reported in the literature. Masia and Cappello et al. in their studies introduced the use of the 3-DoF wrist robot to assess the wrist proprioceptive acuity for flexion-extension, abduction-adduction, and pronation-supination [19–21]. Marini in his study also used a robotic device for three degrees of freedom flexion/extension, radial/ulnar deviation, and pronation/supination to examine physiological mechanisms underlying the position sense of the wrist (Fig. 6.1) [22]. He also presents a robot-aided method to assess joint position sense acuity for the three degrees of freedom of the wrist/hand complex in a cohort of typically developing children [23]. A novel exoskeleton robot called "finger" has also been introduced for quantitatively assessing dynamic position sense in the finger joints (see Fig. 6.1) [24]. Contu introduced "the wrist," a standardized robot-aided method for measuring

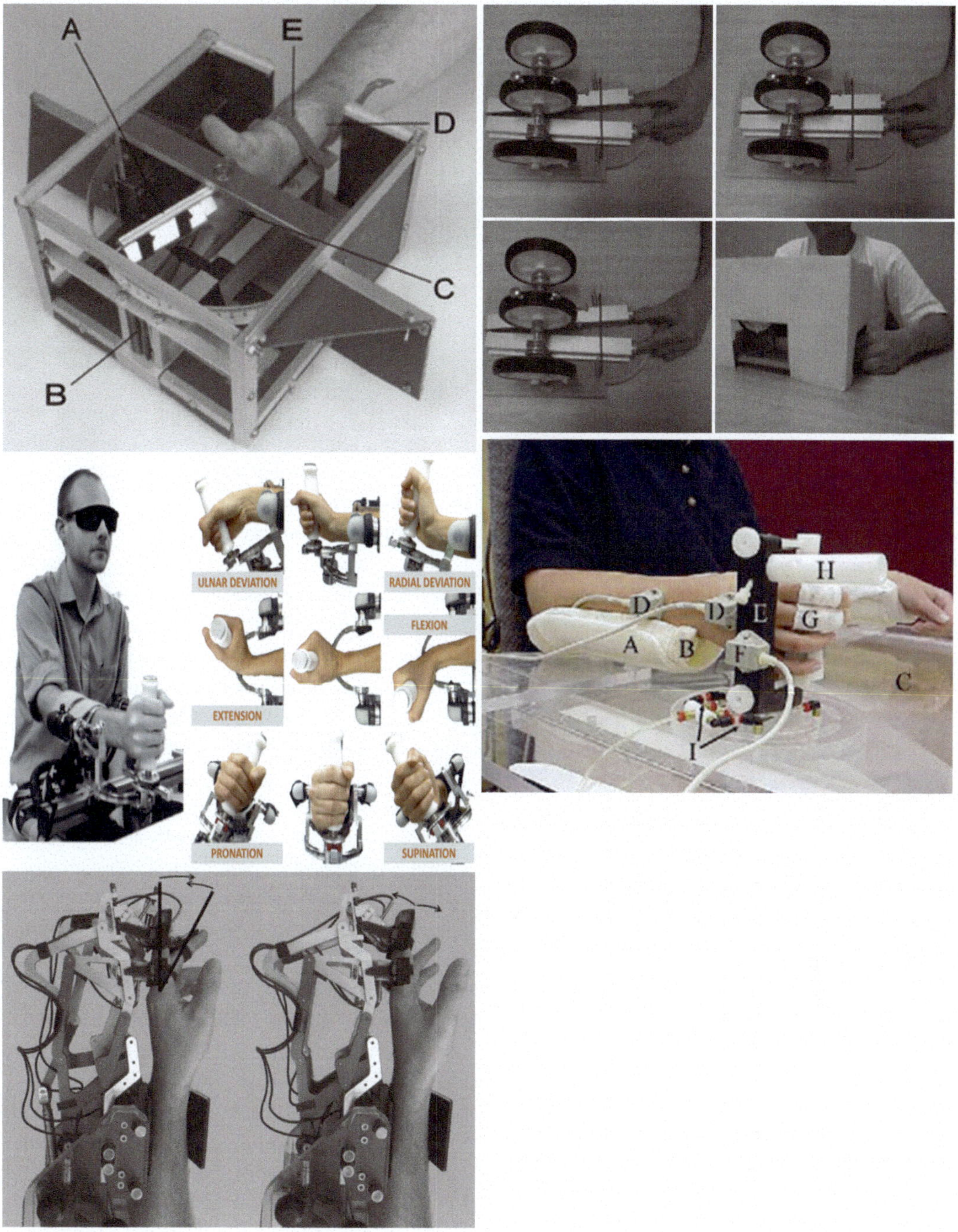

Fig. 6.1 Novel devices described in the literature to assess proprioception of the hand

proprioceptive discrimination thresholds at the wrist to obtain reliable and accurate measures of proprioceptive acuity (Fig. 6.1) [25]. Hosein had also described a simple-to-use and portable novel proprioception measurement technique named "adaptive staircase measurement" for the hand and fingers. There is a tablet-style computer screen over the pronated hand with a white line presented at varying angular increments from the joint being tested. With each stimulus presentation, the subject reports whether he or she feels that the white line is left or right of his or her index fingertip. The psychometric properties of the test (test-retest reliability, inter-rater reliability, and construct validity) are reported as very high [26].

These methods could be summarized as threshold detection of passive motion, displacement perturbations, joint position matching, and reproduction and difference threshold tracking methods [9, 12, 20, 24, 27–32]. Robotic technology can provide a reliable quantitative result to assess proprioception but these systems are mostly experimentally research-oriented methods and really expensive systems so they could not be clinical assessment methods for hand therapy clinics.

In conclusion, there is still lack of single reliable and valid assessment tool which is quick and easy to perform at a clinical setting for the assessment of proprioception of the hand and wrist. Assessments are unreliable and mostly subjective and lack standardization and some of them are expensive and of experimental design.

6.2   Rehabilitation Program in Wrist Proprioception

Evidence-based clinical studies revealing the results of proprioceptive training after wrist injuries are inadequate. For this reason, rehabilitation protocols can be formed within the framework of theoretical principles that are used in the knee and ankle joints [33–35].

Proprioceptive training to be applied to the wrist should be sustained in two phases: Late and early phases post-injury [6].

6.2.1   Early-Phase Rehabilitation Methods

The most important findings that cause impairment are pain, edema, and decrease in the range of active motion which develop in the early period and depend on the severity and type of injury. Immobilization which develops due to injury or surgery may lead to functional deficits. In addition, if there is an accompanying nerve injury, a loss or reduction in the sensation of the wrist and hand may also arise. Therefore, a deficit in conscious proprioception should be taken into consideration in this period.

Proprioceptive exercises done in the early phase could prevent functional demands that may occur due to the prolonged immobilization process. Thus the recovery of functional movement can be facilitated [36–38].

Pain is the most important symptom that causes immobilization in the early period after injury. Proprioceptive losses that occur during the immobilization process are inevitable. By increasing function via early pain management techniques such as cold application and elevation, possible central neuroplastic changes can be corrected or prevented in the early phase. Activity modification, visual feedback methods such as mirror therapy, and desensitization training consisting of methods like tactile stimulation and vibration can be used in the treatment of pain during this period [39, 40]. By using these methods, the input on the peripheral proprioceptive pathways will be increased; thus early sensory reeducation will take place and central reorganization will be restored. Vibration and tactile stimulation applied on the wrist skin and musculotendinous receptors increase the activation of the muscle spindle, kinesthetic motion sensation, and central sensorimotor function. Hence functional movement is achieved [41, 42]. The same mechanism is also applicable for closed kinetic chain exercises of the wrist (e.g., rolling a ball on a table). With these exercises, reduction of pain will be ensured and via controlled loading on the tissue functional joint movement will be established [43].

As mentioned previously, mirror therapy is one of the treatment methods that can be applied in the early phase of wrist injuries. Mirror therapy is a visual feedback method performed by using the position and movement of the healthy limb. With this method, the sensory cortical representation of the affected limb on the other side of the mirror is established and joint position and movement sensations which could not be achieved due to pain are improved leading to a functional active range of motion [44–46].

Passive and active range-of-motion exercises done in the early phase contribute to proprioception. Passive wrist positioning and subsequent active movement performed by the patient are used to treat the impairments of joint position sensation. Active wrist movements may increase proprioceptive input after injury and may also prevent neglect caused by immobilization. Exercises which include active wrist movements such as rolling a small exercise ball on a table and wiping the table with a cloth can be recommended in the early phase (Fig. 6.2). With the use

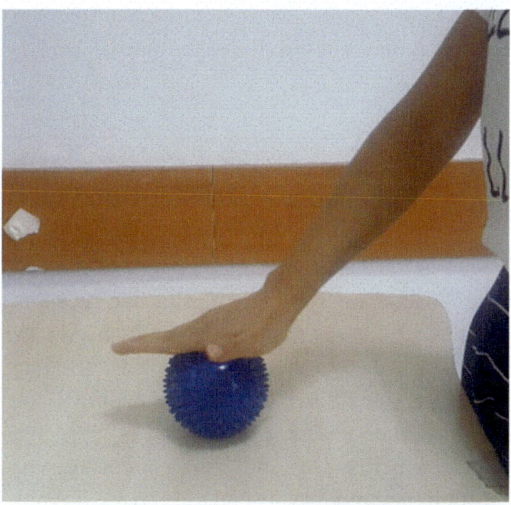

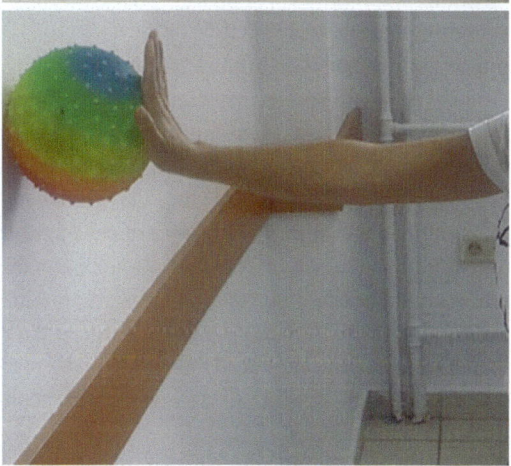

Fig. 6.2 Rolling a ball on a table or wall with different sizes of balls

of such methods, tactile sensory feedback will be provided, and spinal cord reflexes and supraspinal feed-forward efferent pathways and muscles that provide automatic synergistic movement patterns will be stimulated [6].

6.2.2 Late-Phase Rehabilitation Methods

Late-phase rehabilitation methods are particularly used to increase muscle strength and joint stabilization. The factor that will shape the strengthening programs principally is tissue healing.

The healing process and type (bone, connective tissue, tendon, etc.) of the injured tissue, type of surgical intervention (immobilization, surgery, etc.), and patient-related factors (such as bone and soft tissue quality) will differentiate the initiation time of the strengthening exercises. For example, in fractures, the initiation time is 8 weeks. However, depending on the type of intervention (immobilization, type of surgery), type of fracture, and bone quality, this time may vary. For soft-tissue injuries such as ligament injuries, because the healing process will take longer, the initiation of strengthening exercises may extend up to 10–12 weeks [47, 48].

Wrist movements during function include many synergist patterns. For this reason, agonist and antagonist muscles should be included in the strengthening exercises. Isometric exercises are a safe method in the event of an injury with prolonged healing and an immobilization phase. At the same time, isometric exercises performed on the contralateral extremity will contribute to strengthening via bilateral cortical stimulation and stimulation of feed-forward efferent pathways [47, 49, 50].

Isotonic resistance exercises should be used to increase proprioceptive input and to support global stabilization. Isotonic resistance exercises provide concentric and eccentric muscle contractions over a wide range of motion. In this respect, contribution to dynamic joint stabilization is formed by reciprocal and recurrent muscle activation patterns.

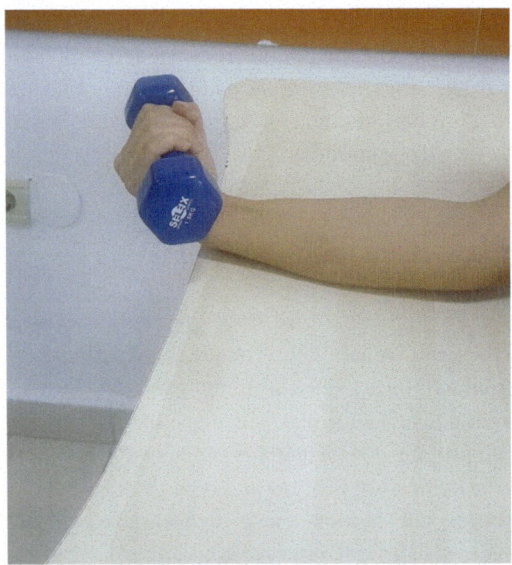

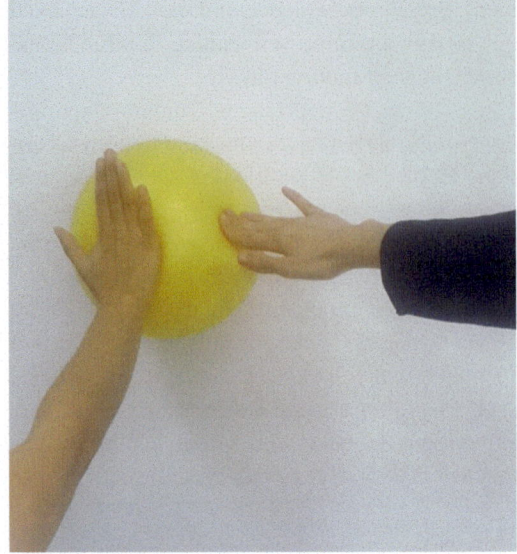

Fig. 6.3 Using weights to improve muscle strength

Fig. 6.4 Perturbation exercises on the wall

Muscle strength and endurance are important in the enhancement of proprioceptive sensation and sensory motor joint control. Different apparatuses such as weights and resistance bands can be used for strengthening exercises (Fig. 6.3). In order to increase muscle endurance, the exercises should consist of many repetitions. Exercise parameters (frequency, number of repetitions, and loads) should be patient specific. Programs should be taught to the patient in detail and a home exercise program must be planned [51, 22].

Perturbation and reactive exercises are also included in late-phase exercises. These exercises often provide unconscious proprioceptive input and provide joint control and stability in activities of daily living. Different materials such as exercise balls and handheld gyroscopes may be used in perturbation and reactive exercises (Fig. 6.4). These exercises have closed kinetic chain and open kinetic chain properties concurrently. During the exercises, not only the wrist but also the entire upper extremity and the whole body contribute actively to the exercise. Thus multiple joint stability is achieved [52].

6.3 Proprioception in Orthopaedics Conditions

The joint mechanoreceptors such as "Ruffini ending," "Pacini's corpuscle," "Golgi-like receptor" and innervation distribution of the wrist and hand play a critical role in order to maintain the joint proprioception. Since the Ruffini ending is the major mechanoreceptor type found in wrist ligaments, which are essential in monitoring wrist positions and motions, Pacini's corpuscle has only been identified occasionally. They have minor importance in wrist neuromuscular stability. The Golgi-type endings are predominantly located in the wrist ligaments and important in monitoring tensile strain in the ligament during ultimate angles of joint motion. Regarding the wrist ligaments, the innervation is most pronounced in the dorsal and triquetral wrist ligaments—the dorsal radiocarpal, dorsal intercarpal, dorsal scapholunate, palmar lunotriquetral, and triquetrocapitate/ hamate ligaments. However the radial and volar wrist ligaments consist of collagen fibers with little to no innervation [53].

Several conditions may impair the proprioception and sensorimotor function of hand and wrist. Especially upper extremity conditions such as carpal tunnel syndrome, distal radius fracture, metacarpal fractures, dislocation, and complex regional pain syndrome are the common causes of the proprioception deficits. To manage these conditions, different modalities are incorporated into practice to enhance proprioception input and restore hand and wrist function [54].

Conclusion

However clinical studies are needed to investigate the effect of proprioception reeducation in patients and individuals with a high demand on wrist function in both preventing and rehabilitating wrist injuries.

References

1. Han J, Waddington G, Adams R, Anson J, Liu Y. Assessing proprioception: a critical review of methods. J Sport Health Sci. 2016;5(1):80–90.
2. Lephart SM, Myers JB, Bradley JP, Fu FH. Shoulder proprioception and function following thermal capsulorraphy. Arthroscopy. 2002;18(7):770–8.
3. Hillier S, Immink M, Thewlis D. Assessing proprioception: a systematic review of possibilities. Neurorehabil Neural Repair. 2015;29(10):933–49.
4. Lincoln NB, Crow J, Jackson J, Waters G, Adams S, Hodgson P. The unreliability of sensory assessments. Clin Rehabil. 1991;5(4):273–82.
5. Riemann BL, Myers JB, Lephart SM. Sensorimotor system measurement techniques. J Athl Train. 2002;37(1):85–9.
6. Hagert E. Proprioception of the wrist joint: a review of current concepts and possible implications on the rehabilitation of the wrist. J Hand Ther. 2010;23(1):2–17.
7. Schmidt L, Depper L, Kerkhoff G. Effects of age, sex and arm on the precision of arm position sense—left-arm superiority in healthy right-handers. Front Hum Neurosci. 2013;24(7):915.
8. Li KZ, Lindenberger U. Relations between aging sensory/sensorimotor and cognitive functions. Neurosci Biobehav Rev. 2002;26(7):777–83.
9. Adamo DE, Martin BJ, Brown SH. Age-related differences in upper limb proprioceptive acuity. Percept Mot Skills. 2007;104(3 Suppl):1297–309.
10. Solgaard S, Carlsen A, Kramhøft M, Petersen V. Reproducibility of goniometry of the wrist. Scand J Rehabil Med. 1985;18(1):5–7.
11. Goble DJ, Coxon JP, Wenderoth N, Van Impe A, Swinnen SP. Proprioceptive sensibility in the elderly: degeneration, functional consequences and

plastic-adaptive processes. Neurosci Biobehav Rev. 2009;33(3):271–8.
12. Gay A, Harbst K, Kaufman KR, Hansen DK, Laskowski ER, Berger RA. New method of measuring wrist joint position sense avoiding cutaneous and visual inputs. J Neuroeng Rehabil. 2010;7(1):5.
13. Leibowitz N, Levy N, Weingarten S, Grinberg Y, Karniel A, Sacher Y, et al. Automated measurement of proprioception following stroke. Disabil Rehabil. 2008;30(24):1829–36.
14. Hewett TE, Paterno MV, Myer GD. Strategies for enhancing proprioception and neuromuscular control of the knee. Clin Orthop Relat Res. 2002;402:76–94.
15. Clark F, Burgess R, Chapin J. Proprioception with the proximal interphalangeal joint of the index finger. Brain. 1986;109(6):1195–208.
16. Wycherley A, Helliwell P, Bird H. A novel device for the measurement of proprioception in the hand. Rheumatology. 2005;44(5):638–41.
17. Han J, Waddington G, Anson J, Adams R. A novel device for the measurement of functional finger pinch movement discrimination. Appl Mech Mater. 2011;66–68:620–5.
18. Cho S, Ku J, Cho YK, Kim IY, Kang YJ, Jang DP, et al. Development of virtual reality proprioceptive rehabilitation system for stroke patients. Comput Methods Prog Biomed. 2014;113(1):258–65.
19. Masia L, Casadio M, Squeri V, Cappello L, De Santis D, Zenzeri J, et al. Enhancing recovery of sensorimotor functions: the role of robot generated haptic feedback in the re-learning process. In: Artemiadis P, editor. Neuro-robotics, Trends in augmentation of human performance, vol. 2. Dordrecht: Springer; 2014. p. 285–316.
20. Cappello L, Contu S, Elangovan N, Khosravani S, Konczak J, Masia L. Evaluation of wrist joint proprioception by means of a robotic device. Ubiquitous Robots and Ambient Intelligence (URAI), 11th International Conference of the IEEE, 2014. p. 531–4.
21. Cappello L, Elangovan N, Contu S, Khosravani S, Konczak J, Masia L. Robot-aided assessment of wrist proprioception. Front Hum Neurosci. 2015;9:198.
22. Marini F, Squeri V, Morasso P, Masia L. Wrist proprioception: amplitude or position coding? Front Neurorobot. 2016;10:13.
23. Marini F, Squeri V, Morasso P, Campus C, Konczak J, Masia L. Robot-aided developmental assessment of wrist proprioception in children. J Neuroeng Rehabil. 2017;14(1):3.
24. Ingemanson ML, Rowe JB, Chan V, Wolbrecht ET, Cramer SC, Reinkensmeyer DJ. Use of a robotic device to measure age-related decline in finger proprioception. Exp Brain Res. 2016;234(1):83–93.
25. Contu S, Marini F, Cappello L, Masia L. Robot-assisted assessment of wrist proprioception: does wrist proprioceptive acuity follow Weber's law? Engineering in Medicine and Biology Society

(EMBC), 38th Annual International Conference of the IEEE; 2016. p. 4610–3.

26. Hoseini N, Sexton BM, Kurtz K, Liu Y, Block HJ. Adaptive staircase measurement of hand proprioception. PLoS One. 2015;10(8):e0135757.

27. Wright ML, Adamo DE, Brown SH. Age-related declines in the detection of passive wrist movement. Neurosci Lett. 2011;500(2):108–12.

28. Simo L, Botzer L, Ghez C, Scheidt RA. A robotic test of proprioception within the hemiparetic arm poststroke. J Neuroeng Rehabil. 2014;11(1):77.

29. Bourke TC, Coderre AM, Bagg SD, Dukelow SP, Norman KE, Scott SH. Impaired corrective responses to postural perturbations of the arm in individuals with subacute stroke. J Neuroeng Rehabil. 2015;12(1):7.

30. Adamo DE, Martin BJ. Position sense asymmetry. Exp Brain Res. 2009;192(1):87–95.

31. Semrau JA, Herter TM, Scott SH, Dukelow SP. Robotic identification of kinesthetic deficits after stroke. Stroke. 2013;44(12):3414–21.

32. Rinderknecht MD, Popp WL, Lambercy O, Gassert R. Experimental validation of a rapid, adaptive robotic assessment of the MCP joint angle difference threshold. In: Auvray M, Duriez C, editors. Haptics: neuroscience, devices, modeling, and applications, lecture notes in computer science. Berlin; Heidelberg: Springer; 2014. p. 3–10.

33. Myers JB, Lephart SM. The role of the sensorimotor system in the athletic shoulder. J Athl Train. 2000;35(3):351–63.

34. Chmielewski TL, Hurd WJ, Rudolph KS, Axe MJ, Snyder-Mackler L. Perturbation training improves knee kinematics and reduces muscle co-contraction after complete unilateral anterior cruciate ligament rupture. Phys Ther. 2005;85(8):740–9.

35. Richie DH. Functional instability of the ankle and the role of neuromuscular control: a comprehensive review. J Foot Ankle Surg. 2001;40(4):240–51.

36. Elbert T, Sterr A, Flor H, Rockstroh B, Knecht S, Pantev C, Wienbruch C, Taub E. Input-increase and input-decrease types of cortical reorganization after upper extremity amputation in humans. Exp Brain Res. 1997;117(1):161–4.

37. May A. Chronic pain may change the structure of the brain. Pain. 2008;137(1):7–15.

38. Price DD, Verne GN, Schwartz JM. Plasticity in brain processing and modulation of pain. Prog Brain Res. 2006;157:333–405.

39. Altschuler EL, Hu J. Mirror therapy in a patient with a fractured wrist and no active wrist extension. Scand J Plast Reconstr Surg Hand Surg. 2008;42(2):110–1.

40. Foell J, Bekrater-Bodmann R, Diers M, Flor H. Mirror therapy for phantom limb pain: brain changes and the role of body representation. Eur J Pain. 2014;18(5):729–39.

41. Cordo P, Gurfinkel V, Brumagne S, Flores-Vieira C. Effect of slow, small movement on the vibration-evoked kinesthetic illusion. Exp Brain Res. 2005;167(3):324–34.

42. White O, Proske U. Illusions of forearm displacement during vibration of elbow muscles in humans. Exp Brain Res. 2009;192(1):113–20.

43. Watson HK, Carlson L. Treatment of reflex sympathetic dystrophy of the hand with an active "stress loading" program. J Hand Surg. 1987;12(5):779–85.

44. Rosén B, Lundborg G. Training with a mirror in rehabilitation of the hand. Scand J Plast Reconstr Surg Hand Surg. 2005;39(2):104–8.

45. Ezendam D, Bongers RM, Jannink MJ. Systematic review of the effectiveness of mirror therapy in upper extremity function. Disabil Rehabil. 2009;31(26):2135–49.

46. Deconinck FJ, Smorenburg AR, Benham A, Ledebt A, Feltham MG, Savelsbergh GJ. Reflections on mirror therapy: a systematic review of the effect of mirror visual feedback on the brain. Neurorehabil Neural Repair. 2015;29(4):349–61.

47. Skirven TM, Osterman AL, Fedorczyk J, Amadio PC. Rehabilitation of the hand and upper extremity, 2-volume set E-book: expert consult. London: Elsevier Health Sciences; 2011.

48. Handoll H, Madhok R, Howe T. Rehabilitation for distal radial fractures in adults. Cochrane Database Syst Rev. 2006;19:3.

49. Prosser R, Herbert R, LaStayo PC. Current practice in the diagnosis and treatment of carpal instability results of a survey of Australian hand therapists. J Hand Ther. 2007;20(3):239–43.

50. Lee M, Gandevia SC, Carroll TJ. Unilateral strength training increases voluntary activation of the opposite untrained limb. Clin Neurophysiol. 2009;120(4):802–8.

51. Leger AB, Milner TE. Muscle function at the wrist after eccentric exercise. Med Sci Sports Exerc. 2001;33(4):612–20.

52. Balan SA, Garcia-Elias M. Utility of the Powerball® in the invigoration of the musculature of the forearm. Hand Surg. 2008;13(02):79–83.

53. Hagert E, Forsgren S, Ljung BO. Differences in the presence of mechanoreceptors and nerve structures between wrist ligaments may imply differential roles in wrist stabilization. J Orthop Res. 2005;23:757–63.

54. Hagert E, Garcia-Elias M, Forsgren S, Ljung BO. Immunohistochemical analysis of wrist ligament innervation in relation to their structural composition. J Hand Surg [Am]. 2007;32(1):30–6.

Proprioception After Spine Injury and Surgery

7

Burcu Akpunarli, Caglar Yilgor, and Ahmet Alanay

7.1 Introduction

Proprioception is an important component of the somatosensory system of the human body. It is a fundamental sense that provides postural control, balance, and movement precision. It consists of movement sense (kinesthesia), joint position sense (conscious or unconscious), and force sense [1]. It perceives the force, weight, and timing of the muscle contractions [2, 3]. Spinal proprioception plays a significant role in somatosensory system. Cervical proprioception not only gives information about neck proprioception and position changes in shoulder girdle, but it is also associated with vestibular and visual systems [1, 3]. Trunk provides proprioceptive information on the extremity girdles, and supplies dynamic and static stabilization of the body. A decrease in position sense will cause a decrease in control of the middle-layer muscles of the spine, leading to spinal instability [3]. Various studies have

proven that a decrease in spinal proprioception and balance leads to sensorimotor dysfunction and impaired motor control which are risk factors for traumas, pain disorders, and deformities such as scoliosis. Although the studies are limited in number, they reveal that an intact spinal proprioception is fundamental for static and dynamic balance [3], after spinal surgery. Hence, in order to protect this precious "sixth sense" of the human body, a precise understanding of the anatomy, assessment, etiological factors of disruption, consequences, and management of these disorders is required.

7.2 Description

Proprioception contributes to awareness of body parts, their movement, and position [4]. It is a crucial sense for maintaining verticality. Static proprioception gives the information on position and dynamic proprioception gives the information on movement to central nervous system. Thus, it is the most valuable sense in internal representation of the adult body map, also known as body schema, which is needed for appropriate motor commands [1, 4, 5]. Additionally, proprioception provides information at the end of the movement; this is needed to compare intended, predicted, and actual movements, and is therefore essential for motor learning [1].

B. Akpunarli, M.D.
School of Medicine, Acibadem Mehmet Ali Aydinlar University, Istanbul, Turkey
e-mail: burcu.akpunarli@acibadem.edu.tr

C. Yilgor, M.D. • A. Alanay, M.D. (✉)
Department of Orthopedics and Traumatology, School of Medicine, Acibadem Mehmet Ali Aydinlar University, Istanbul, Turkey
e-mail: caglaryilgor@gmail.com; aalanay@gmail.com

© Springer International Publishing AG, part of Springer Nature 2018
D. Kaya et al. (eds.), *Proprioception in Orthopaedics, Sports Medicine and Rehabilitation*, https://doi.org/10.1007/978-3-319-66640-2_7

Proprioception continuously works in interaction and coordination with visual and vestibular inputs [6], which are integrated and processed in the central nervous system. This results in an adapted final motor command that coordinates activation patterns of skeletal muscles. It is important to take these interactions into consideration when performing tests to measure one between visual, vestibular, and proprioceptive sense. Cervical proprioceptive information plays a particularly important role in head and eye movement control through its connections with vestibular nuclei. Cervical proprioception is involved in cervico-collic, cervico-ocular, and tonic neck reflexes [1].

7.3   Anatomy

Proprioceptive information is sensed by a combination of different structures in the body, which are termed as proprioceptors/mechanoreceptors. Spinal proprioceptors consist of fascial/joint proprioceptors, muscular proprioceptors, skin proprioceptors, and graviceptors [3, 7].

Muscular proprioceptors are considered the most important source of proprioceptors [7]. There are two forms of muscle receptors: muscle spindles and Golgi tendon organs. The density of muscular proprioceptors varies throughout the body, according to demand. An example is the high density of muscle spindles at suboccipital muscles of the neck due to cervical spine's role in head and eye movement control mechanism [1, 8].

Fascial and joint proprioceptors are located in joint capsules and deep muscular fascia. They contribute to both static and dynamic position senses. Changes in joint positions create tension and compression leading the facet joint mechanoreceptors to send signals to central nervous system (CNS) [3]. Joint proprioceptors sense the entire range of motion and are vital for joint stability [1, 9, 10].

Skin mechanoreceptors are categorized into four: Meissner's corpuscles, Pacinian corpuscles, Merkel endings, and Ruffini endings. The proprioceptive information from skin contributes to both dynamic position and velocity sense according to the location in the body [7, 11]. Skin plays a significant role in kinesthesia and contributes to movement sensation in most joints [7].

Graviceptors also help perception of postural verticality [12]. They are divided into two groups, vestibular and extra-vestibular, and they are mostly found in the head and trunk [13, 14]. They provide information on changes in the body with respect to gravity line [3].

The proprioceptors of the spine are located in the intervertebral discs, facet joints, spinal ligaments, and spinal muscles [3, 15]. Muscle spindles are the most important structures responsible for proprioceptive sensory perception, and the most powerful stimulus is muscle-tendon vibration [3]. Animal studies have demonstrated that the viscoelastic and ligamentous structures of the spine have a major role in kinesthetic perception within the sensory cortex and in spinal muscle control [16]. The proprioceptors in ligaments become activated when stretched and contribute to both static and dynamic spinal proprioception [3], as well as the ligamento-muscular reflex of the lumbar spine [17]. Intervertebral disc receptors are found in the external layers of annulus fibrosus and their location varies with age. The proprioceptors of facet joints are mostly found in the cervical spine due to its higher mobility [14].

The conscious proprioceptive information reaches the CNS via three connections. First, it is delivered to medulla spinalis via peripheral neurons through dorsal root ganglions. The axons connect to nucleus cuneatus and nucleus gracilis. From there, the information is sent to ventral posterolateral nucleus of thalamus. Finally, the axons terminate in the somatosensory cortex. On the other hand, the unconscious proprioceptive information is delivered to cerebellum via spinal nucleus [1, 3].

7.4   Assessment of Spinal Proprioception

Clinical assessment of proprioception can be generally divided into specific and nonspecific tests. Specific assessment comprises measurement of kinesthesia, joint position sense, and force sense. Nonspecific tests measure the balance of the body and include visual, vestibular, and proprioceptive senses, as well as central nervous system and motor function. Different variables can be calculated while the subject reproduces a predetermined target, which are constant error, variable error, and absolute error. Constant error corresponds to deviation from the target and shows accuracy and error as in overshooting or undershooting the target. Absolute error also provides an estimate of accuracy, but unlike constant error the direction of the error is not considered in the calculation. Variable error indicates precision of movement. Hence, with these variables, precision and accuracy of joint position sense and threshold to detection of passive motion can be described [1].

In order to get the most accurate results as in the means of power of the study, spinal proprioception tests should include at least six trials, since this is the point where precision tends to stabilize [18]. Spinal proprioception depends on the position of the body, as in means of standing and lying [3]. Experiments have revealed that the best position for the accuracy of proprioceptive sense is vertical [19]. Also, specific perturbations of sensory information during the tests must be used to differentiate the proprioceptive information [1, 20]. It has been demonstrated through various experiments that visual stimuli result in visually evoked potentials and can initially override vestibular and proprioceptive signals. The occlusion of visual sensation results in upregulation of vestibulo-proprioceptive information in the central nervous system [6]. The size and speed of the movements should be standardized between trials and subjects [1]. It must be kept in mind while choosing subjects that adolescents and adults have different levels of body schema and adolescents underuse proprioception due to sudden growth-related changes in the body [4, 5].

Cervicocephalic relocation test/joint position sense is a specific test to study cervical spine proprioception in routine practice. The subject is seated on a chair with high back (to limit the trunk rotations) 90 cm from a wall in neutral head position, wearing a headband with laser pointer on sagittal plane. The laser emitter should be in the plane of ear's tragus. The subject first faces the wall in neutral position, and the starting point is marked. The subject wears opaque glasses to fully obstruct visual sense, and performs an active neck movement, and then returns to starting point. The final position is measured against the starting point. Cervical extension, flexion, and rotation are performed by the subject. The results show if there is any deficit in cervical proprioception [21–23]. The mean of eight trials is sufficient to give reliable measurements [24]. The joint position errors are calculated and the ones greater than $4.5°$ are considered abnormal. If overshooting the starting point, jerky movements, or dizziness is present during the procedure, cervicocephalic relocation test can be used to interpret the impairment [25].

Lumbar proprioception can be assessed via lumbar motion sense or motion perception threshold. The subject sits on a seat with a stepper motor underneath, while upper body is fixed to backrest to minimize vestibular feedback, crossing arms over the chest, wearing eye coverage and noise canceling headphones. Lumbar spine is rotated in the transverse plane, including an axial rotation of the lumbar spine, by rotating the seat via stepper motor at steady and slow rate. Vibration should be minimized by positioning a ball bearing under the seat. As the motion is sensed, the subject presses a switch that stops motion, and states the direction of motion (to minimize biased trials). The motion perception threshold of the subject is then calculated to evaluate lumbar proprioception [26, 27].

Cervical kinesthesia can be measured with the acuity of a tracking task. A sensor on the forehead of the subject and another on the back of the head is placed in the same sagittal plane. The subject is then seated in front of a computer monitor at a distance of 100 cm. A marker moves on the monitor and the patient is asked to trace the unpredictable movement pattern of the marker. The mean displacement and time on the target are calculated, and the kinesthesia of the cervical spine is thus assessed [1, 20, 28].

Force sense of a subject can be measured by comparing a force generated by the subject to the target force via pressure biofeedback devices. Cranio-cervical flexion test is an example for assessing force sense in cervical spine. Electromyographic muscle activity and change in position and pressure are measured by a sensor. The precision accuracy of the pressure and the ability to maintain it are used to evaluate the subject's force sense [20, 29].

Fukuda-Unterberg stepping test is a nonspecific dynamic test and is originally developed to measure the vestibular input, but it reveals the overall combination of somesthetic and vestibular information [5, 30]. It stimulates the activation of dynamic proprioceptive input and its central integration. The patient closes his/her eyes to eliminate visual afferents, and walks in place, with 45° hip flexion in every step, while arms are outstretched at 90°. A foot is chosen and its heel position and axis at the beginning are marked over the standing surface via drawing two separate rays. After 50–100 steps, the rotation of the chosen foot is measured by measuring the angle between the axis of the foot in the beginning and in the end. Also, the distance between start and end positions of the heel is calculated. Due to its dynamic property, it can be used to assess the proprioception in adolescent idiopathic scoliosis, where dynamic proprioception is disrupted [3].

Oculomotor and eye-head coordination tests are nonspecific proprioception tests that can be used in patients with cervical pain disorder. The neurophysiological connections of cervical spine proprioceptors and visuo-vestibular organs make the test important. Maintaining gaze while moving head, coordination of eye and head movement, and eye follow while keeping the head still in neutral neck position compared to neck torsion are some of the abilities that can be assessed to evaluate proprioception [1, 20].

Muscle-tendon vibration is another evaluation method of proprioception where transcutaneous vibration is performed to muscles or tendons. Action potentials created by specific frequency of vibrations cause kinesthetic illusion where CNS interprets the illusory sensation as muscle contraction. This leads to compensatory postural responses in the body, and therefore perturbs proprioception [4]. Vibration of the trunk and neck elicits a tilt in body orientation both during quiet stance and walking [31]. This method can be used to evaluate the proprioception sense deprivation in balance control [32].

7.5 Spinal Proprioception Disturbances

Pain, fatigue, and trauma can cause proprioception disturbances [1]. Spinal proprioception can also be altered due to disc herniation, canal stenosis, and deformity [33, 34].

Pain can affect proprioception at both peripheral and central levels of nervous system. Acute and chronic musculoskeletal pain disorders lead to impairments in cervical and lumbar proprioception [1]. It has been shown that spinal proprioception is affected not only during the pain, but also after the pain subsides [35]. In the presence of pain, the reflex activity is altered and nociceptors are activated which leads to sensitivity of gamma muscle spindles. It can also affect the perception in the central nervous system that leads to reorganization of the somatosensory cortex [1].

Cervical pain alters cervical joint position sense and sensorimotor control of the neck [35]. A disrupted cervical proprioception results in dizziness, visual disturbance, and altered head and eye movement control. Balance is disturbed in the short term, while other musculoskeletal disturbances might be observed in the long term [1].

Low back pain disrupts proprioceptive postural control, and leads to impairments in lumbar joint position sense and kinesthesia [15, 19, 35–37]. Poor spinal joint position sense leads to joint instability and chronic pain, and the pain itself impairs proprioception, forming a vicious cycle [26, 34].

Impaired lumbar proprioception has been observed previously in lumbar spinal stenosis (LSS) patients. LSS patients have paraspinal muscle denervation, which is highly correlated with static and dynamic balance disruption, and an impairment in paraspinal muscle reflex activation [33, 38]. They have difficulties sensing lumbar rotational movements, and this shows impairment in proprioception [39]. This may be due to a sensory loss or deficit in information processing. Their preparatory muscle activation is also impaired, which indicates a central control mechanism involvement [33].

Trauma causes loss of musculoskeletal tissue and mechanoreceptors and thus results in persistent impairment of proprioception [1]. Parkhurst et al. did the first research to evaluate lumbar proprioception deficit and low back injury. They concluded that proprioceptive asymmetries were associated with injuries, and that proprioception deficits due to those injuries were mostly seen in sagittal and coronal planes. They also found that the risk of a low back injury was mostly correlated with a preexisting spinal disorder [2]. This again creates a cycle where an injury would affect proprioception, and thus lumbar motor function, and consequently increase the risk of reinjury. Alteration in proprioception leads to impaired motor control and disruption in regulation of muscle stiffness [1]. Degraded motor function increases patient's risk of trauma [2].

In the case of cervical spine trauma, sports concussions and motor vehicle accidents are major risk factors for whiplash injury. Cervical kinesthesia is impaired as a result of whiplash injury [40]. It has been suggested that risk groups such as rugby players should be tested for cervical proprioception following an injury and that cervical kinesthesia patients should be monitored and treated early [41, 42].

Spinal proprioception impairment can also accompany spinal deformities such as scoliosis. Neurological deficit due to scoliosis has first been suggested by Barrack et al. [43]. Later on, researchers have found correlations between adolescent idiopathic scoliosis (AIS) and proprioception impairment. Guyot et al. showed in their study that some of the AIS patients had alterations in their cervical joint position senses. The postural control is perturbed in AIS due to alterations in sensory input, altered sensory re-weighting, central integration, and motor response [5]. Due to these disturbances, patients' dynamic proprioception is impaired, yet they still have the same static proprioception level with healthy adolescents [5, 44]. Postural disturbance due to impaired proprioception may lead to progression of scoliosis [5, 21].

7.6 Prevention, Early Detection, and Management of Spinal Proprioception Disturbances

To prevent lumbar proprioception disturbances, the etiologies such as trauma should be avoided. Algahir et al. showed that sitting posture and shoulder position have effects on proprioception, which led them to the conclusion that seats with arm support should be preferred by risk groups such as office workers in order to prevent cervical proprioceptive disturbances [34].

Considering the potential complications of spinal proprioception disturbances, various studies have suggested screening in high-risk groups such as AIS patients, or patients with a history of spinal trauma [21, 41, 42]. An evaluation would be useful in early detection of proprioceptive disturbance and timely management, preventing vicious cycles of reinjury and further deterioration of deformities.

Physical therapy choices might be considered while managing proprioception disorder. Passive joint movement techniques have also been reported to have beneficial effects on spinal proprioception [20]. To improve muscle strength and resolve fatigue, which is another cause of proprioception impairment, specific proprioceptive trainings should be performed without provoking pain, effusion, or significant fatigue [1]. Vibration training is a method to alter spine proprioception, and an example is that isometric neck extension using a sling system with superimposed vibration stimuli significantly enhances force sense of cervical spine [20, 37]. Oculo-cervical programming is a treatment option in improving cervical spine proprioception [21]. Case–control studies have shown that lumbar stabilization exercise has beneficial effects on lumbar proprioception [27].

7.7 Proprioception and Spine Surgery

Spinal proprioception can be altered after spinal surgery. Janssens et al. showed that, 2 weeks after lumbar microdiscectomy, patients rely on their ankle proprioception rather than lumbosacral proprioception to maintain their balance. This maladaptation is more pronounced in paramedian approach compared to transmuscular. This may account for the disability seen in patients after lumbar microdiscectomy. Early physiotherapy may help resolve this impairment [45].

On the contrary, surgical restoration of spinal proprioception is a subject that is still under investigation. Kaariainen et al. evaluated the effects of spinal decompression surgery on 30 LSS patients. They have undergone total and hemilaminectomies, mostly on L3/L4 and L4/L5 levels. The results demonstrated that lumbar proprioception improved shortly after the decompression surgery, but deteriorated again with 2-year follow-up. Further studies must be performed to investigate surgical methods of proprioception restoration [33].

7.8 Future Directions

Proprioception in spinal surgery is a subject that requires further research. Studies on proprioceptive outcomes with different surgical approaches, pathophysiology of the proprioception disturbances in spinal disorders, and surgical treatment options for spinal proprioception disturbances are warranted. A better understanding and quantification of spinal proprioception may help prevent spinal proprioception disturbances and vicious cycles that aggravate pathologies.

References

1. Roijezon U, Clark NC, Treleaven J. Proprioception in musculoskeletal rehabilitation. Part 1: basic science and principles of assessment and clinical interventions. Man Ther. 2015;20(3):368–77.
2. Parkhurst TM, Burnett CN. Injury and proprioception in the lower back. J Orthop Sports Phys Ther. 1994;19(5):282–95.
3. Karakaya MG. Spine and proprioception. In: Kaya D. Ed., Proprioception: The forgetten sixth sense. USA: OMICS Group eBooks; 2016. pp. 89–105. ISBN: 978-1-63278-018-8.
4. Assaiante C, Barlaam F, Cignetti F, Vaugoyeau M. Body schema building during childhood and adolescence: a neurosensory approach. Neurophysiol Clin. 2014;44(1):3–12.
5. Le Berre M, Guyot MA, Agnani O, Bourdeauducq I, Versyp MC, Donze C, et al. Clinical balance tests, proprioceptive system and adolescent idiopathic scoliosis. Eur Spine J. 2017;26(6):1638–44.
6. Bronstein AM. Multisensory integration in balance control. Handbook Clin Neurol. 2016;137:57–66.
7. Proske U, Gandevia SC. The proprioceptive senses: their roles in signaling body shape, body position and movement, and muscle force. Physiol Rev. 2012;92(4):1651–97.
8. Liu JX, Thornell LE, Pedrosa-Domellof F. Muscle spindles in the deep muscles of the human neck: a morphological and immunocytochemical study. J Histochem Cytochem. 2003;51(2):175–86.
9. Sojka P, Johansson H, Sjölander P, Lorentzon R, Djupsjöbacka M. Fusimotor neurones can be reflexly influenced by activity in receptor afferents from the posterior cruciate ligament. Brain Res. 1989;483(1):177–83.
10. Needle AR, Charles BBS, Farquhar WB, Thomas SJ, Rose WC, Kaminski TW. Muscle spindle traffic in functionally unstable ankles during ligamentous stress. J Athl Train. 2013;48(2):192–202.
11. Cordo PJ, Horn JL, Kunster D, Cherry A, Bratt A, Gurfinkel V. Contributions of skin and muscle afferent input to movement sense in the human hand. J Neurophysiol. 2011;105(4):1879–88.
12. Barbieri G, Gissot AS, Fouque F, Casillas JM, Pozzo T, Perennou D. Does proprioception contribute to the sense of verticality? Exp Brain Res. 2008;185(4):545–52.
13. von Gierke HE, Parker DE. Differences in otolith and abdominal viscera graviceptor dynamics: implications for motion sickness and perceived body position. Aviat Space Environ Med. 1994;65(8):747–51.
14. McLain RF, Raiszadeh K. Mechanoreceptor endings of the cervical, thoracic, and lumbar spine. Iowa Orthop J. 1995;15:147–55.
15. Hobbs AJ, Adams RD, Shirley D, Hillier TM. Comparison of lumbar proprioception as measured in unrestrained standing in individuals with disc replacement, with low back pain, and without low back pain. J Orthop Sports Phys Ther. 2010;40(7):439–46.
16. Holm S, Indahl A, Solomonow M. Sensorimotor control of the spine. J Electromyogr Kinesiol. 2002;12(3):219–34.
17. Stubbs M, Harris M, Solomonow M, Zhou B, Lu Y, Baratta RV. Ligamento-muscular protective reflex in the lumbar spine of the feline. J Electromyogr Kinesiol. 1998;8(4):197–204.
18. Allison GT, Fukushima S. Estimating three-dimensional spinal repositioning error: the impact of

range, posture, and number of trials. Spine (Phila Pa 1976). 2003;28(22):2510–6.

19. Lee AS, Cholewicki J, Reeves NP, Zazulak BT, Mysliwiec LW. Comparison of trunk proprioception between patients with low back pain and healthy controls. Arch Phys Med Rehabil. 2010;91(9):1327–31.

20. Clark NC, Roijezon U, Treleaven J. Proprioception in musculoskeletal rehabilitation. Part 2: clinical assessment and intervention. Man Ther. 2015;20(3):378–87.

21. Guyot MA, Agnani O, Peyrodie L, Samantha D, Donze C, Catanzariti JF. Cervicocephalic relocation test to evaluate cervical proprioception in adolescent idiopathic scoliosis. Eur Spine J. 2016;25(10):3130–6.

22. Mallau S, Bollini G, Jouve JL, Assaiante C. Locomotor skills and balance strategies in adolescents idiopathic scoliosis. Spine (Phila Pa 1976). 2007;32(1):E14–22.

23. Revel M, Andre-Deshays C, Minguet M. Cervicocephalic kinesthetic sensibility in patients with cervical pain. Arch Phys Med Rehabil. 1991;72(5):288–91.

24. Pinsault N, Fleury A, Virone G, Bouvier B, Vaillant J, Vuillerme N. Test-retest reliability of cervicocephalic relocation test to neutral head position. Physiother Theory Pract. 2008;24(5):380–91.

25. Treleaven J. Sensorimotor disturbances in neck disorders affecting postural stability, head and eye movement control. Man Ther. 2008;13(1):2–11.

26. Boucher JA, Roy N, Preuss R, Lariviere C. The effect of two lumbar belt designs on trunk repositioning sense in people with and without low back pain. Ann Phys Rehabil Med. 2017;60(5):306–11.

27. Boucher JA, Preuss R, Henry SM, Dumas JP, Lariviere C. The effects of an 8-week stabilization exercise program on lumbar movement sense in patients with low back pain. BMC Musculoskelet Disord. 2016;17:23.

28. Kristjansson E, Hardardottir L, Asmundardottir M, Gudmundsson K. A new clinical test for cervicocephalic kinesthetic sensibility: "the fly". Arch Phys Med Rehabil. 2004;85(3):490–5.

29. Jull GA. Deep cervical flexor muscle dysfunction in whiplash. J Musculoskelet Pain. 2010;8(1–2):143–54.

30. Honaker JA, Boismier TE, Shepard NP, Shepard NT. Fukuda stepping test: sensitivity and specificity. J Am Acad Audiol. 2009;20(5):311–4.

31. Courtine G, De Nunzio AM, Schmid M, Beretta MV, Schieppati M. Stance- and locomotion-dependent processing of vibration-induced proprioceptive inflow from multiple muscles in humans. J Neurophysiol. 2007;97(1):772–9.

32. Simoneau M, Richer N, Mercier P, Allard P, Teasdale N. Sensory deprivation and balance control in idiopathic scoliosis adolescent. Exp Brain Res. 2006;170(4):576–82.

33. Kaariainen T, Taimela S, Aalto T, Kroger H, Herno A, Turunen V, et al. The effect of decompressive surgery on lumbar paraspinal and biceps brachii muscle function and movement perception in lumbar spinal stenosis: a 2-year follow-up. Eur Spine J. 2016;25(3):789–94.

34. Alghadir A, Zafar H, Iqbal Z, Al-Eisa E. Effect of sitting postures and shoulder position on the cervicocephalic kinesthesia in healthy young males. Somatosens Mot Res. 2016;33(2):93–8.

35. Malmstrom EM, Westergren H, Fransson PA, Karlberg M, Magnusson M. Experimentally induced deep cervical muscle pain distorts head on trunk orientation. Eur J Appl Physiol. 2013;113(10):2487–99.

36. Claeys K, Brumagne S, Dankaerts W, Kiers H, Janssens L. Decreased variability in postural control strategies in young people with non-specific low back pain is associated with altered proprioceptive reweighting. Eur J Appl Physiol. 2011;111(1):115–23.

37. Brumagne S, Cordo P, Lysens R, Verschueren S, Swinnen S. The role of paraspinal muscle spindles in lumbosacral position sense in individuals with and without low back pain. Spine (Phila Pa 1976). 2000;25(8):989–94.

38. Ozcan-Eksi EE, Yagci I, Erkal H, Demir-Deviren S. Paraspinal muscle denervation and balance impairment in lumbar spinal stenosis. Muscle Nerve. 2016;53(3):422–30.

39. Leinonen V, Maatta S, Taimela S, Herno A, Kankaanpaa M, Partanen J, et al. Impaired lumbar movement perception in association with postural stability and motor- and somatosensory-evoked potentials in lumbar spinal stenosis. Spine (Phila Pa 1976). 2002;27(9):975–83.

40. Oddsdottir GL, Kristjansson E. Two different courses of impaired cervical kinaesthesia following a whiplash injury. A one-year prospective study. Man Ther. 2012;17(1):60–5.

41. Hides JA, Franettovich Smith MM, Mendis MD, Smith NA, Cooper AJ, Treleaven J, et al. A prospective investigation of changes in the sensorimotor system following sports concussion. An exploratory study. Musculoskelet Sci Pract. 2017;29:7–19.

42. Kristjansson E, Bjornsdottir SV, Oddsdottir GL. The long-term course of deficient cervical kinaesthesia following a whiplash injury has a tendency to seek a physiological homeostasis. A prospective study. Man Ther. 2016;22:196–201.

43. Barrack RL, Wyatt MP, Whitecloud TS, Burke SW, Roberts JM, Brinker MR. Vibratory hypersensitivity in idiopathic scoliosis. J Pediatr Orthop. 1998;8:389–95.

44. Assaiante C, Mallau S, Jouve JL, Bollini G, Vaugoyeau M. Do adolescent idiopathic scoliosis [AIS] neglect proprioceptive information in sensory integration of postural control? PLoS One. 2012;7(7):e40646.

45. Janssens L, Brumagne S, Claeys K, Pijnenburg M, Goossens N, Rummens S, et al. Proprioceptive use and sit-to-stand-to-sit after lumbar microdiscectomy: the effect of surgical approach and early physiotherapy. Clin Biomech (Bristol, Avon). 2016;32:40–8.

Proprioceptive Rehabilitation After Spine Injury and Surgery

8

Yildiz Erdoganoglu and Sevil Bilgin

8.1 Spine Anatomy, Pathomechanics, Injury

8.1.1 Columna Vertebralis

The human spine consists of 7 cervical, 12 thoracic, and 5 lumbar vertebra bodies, as well as 5 fused sacral vertebrae and 5 fused coccygeal vertebrae. In each region, the vertebrae have unique features that support them in performing main functions. They are connected to each other by fibrocartilaginous structures and ligaments called discus intervertebralis. The sizes of the vertebrae and discs increase from top to bottom. Approximately 71 cm in an adult man, the size of the spine is 61 cm in the adult female. ¼ of this length is produced by discs, and ¾ is formed by vertebrae. The spinal cord runs in the central canal and commonly ends at the L1–2 level. Nerve roots come from the neural foramina. The spine has a complex mechanical structure: the facet joints and discs function as pivotal ligaments while passive muscles, acting as active elements, contribute to formation [1].

Three basic biomechanical functions of the spinal column are as follows [2, 3]:

1. Head, upper part of the body, and external load carried as well as their associated bending moments to the pelvis, stabilization of the body
2. Providing body and head movement
3. Protection of vertebrae integrity, prevention of forces and movements that may result in potential damage

Functional spine unit: Functional unit of the spine is the one that carries biomechanical properties of the entire spinal cord that refers to the smallest segment. This structure consists of two adjacent vertebrae and soft tissues combining them. The front part of the functional unit is mainly capable of carrying loads, shock absorbers. The anterior part consists of vertebral bodies, intervertebral disc, and longitudinal ligaments. Vertebral arches, intervertebral joints, transverse and spinous processes, and ligaments form the posterior part of the functional unit. The back part protects neural structures and guides the movement of the units during flexion and extension [4, 5].

Y. Erdoganoglu, P.T., Ph.D. (✉)
Department of Physiotherapy and Rehabilitation, Faculty of Health Sciences, Uskudar University, İstanbul, Turkey
e-mail: yildiz.erdoganoglu@uskudar.edu.tr

S. Bilgin, P.T., Ph.D.
Department of Physiotherapy and Rehabilitation, Faculty of Health Sciences, Hacettepe University, Ankara, Turkey
e-mail: sevilcuvalci@yahoo.com

© Springer International Publishing AG, part of Springer Nature 2018
D. Kaya et al. (eds.), *Proprioception in Orthopaedics, Sports Medicine and Rehabilitation*,
https://doi.org/10.1007/978-3-319-66640-2_8

8.1.2 Cervical Spine Anatomy

Cervical vertebrae are located between the skull and thorax. The smallest and most mobile vertebrae in the presacral vertebrae are in this region. Seven cervical vertebrae, 5 intervertebral discs, 14 facet joints, ligaments, and muscles allow this region to have a wide range of motion. Structurally, the 1 [C1 = atlas] and 2 cervical vertebra [C2 = axis] are different from the others. The seventh cervical vertebra is a transitional vertebra. The cervical spine may be divided into upper and lower parts [6].

Upper cervical spine: The upper cervical region consists of C1 [atlas] and C2 [axis] jointed with occiput condyles. This zone joints are quite mobile. Approximately 30% of the cervical flexion/extension movement and more than 50% of the axial rotation are in this region. In this region, there are synovial joints instead of intervertebral discs [7, 8].

Lower cervical spine: Five spines that form lower cervical vertebrae are similar to one another but they are different from C1 and C2. Compared to the upper part, the alignment is more stable and contributes to overall mobility. Spinal canal is narrower, and any pathologies in this part lead to more damages because there is less space remaining for the spinal cord [6].

In cervical spine neuroanatomy, the cord is enlarged with lateral extension of the gray matter that consists of anterior horn cells. The lateral dimension spans 13–14 mm, and anterior-posterior extent measures 7 mm. An additional 1 mm is needed for cerebrospinal fluid both anteriorly and posteriorly, in addition to 1 mm for the dura. A total of 11 mm is needed for the cervical spinal cord. The spinal nerve that exits at each vertebral level results from the anterior and posterior nerve root union [9].

The foramina are largest at C2–C3 and their size progressively decreases to C6–C7. The spinal nerve and spinal ganglion take up 25–33% of the foraminal space. The neural foramen is bordered anteromedially by the uncovertebral joints, posterolaterally by facet joints, superiorly by the pedicle of the vertebra above, and inferiorly by the pedicle of the lower vertebra. The edge of the end plates and the intervertebral discs form the foramina medially [7].

There are interconnections between the sympathetic nervous system and the spinal nerves. The latter exits the cervical spine above their correspondingly numbered vertebral body from C2 to C7. Since the numbering of cervical spinal nerves starts above the C1 level, eight cervical spinal nerves exist: the first one exits between the occiput and C1while the eighth exits between C7 and T1 [9, 10].

8.1.3 Cervical Spine Joints

The *atlanto-occipital joint* occurs between the massa lateralis of the atlas and the condyles of the occipital bone. It is a synovial type joint. In the atlanto-occipital joints, the head tilts backwards and forwards. This joint also allows the lateral flexion of the head. The primer movement is flex*ion* [10].

Atlantoaxial joint consists of two joints of atlantoaxialis lateralis and one joint of atlantoaxialis medialis. These are synovial joints. The primer movement is rotation.

Intervertebral joints occur as of below the second cervical vertebra whereby each body of vertebra forms symphysis through intervertebral discs. These joints come with a design capable of carrying body weight and pressure onto vertebrae.

Uncovertebral [Luschka's] joints: Lateral aspect of the vertebral bodies has superior projections known as the uncinate process.

Facet [zygapophyseal] joints are a set of synovial joints between the articular processes of two adjacent vertebrae. They have a fine joint lining and adsorb onto the articular surface.

8.1.4 Cervical Spine Ligaments

Apex [tip] dens are the origin of *apical ligament* and the insertion is the occiput. It stretches when traction is applied to the head. *Transverse ligament* is a strong band extending between the inner surfaces of atlas mass lateralis. When dens move backwards, it prevents it from impacting the spinal cord, causing damages. The atlanto-occipital joint is mainly stabilized with transverse and apical ligaments. The two ligaments constitute the cruciate ligament together. *Alar ligament* commences at lateral aspects of the dens axis, and adsorbs onto external aspect of the foramen magnum. This particular ligament controls rotation of the head and lateral flexion on the atlanto-occipital joint. It also forms major part of the stabilization system for the upper cervical spine.

Anterior and posterior longitudinal ligaments [ALL vs. PLL] are situated on the anterior and posterior aspects of the corpus vertebrae, running down along all vertebral column. ALL is responsible for stability of the joints in between the vertebrae, and helps to prevent vertebral column hyperextension. PLL helps to prevent hyperflexion of columna vertebralis, and invertebral disc from backward bending. Tectorial membrane is a strong band that extends upwards off from PLL, and becomes stretched with the head flexion movement. *Ligamentum flavum* extends between the reverse aspect of the laminae of lower vertebrae and front aspect of the laminae of upper vertebrae. It prevents laminae from being parted in case of flexion and assists extension in resuming its anatomic position. *Supraspinal ligaments* extend from the seven cervical vertebra to sacrum and interconnect the tips of spinous process. These ligaments are superiorly bordered by *ligamentum nuchae* and inferiorly by *ligamentum interspinale*. It counteracts the flexion and supports head in resuming anatomic position. Also, *ligamentum nuchae* supports the head. *Intertransverse ligaments* interconnect transverse projections of adjacent vertebrae [6, 8, 11].

8.1.5 Cervical Muscles

They are treated in two groups as anterior-lateral and suboccipital muscles. Muscles on the anterior side were located in three positions, superficial, middle, and deep. Superficial neck muscles: M. platysma, M. sternocleidomastoideus, and M. trapezius. Cervical muscles in the deep plane:

scalene muscles and prevertebral muscles [M. longus colli, M. longus capitis]. Suboccipital muscles are M. rectus capitis anterior, M. rectus capitis lateralis, M. rectus capitis posterior major, M. rectus capitis posterior minor, M. obliquus capitis superior, and M. obliquus capitis inferior [12].

8.1.6 Cervical Spine Pathologies

Cervical region is a strong structure that houses the spinal cord and flexibly allows movement of the head and body. The mobility has other functions, namely it protects neural structures [spinal cord and roots] thanks to the median canal, as well as contralateral vertebral artery. The conflicting functions are provided by the strong and delicately moving structure of the cervical spine. It is as strong as to carry a 3.5–5.5 kg head, and the strength is driven by the vertebral corpus anteriorly and facet joints [articular column] posteriorly [13]. Its mobility is provided by ligamentous intervertebral discs, a set of synovial joints superiorly, and an inferiorly complex system of joints that, in turn, are composed of a pair of facet joints situated posteriorly on each level [37 joints in total], and 50 pairs of muscles [14]. The complex is in constant movement, and the neck moves 600 times per hour, that is, once every 6 s [10]. For its complex structure and functional versatility, cervical spine is known as an area that frequently encounters instability and complaints of pain due to age-related degenerative processes and trauma.

8.1.6.1 Torticollis

Torticollis defines a condition of ipsilateral head tilt, and contralateral face and chin rotation due to sternocleidomastoid [SCM] muscular contraction mostly in affected direction. It may be congenital or may be developed posteriorly. The most common reason for congenital torticollis is muscular torticollis due to unilateral fibrosis of the SCM muscle. Normal position of the head is provided by signals from otolith apparatus, semicircular canals, and neck and retina proprioceptors [15]. Otolith apparatus is responsible for static position of the head. Stimulus from these sources is transmitted to vestibular cerebral trunk nuclei. Upon system integration of the stimulus from retina, head position is provided delicately to the smallest detail. Primary trapezius that supports the head and is responsible for upright position is the SCM muscle and paravertebral muscles. Factors that result in abnormality there do lead to torticollis by triggering problems at spinal column [15]. If not treated, torticollis may result in plagiocephaly, hemifacial hypoplasia, and compensatory scoliosis at later ages.

8.1.6.2 Cervical Spondylosis

Cervical spondylosis relates to a nonspecific spinal degenerative process and it is likely to result in varying degrees of stenosis at both central spinal canal and root canals. Hypertrophy of lamina, articular facets, ligamentum flavum, osteophyte, degenerative disc, and posterior longitudinal ligament are among the factors that contribute to narrowing. Among other pathological processes are the cervical lordosis and vertebral body subluxation. A congenitally narrow canal paves the way for early development of symptoms. A limited number of changes may be observed in the first 20 years of life but degeneration becomes more evident as of the third decade [16]. Degeneration often starts on disc level and it is most commonly seen at C5/C6 and C6/C7. Majority of cases over 50 tend to show radiological evidence of degenerative disease while neurological symptoms or signs are limited to minority only [17].

8.1.6.3 Cervical Sprain [Whiplash]

Whiplash is an injury from breakaway thrust and slowdown thrust due to hits and cracks in accidents involving vehicles. It is a traumatic injury to soft-tissue structures in the cervical spine region caused by hyperflexion, hyperextension, or rotation injury without fractures, dislocations, or intervertebral disc herniations. Symptoms may be seen immediately or delayed. Headaches, cognitive problems, and back pain are the associated complaints of uncertain pathophysiology. Patients with neck pain and stiffness are advised to undergo cervical spine flexion and extension views. No further investigations are indicated if a satisfactory range of movement is achieved [18].

8.1.7 Thoracic Spine

The thoracic spine consists of 12 cervical vertebrae between the cervical spine and the lumbar spine. All thoracic vertebrae join with ribs. Ribs, sternum, and thoracic spine together form the rib cage. The rib cage contains the heart, main vessels, and lungs, supporting the shoulder belt. According to the lumbar spine, it is less affected by mechanical stresses and can make more rotation [1].

The thoracic vertebral body's transverse and anterior-posterior lengths are equal to one another. Superior costal joint is situated at posterolateral aspect of the vertebral body superior while inferior costal joint is situated at the lower posterolateral aspect thereof. At the sides of the first thoracic neurocentrum, a full facet and semi-facet exist for the first and second costal cartilage, respectively. Pedicles are followed by superior costal joint ligaments and laminae. There are superior joint aspects on the upper part of where laminae and pedicles join, and inferior joint aspects on the lower part of the same area. The superior joint aspects are in dorsal and lateral direction; inferior joint aspects are ventral, inferiorly and medially. Likewise transverse projections are extended laterally to the joint points of pedicles and laminae. The rib tuberculum and articulating transverse costal joint exist on transverse projection [19, 20]. Facet joint of the thoracic vertebrae has a 60-degree angle on sagittal plane and 20-degree angle on frontal plane. The structure limits flexion and extraction, and allows lateral rotation [21].

8.1.8 Thoracic Spine Joints

Thoracic spine joints can be divided into two groups: One group is represented by those present throughout the vertebral column, and the other are the ones unique to the thoracic spine [22, 23].

There are two types of joints with the first group:

Between vertebral bodies—adjacent vertebral bodies are joined by intervertebral discs, made of fibrocartilage. This is a type of cartilaginous joint, known as a symphysis.

Between vertebral arches—formed by the articulation of superior and inferior articular processes from adjacent vertebrae. It is a synovial type joint.

8.1.9 Thoracic Spine Ligaments

Ligaments are specific to thoracic spine. Also, a number of small ligaments come to support the costovertebral joints [24, 25]:

Radiate ligament of head of rib fans outwards from the head of the rib to the bodies of the two vertebrae and intervertebral disc. *Costotransverse ligament* connects the neck of the rib and the transverse process. *Lateral costotransverse ligament* extends from the transverse process to the tubercle of the rib. *Superior costotransverse ligament* passes from the upper border of the neck of the rib to the transverse process of the vertebra superior to it.

8.1.10 Major Muscles of the Thoracic Spine

The major muscles on thoracic region are shown in Table 8.1.

8.1.11 Thoracic Spine Pathologies

8.1.11.1 Hyperkyphosis

Upright position involves a natural kyphosis angle of approximately 40–45° but angular increase results in hyperkyphosis. Trauma, spinal instability, developmental and growth anomaly in vertebrae, severe degenerative disc disease,

marked osteoporosis, and osteoporosis-based fractures may be cited as reasons for hyperkyphosis [26]. One common reason for progressive thoracic kyphosis is Scheuermann's disease and osteoporosis, while Scheuermann's disease and juvenile disorder are the reasons for adolescence thoracic hyperkyphosis. The reason is not precisely known though. Primarily it is considered that the reason is abnormal speed of development of different parts of the vertebra that in turn results in extreme anterior curvature at thoracic area and upper lumbar vertebral bodies. Age-related hyperkyphosis is an exaggerated anterior curvature in the thoracic spine that occurs commonly with advanced age. It is shown by epidemiologic studies that elderly population is commonly affected by age-related hyperkyphosis with estimated range of 20–40% [27]. Osteoporosis-based thoracic hyperkyphosis progression often results in compression fracture in elderly women [28].

8.1.11.2 Scoliosis

Scoliosis is a medical condition of three-dimension deformity on the vertebral column due to lateral deviation on frontal plane, torsion n horizontal plane, and irregularity on sagittal plane [hyperlordosis, hypolordosis, hyperkyphosis, and hypo/hyperkyphosis] [29]. A normal spine shows physiological deviations when looked at from the side [cervical lordosis, thoracic kyphosis, and lumbar lordosis] even though it shows none frontally-posteriorly. In case of direct graph of upright posture, any lateral curvature for and above 10° is defined as scoliosis. The Cobb method is accepted as the method of standard measurement for measuring the degree of curvature [30, 31]. Scoliosis is recognized to be idiopathic by 80% but the reason for deformity is not known [32]. Quite a number of factors are considered to be

Table 8.1 Major muscles of the thoracic spine

Superficial layer	Intermediate layer	Deep layer
• Trapezius • Latissimus dorsi • Rhomboids • Serratus posterior superior • Serratus posterior inferior	• Thoracic erector spinae	• Transversospinalis muscles Semispinalis Multifidus Rotatores

responsible in etiology. Genetics, central nervous system, melatonin, postural balance factors and postural nine mechanism, vestibular mechanisms, metabolic and chemical factors, platelet anomalies, and ligament anomalies are held responsible [33, 34].

Scoliosis causes deformation in the body and is likely to end up with cardiopulmonary complications at later decades. Recurring pulmonary infections, hypoxic conditions, increased pulmonary resistance, and right ventricle failure due to pulmonary hypertension are named among the important diseases it is responsible for. Apart from the foregoing, it leads to certain psychological disorders and cosmetic concerns [35, 36].

8.1.12 Lumbar Spine

The lumbar vertebral column from five active vertebrae forms 25% of the entire spine length. Functionally, the lumbar vertebrae rest on the sacrum and are treated as a lumbosacral spine with the sacrum as it is in close contact with the sacrum [37].

8.1.13 Lumbar Spine Joints

The lumbar spine delicately houses two types of joint [38]. Not both of these articulations are unique to the lumbar vertebrae; they are present throughout the vertebral column.

Between vertebral bodies, adjacent vertebral bodies are joined by intervertebral discs that are made of fibrocartilage. This is a type of cartilaginous joint, and it is known as a symphysis.

Between vertebral arches, formed by the articulation of superior and inferior articular processes from adjacent vertebrae. It is a synovial type joint.

Facet joints of the lumbar area have a 45° angle on the frontal plane while the angle on the axial plane is 90°. This allows flexion and extension movements and limits rotation [39].

Table 8.2 Lumbar spine ligaments

Lumbar spine ligaments
• Anterior longitudinal ligament
• Posterior longitudinal ligament
• Ligamentum flavum
• Supraspinous ligament
• Interspinous ligament
• Intertransverse ligaments
• Fibrous capsules of the facet joints
• Annulus fibrosus of the disc joints
• Nuchal ligament

8.1.14 Lumbar Spine Ligaments

The ligaments play an important role in the stabilization of the spinal column by showing resistance to stretching (Table 8.2). The posterior ligaments counteract the flexion, while the anterior ligaments counteract the extension [40].

8.1.15 Lumbar Spine Muscles

Muscles are the active stabilizing elements of the spinal column (Table 8.3) [41]. The lumbar dorsal muscles provide the extensor. Taking the support from the sacrum, they perform tasks in the lumbar and thoracic region. They contribute to muscle tones and lordosis [42]. The rectus abdominis and psoas muscles in front of the abdominal wall work as antagonists of the posterior respiratory spines. Side abdominal muscles rotate to the spine.

Muscle groups that are also named as core muscles and actively play a role in sensory-motor control of the spine can be grouped as follows by their property [43–45].

8.1.16 Intervertebral Disc

Intervertebral discs are flexible hydrodynamic structures between two adjacent vertebral bodies. The lower and upper faces of the discs are

Table 8.3 Lumbar spine muscles

Local paravertebral muscles	Global polysegmental paravertebral muscles	Affective muscles on intra-abdominal pressure
• Intertransversarii • Interspinous • Multifidus • Longissimus thoracis pars lumborum • Iliocostalis lumborum pars lumborum • Quadratus lumborum, medial fibers • Transversus abdominis • Obliquus internus abdominis [fiber insertion into thoracolumbar fascia]	• Longissimus thoracis pars thoracis • Iliocostalis lumborum pars thoracis • Quadratus lumborum lateral fibers • Rectus abdominis • Obliquus externus abdominis • Obliquus internus abdominis	• Abdominal muscles • Pelvic floor • Diaphragma

associated with the vertebra corpus. Thickness varies according to where they are and the same places of the disc. The anterior part of the cervical and lumbar discs is thicker than posterior. Thus, they contribute to cervical and lumbar lordosis formation [46, 47]. The peripheral parts are fed from adjacent vessels, and there is no blood vessel in the central part. Feeding of this part is by way of diffusing from spongiose bone tissue. Therefore, peripheral part containing the vascular structure and the veinless central part reacts to injury differently.

The disc columna vertebralis allows the absorption and distribution of loads carried onto. Discs do not contain joint space, synovial membrane, veins, or nerves. As they are fed by diffusion, diseases are different from those of other synovial joints. In the center there is a nucleus of gel consistency called nucleus pulposus, and a capsule consisting of collagen fibers called annulus fibrosus around it. The hydrostatic pressure generated by the loads is radially distributed evenly across the annulus by the nucleus pulposus. The surfaces of the vertebrae between the nucleus pulposus are covered with a microporous cartilage. This cartilage is permeable to liquid for its porous structure. When standing, the axial load allows water in from the gelatinous matrix of the nucleus to the cartilage [48, 49]. Due to ongoing loading during the day, the nucleus shrinks significantly at the end of the day.

Having studied intervertebral disc innervations, researchers suggest that mechanoreceptors in the outer annulus, as well as the posterior and anterior longitudinal ligaments, have proprioceptive functions that provide sensation of movement and posture [50, 51].

8.1.17 Lumbar Spine Pathologies

8.1.17.1 Spondylosis

Spondylosis is a broad term meaning degeneration of the pars interarticularis of vertebra [52]. Spondylosis may be as prevalent as with 60% of the public and transforms to spondylolisthesis by 75% in case of bilateral phenomena. Lumbar stenosis is most commonly seen at the L4/5 level; L3/4 is, however, the next most frequently involved level. Lumbar stenosis is usually seen in patients that are known to have a developmentally shallow spinal canal related to small neural arches and short pedicles. If stenosis is severed by acquired degenerative changes including without limitation facet joint/ligamentous hypertrophy, disc protrusion, instability, or spondylolisthesis, patients may present it later in life [53].

Even though recurrent hyperextension traumas on an immature spine are considered as the most common reason for spondylosis, micro traumas due to congenital weakness or pars interarticularis displacement as well as multifactorial reasons are the defined mechanisms for spondylosis [53, 54].

Spondylosis is often seen in adolescence, and the course of disease may come symptom free [52]. Patients suffer from increased pain in hyperextension position and the pain diminishes in rest position. It may be seen in cases that neurologic symptoms are often accompanied by spondylolisthesis.

8.1.17.2 Spondylolisthesis

Spondylolisthesis is defined as the anterior displacement or one vertebra over another [55]. Most cases are considered to result from minor overuse trauma, particularly repetitive hyperextension of the lumbar spine. Spondylolysis, which is defined as a break in the vertebra typically in the region of the pars interarticularis, may or may not be associated with a spondylolisthesis. If the pars defect is bilateral, it may allow slippage of the vertebra, typically L5 on S1, and this leads to spondylolisthesis [56, 57].

The most commonly adopted method of grading is the Meyerding classification, which divides lower vertebra surface into four segments of 25% each and enables slippage grading accordingly.

8.1.17.3 Spinal Stenosis

Spinal stenosis is an abnormal narrowing of the spinal canal [58]. This narrowing limits the amount of space available for the spinal cord and for the nerves. Spinal stenosis can occur anywhere in the spinal canal but is most commonly encountered in the cervical and lumbar spine. Lumbar spinal stenosis is often accompanied by lower extremity pain and weakness. Stenosis may be located centrally, laterally, or in combination. When narrowing is present in the spinal canal in case of central spinal stenosis, it comes along with lateral recess in lateral spinal stenosis or with narrowing in intervertebral foramina. Lateral recess is limited with lateral pedicle, superior facet joint projection on the posterior, posterolateral face on the vertebral body, and intervertebral disc on the anterior. Lateral spinal stenosis often develops due to superior facet joint projection, revealing a root pressure [58, 59].

Degenerative arthritis and age-related bony and soft-tissue changes are the most common reasons for developing spinal stenosis. Patients over 50 are the common ground of spinal stenosis and the condition tends to become progressively severe with age. Anticipated consequences of ageing may cause spinal arthritis and this, in turn, results in spinal stenosis. The reason for this can be bone spurs [a.k.a. osteophyte], bulging, intervertebral disc deformity with age, and ligaments thickening between the vertebrae [60].

The symptoms of spinal stenosis depend on the location of the stenosis in the spinal canal, as well as the severity of the condition. Pain, cramp, weakness, and loss of sensations are among the complaints arising out of spinal cord and/or nerve root compression. The symptoms usually commence at a slower pace and deteriorate over time.

8.2 What Is Proprioception in the Spine?

Proprioception is a complex task of interaction between afferent and efferent inputs for controlling body motions and relative position of the limbs [61]. It covers two aspects of the sense of location both statically and dynamically. It is a component of the somatic sense of mechanoreceptors that enable stability of the body between static and dynamic loads, and also enable it to preserve orientation [61]. Proprioception is composed of three primary parameters: position and sense of motion of the joints; force related to muscular contraction, sense of effort, and weight; and perceived timing of muscular contraction [62].

Proprioception is the fundamental component of sensorimotor system, and is responsible for providing afferent information for central nervous system.

8.2.1 Structures Responsible for Proprioception

• Muscle spindles • Golgi tendon organs • joint receptors • informing the cerebellum of position sense, force, effort. • a role in the neural control of movement.

Mechanoreceptor afferents are isolated in the paraspinal muscles; interspinous, supraspinous, flaval, and anterior longitudinal ligaments; thoracolumbar fascia; capsule; lumbar intervertebral discs; and cervical, thoracic, and lumbar facet joints in the spine. Mechanoreceptors have information about reflex regulation of muscle tone as well as about awareness of position sense and movement sense [63]. Recent studies demonstrate that muscle afferents are the primary mechanoreceptors for position and movement sense and joint afferent receptors are most active at the limits of joint movement. Joint movements cause tissues to get deformed and this, in turn, leads to excitation of mechanoreceptor neurons that innervate the area and to initiation of action potentials. These action potentials are afterwards directed to the spinal cord for muscle tone reflex regulation or to higher centers of the central nervous system for signal processing, and eventually for a suitable reaction. In the central nervous system, proprioceptive signals are construed against the background input received from other sources including visual, audio, and vestibular systems [62]. Central nervous system also generates command signals for timing, grading, and destination of the motor output in addition to these afferent data.

Cervical spine plays an important part in providing proprioceptive impulse. Cervical proprioceptive system houses sensitive fibers that connect and bridge over cervical intervertebral joint mechanoreceptors, trapezius and ligament mechanoreceptors, muscle spindle located at deep-seated muscles of cervical spine, cornu posterior neurons of the spinal cord, and neck proprioceptors. For reason of central and reflective link intensity of mechanoreceptors, cervical spine plays an important part also in generating proprioceptive input. In neck pathologies, sensorimotor disorders based on proprioceptor receptor dysfunction are common. In neck disorders, cervical receptor dysfunction affects sensorimotor control union combination, timing, and conversion, leading to afferent input changes [13].

Cervical mechanoreceptor functions get deformed depending on direct trauma, functional disability of muscles [increased fatigue], or degenerative muscular transformation [fiber transformation, fat infiltration, muscular atrophy]. In addition, muscle spindle sensitivity at many levels of the nervous system, cortical presentation, and cervical afferent "input" modulation may change due to pain effect. In nonspecific cervical pathologies, proprioception sense may be affected or kinesthetic sensitivity may be changed depending on muscular and articular receptor lesion or functional disability. Also psychosocial factors cause change in muscle spindle activity, activating sympathetic nervous system [64, 65].

Cervical spine injuries may cause damages in sensory receptors that surround and innerve cervical structures. These sensors are muscle spindle located at intervertebral and dorsal muscles that provide central nervous system [CNS] with information about any changes in muscular length. Evidence is present that gamma motor neurons are inhibited due to pain after injuries that result in incorrect proprioceptive sensation not from muscular movements to MSS. This is crucial for everyday activities because moving an object involves significant motion of head and neck.

Structures in the lumbar spine, more specifically fibers [i.e., supraspinous, interspinous, and ligamentum flavum], intervertebral discs, facet joints, and interspinous muscles have mechanoreceptor afferents that are capable of proprioception [66, 67].

A number of studies have analyzed the role of proprioception in chronic low back pain, and proprioception has been found to have decreased with the spine of patients that suffer from chronic low back pain both when standing and in crawling position [68]. It is hypothesized that overloads on the spine or on body muscle may result in muscle spindle damages or disability. Muscle-tendon vibration and microneurography studies reveal the important role of muscle spindles in proprioception [69]. Introducing a vibratory stimulus like the one from a tuning fork is considered to cause perceived lengthening of a trunk muscle [if over 40 Hz], as well as a perceived shortening of trunk muscle [if under 40 Hz] [69]. This leads to an increased righting error, such that when a patient tries to return to neutral position, they can overshoot or undershoot their target. Spinal joints between adjacent vertebrae are rich in mechanoreceptor nerve fibers that supply information to the brain. This reflex pathway is necessary for vestibular and ocular righting reflex actions, normal spinal coupling motions, balance, and proprioception [70]. When a joint is compressed, inflammation results; hence, decreased mobility of nutrients gets into the joint. Joints are not lubricated or nourished as efficiently, and joint pathology results which destroys the reflex arc to the brain. As the arc is destroyed, the patient gradually loses its expected coupling motion, righting reflex actions, and ability to maintain balance and upright posture under gravity [70]. This may possibly explain the finding of increased postural sway. The joint capsules are also richly endowed with sensory nerve endings [nociceptors], which are sensitized and eventually synapse in the thalamus: Here, they spill over to the segment's motor neurons that cause reflexive muscle spasm of that segment, consequently causing pain. It can therefore be concluded that decreased muscle spindle input may impair spinal proprioception and segmental stability [71].

When a joint is injured, mechanoreceptor function adversely affects the coordinated muscle contraction and results in changes in the perception of body-space relation [70], which, in turn, results in chronic low-back problems.

Studies show that muscle spindle input of the multifidus is significant for accurate positioning of the pelvis and lumbosacral spine in a sitting posture [72]. Accordingly it is hypothesized that proprioceptive deficits from an inhibited multifidus may cause muscle dysfunction and altered spinal stability [72]. Also, clinical trials show that focused retraining of the deep muscle co-contraction is likely to reverse multifidus inhibition.

8.3 Clinical Interventions to Improve Proprioception After Surgery

At all levels of the CNS, proprioception is processed and integrated with other somatosensory and visual and vestibular information before culminating in a final motor command, which coordinates skeletal muscles' activation patterns [73]. Proprioception is the process of formation of reactions whereby body parts are safest, and the proprioceptive process is administered by deep senses. Deep senses are position senses, muscular and tendon sensorial vibration, as well as pressure, balance, and other senses that provide information about overall body and extremities. These senses are perceived by special sensors inside tissues which are named mechanoreceptor, from where they are transmitted to the central nervous system. Central nervous system organizes and analyzes the senses, forming a response for keeping joints in the safest possible position as it may be. Thus created, the responses are transmitted to the target joint and to the target area through the neural network. This is how necessary precautions are taken to ensure the safest possible maneuver for the joint or for extremities [74].

By specifically contributing to proprioception, mechanoreceptors are termed proprioceptors and these are present in muscle, tendon, joint, and fascia receptors in the skin and these, too, may contribute to proprioception [75, 76].

As it will be seen here, the proprioceptive process is of great significance for protecting joints, organs, extremities, and organelles in the body against injuries. For this reason, a number of internal and external factors that are likely to affect the proprioceptive process positively or negatively—as the case may be—and may intervene in the process are and have been studied by various researchers. Though with functional issues, proprioception and compensatory mechanisms have become known quite recently.

Consequently, their importance for postoperative stability has become prominent [77].

It has been stated that proprioception makes significant contributions in keeping postural control in postspinal surgeries, or structures that contribute to proprioception during a disc replacement surgery are vulnerable [78]. Having conducted studies on the innervation of the intervertebral disc, researchers suggest that mechanoreceptors in outer annulus and also posterior and anterior longitudinal ligaments function as proprioceptors, and they provide sensation of movement and posture. A disc replacement surgery takes from a substantial portion of annulus and also from the anterior and posterior longitudinal ligaments to a certain extent; therefore it is likely that the proprioceptive input at the segment is actually affected [50, 51]. For this reason, practices to support proprioception should be added as early as possible when planning a treatment program for postoperative pain, muscular spasm, restricted joint mobility, muscular weakness, lack of balance, and similar symptoms. Using passive techniques such as manual therapy, soft tissue techniques and taping or braces for augmenting the somatosensory information may be worthwhile because these techniques trigger mechanoreceptors in joints, soft tissues, and skin so as to transmit sensory information to CNS. If manual therapy is to be preferred, then involve plastic changes in sensory integration within CNS [79]. Exercise therapy also plays a significant role in enhancing proprioception.

8.3.1 Exercise

Exercise can be considered as "proprioceptive training" since it creates an afferent input from the joint and muscle-tendon mechanoreceptors to the central nervous system. Any type of exercise will activate the proprioceptors; however what is important is that these exercises generate certain changes, particularly in the nervous system,

through different ways. For example, through motor control exercises it is aimed to generate changes in the motor cortex and prevent repeated injury and obtain a healthy spine structure [73, 80]. It is stated that motor control training aimed at lumbar region stimulates synaptogenesis, synaptic potential, and reorganization of movement representation in the motor cortex [81, 82].

8.3.2 Motor Control Exercises

8.3.2.1 Lumbopelvic Motor Control Exercise

Lumbopelvic motor control is based on a special connection between the musculoskeletal system and the central nervous system circuits [83]. The local muscles including multifidus, pelvic floor, transversus abdominis, and diaphragm muscles under the central nervous system's control play an important role in establishing healthy motor control [84]. The healthy relationship between synergic co-contraction of local muscles and central nervous system is necessary for establishing lumbopelvic stability. The stability in the lumbopelvic region is obtained through the activation of the local muscles before any perturbation that occurs in the body. Changes observed in the local muscles due to the disruption of the motor control in this region [pain, acute inflammation of spinal ligaments [85], or lessened stiffness of soft tissues] due to elongated or repetitive forward-bent posture [86, 87], and surgical applications [88, 89] that result in delayed activation, disrupt the stability in the region and set the stage for injuries and threaten healthy waist and spine structure [90]. This unfavorable process adversely affects the lumbar region's proprioception [91, 92].

For this reason, exercise programs aimed at strengthening the specifically selected muscles should be started as soon as possible post-surgery, in order to reduce structural and functional disorders, lessen pain, and as well as increase proprioception.

Special exercises related with segmental stabilization were created based on a number of aspects. These are

- Improving the motor control aspect of muscle function
- Establishing neutral spine posture
- Co-contraction of body muscles (including multifidus and TA)
- Tonic contractions that continue at a reduced level
- Full co-contraction of TA and multifidus, independently from global muscles
- Benefiting from methods that reduce global muscle activation allowing for deep-muscle co-contraction
- Benefiting from new facilitation strategies in order to provide deep-muscle co-contraction
- Selection of personalized treatment strategies

Co-contraction exercises are defined like special motor skills. While those without any waist problem stories perform such exercises with a good figure, people with waist problems encounter great difficulty in performing this skill. For this reason this motor skill is better rehabilitated through motor learning method instead of motor skill strength and endurance-increasing exercises.

8.3.3   Special Exercise Concept

Special exercise concept is based on succeeding in co-contraction of key local muscles (TA, MU, diaphragm, pelvic floor muscles). The aim is for these muscles to directly rest against the lumbar vertebra, and to influence the local spinal segmental support by increasing the intra-abdominal pressure and the tension in TLF. Explaining the cylinder-like effect of these muscles to the patient, the understanding of the use of these muscles plays a very important role in the facilitation strategies of these muscles. Actually, each of the four muscles is used to facilitate the other. For example if the patient is unable to activate TA, the activation is attempted through the facilitation of lumbar MU or pelvic floor muscles [93].

Activation of TA through "abdominal hallowing" (pulling the abdomen up and in) movement: TA is activated through the "abdominal hallowing" movement, without causing the global muscles to contract, by pulling "the abdominal wall in and up during normal breathing in and out pattern, without moving the spine and pelvis" [94, 95]. This motor skill is unfamiliar to the patient. For this reason a good learning is an important part of the treatment. The movement of the TA is the pulling in of the abdominal wall and the narrowing of the waist. For this reason the principle behind teaching contraction is finding a way that teaches how to pull in the abdominal wall. The most successful method is to ask the patient to focus on the lower abdominal segment. In the recent studies it is stated that the lower segment of TA is the most fundamental part for spinal stabilization.

Breathing in-out pattern (diaphragm): In expiration, TA is used to activate this muscle. During expiration, the isolated operation of TA is achieved through hyperoxic-hypercapnic conditions and an inspiratory load that leads to increase in expiratory air outlet. In both cases, TA activation increases involuntarily and selectively. In order to teach this to the patient in an effective figure, the patient is asked to breathe in the external air and to move the abdomen upwards during expiration [96]. Patients who frequently utilize obliquus externus will cause frequent displacement with expiration. First of all, the patient's attention must be brought to loose diaphragmatic respiration. When we observe comfortable breathing of the patient, the TA contraction must be started.

Pelvic floor: Using pelvic floor muscles' contraction is the most effective method of achieving isolated contraction of TA. What's fundamental to TA's contribution to the stabilization in the spine is the contraction of the diaphragm and the pelvic floor muscles. Utilization of pelvic floor contraction is beneficial for patients who need to facilitate TA contraction and are having difficulty in understanding the movement. Furthermore, it is a primary technique for those people who cannot relax the obliquus externus muscle in the "abdominal hallowing" movement. Description of the muscle anatomy between the sacrum and the front of the pelvis will help the patient in visualizing this muscle's contraction. Lying on one's back with bent knees or side-lying position is the best position to teach the pelvic floor contraction in the beginning. Clinician or the patient slowly and deeply palps the lower abdomen and the patient is asked to breathe comfortably, slowly let his/her breath out, and slowly and gently pull the pelvic floor muscles. Co-activation of pelvic floor and TA results in feeling a deep tension inside the abdominal wall [97]. Pelvic floor muscles' contraction is also used for teaching and facilitating the isometric contraction of segmental MU. It is particularly helpful if the patient feels a weak awareness in the MU muscle [98].

8.3.4 Including Motor Skills in Light Functional Activities

At this phase, the aim is to attempt the continuation of deep muscle co-contraction with light loading. At this level, deep muscle co-contraction is maintained in the presence of global muscle system activity, while the normal breathing in-out pattern continues. At this phase, two functional conditions are practiced. These are the following:

1. Using deep muscles in order to maintain lumbopelvic support function in harmony with the global muscle system while breathing in and out normally under light load in static conditions, for example slow and controlled movements of lower and upper extremities
2. Using deep muscles in order to maintain lumbopelvic support function during body movements around neutral position while the global muscle system is phasic active: This is a difficult level where the deep system muscles' control is practiced. Therefore, it must be performed with care and control. At this phase the deep and global muscle systems will work in both interdependent and independent roles.

8.3.5 Combining Heavy Functional Work with Motor Skill

At this phase of the program, the aim is to sustain the contraction of local muscles which are sufficient for controlling the lumbar spine position, under increasing load. The load level varies from between patients and the patient's needs and requirements in work and private life should be monitored. This program includes a functional exercise program related with the persons' daily life, job, and sports activities.

8.3.6 Early-Period Lumbopelvic Motor Control Exercises Spinal Surgery (Day 2 to Week 6 Post-operation)

In this phase, the aim is to teach the patient the "abdominal hallowing" basic movement that allows for the activation of deep muscles. Once the patient correctly learns the movement the endurance training of these muscles is started. While initially the "abdominal hallowing" basic movement is maintained for 5–10 s, the aim is to reach 30–45 s of protection period. This process varies for each person; however it can be achieved in 2–3 weeks. In the second stage of this phase, the aim is to continue conscious activation of the deep muscles during the performing of the exercises. The attention should always be on control, and progress should not be too rapid. Since pain and fatigue will have negative impact on proprioception, the training should be conducted without creating pain or fatigue [99] (Figs. 8.1, 8.2, 8.3, 8.4, 8.5, 8.6, 8.7, 8.8, 8.9, 8.10, 8.11, and 8.12).

8.3.7 Late-Period Postspinal Surgery (6–12 weeks)

During this period, while the contraction of deep muscles continues, the loading of the exercises also increases. The patient switches from stationary ground to moving ground and from simple extremity movements to complex movements

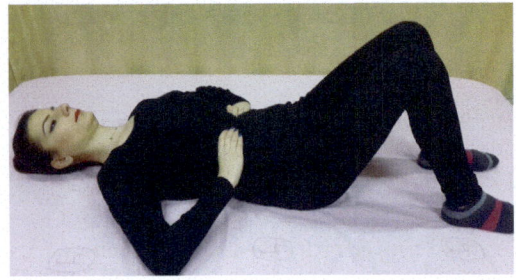

Fig. 8.1 Diaphragmatic breathing

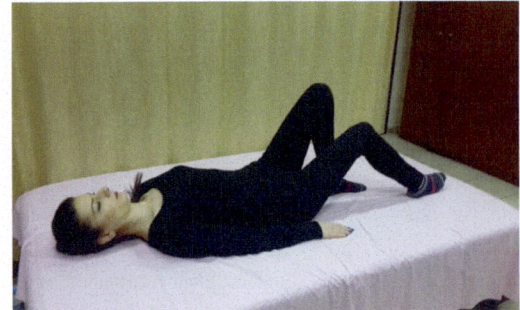

Fig. 8.4 TrA&MF-heel slide

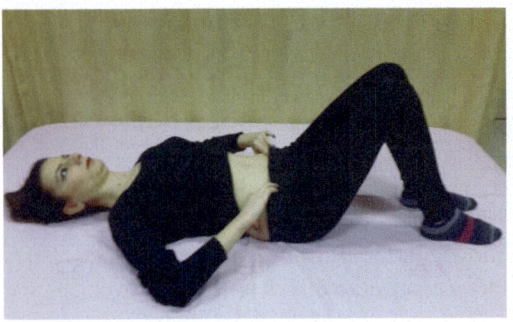

Fig. 8.2 Basic TrA&MF activation

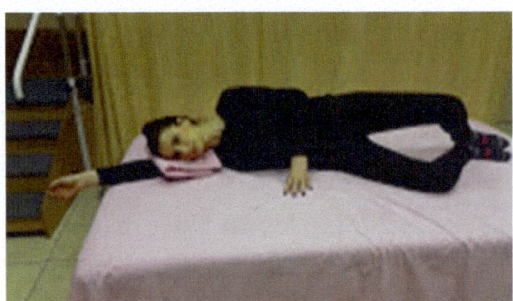

Fig. 8.5 TrA&MF-side lying-bent knee fallout

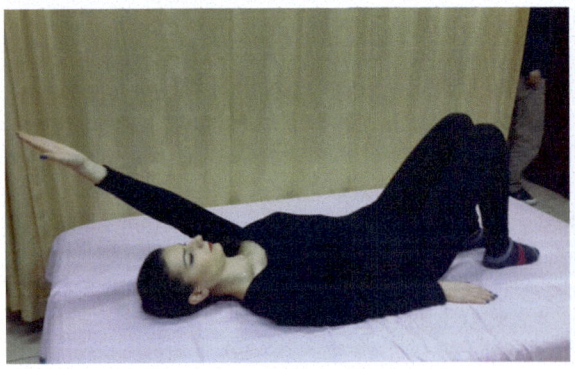
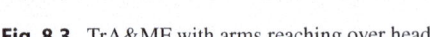
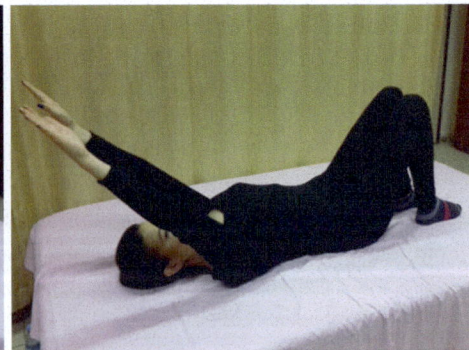

Fig. 8.3 TrA&MF with arms reaching over head

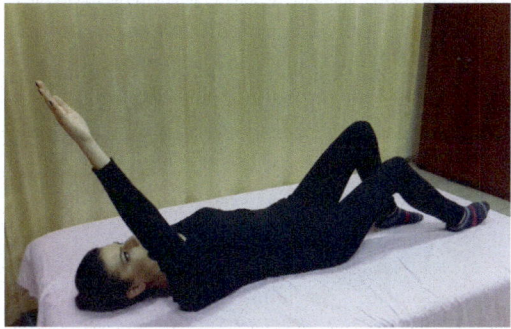

Fig. 8.6 TrA&MF-heel slide and same side or opposite arm overhead

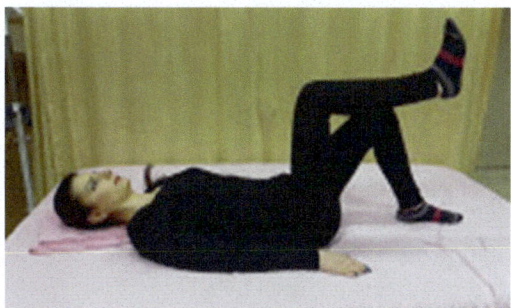

Fig. 8.7 TrA&MF-single knee lift

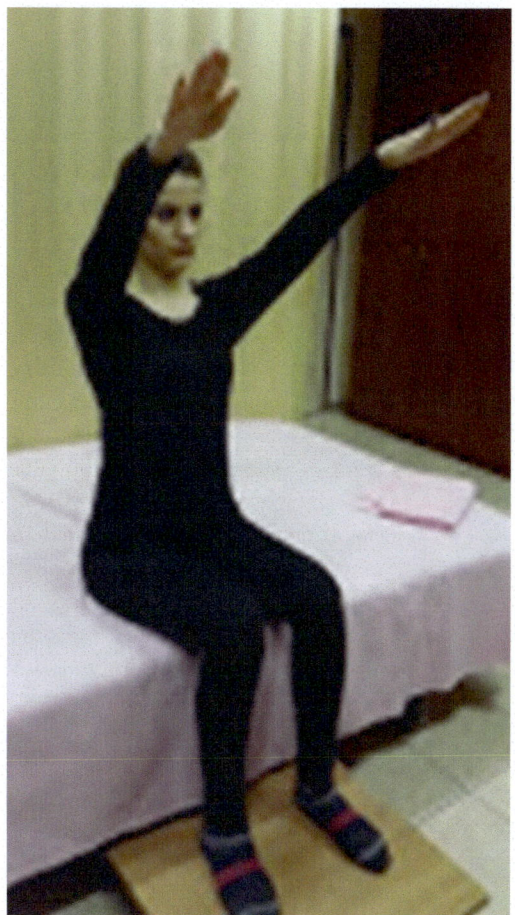

Fig. 8.9 TrA&MF-sitting-eyes closed, arm movement

to help develop position awareness and balance (Figs. 8.13, 8.14, 8.15, 8.16, 8.17, 8.18, 8.19, 8.20, and 8.21).

8.3.8 Cervical Stabilization Exercise

Cervical stabilization exercises are developed to increase motor control of cervical spine. The special muscles which are the focus in this program

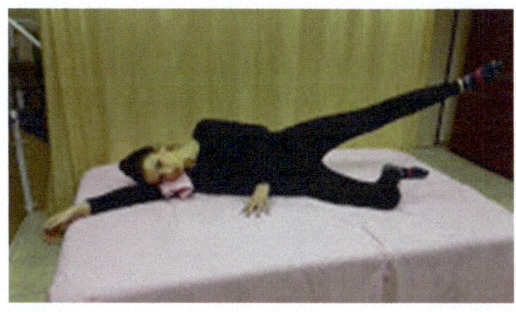

Fig. 8.8 TrA&MF-hip abduction

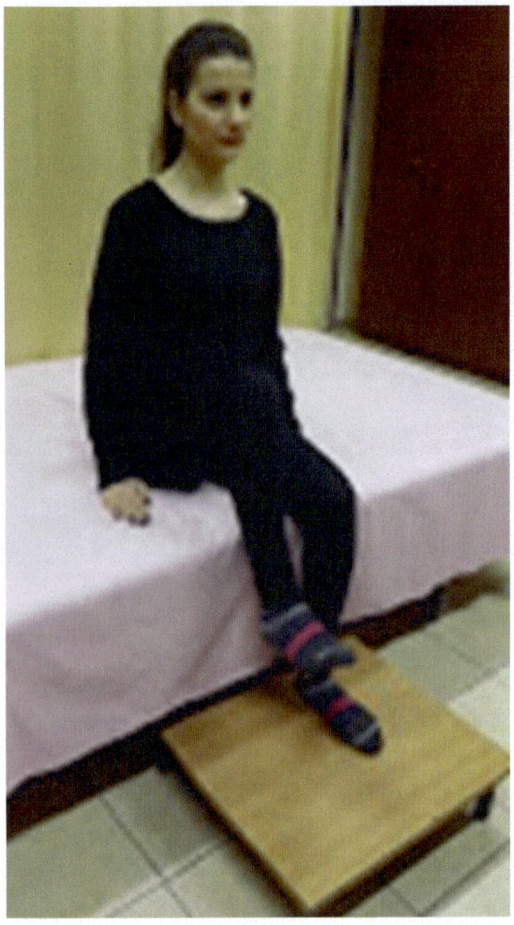

Fig. 8.10 TrA&MF-sitting-eyes open, single knee lift

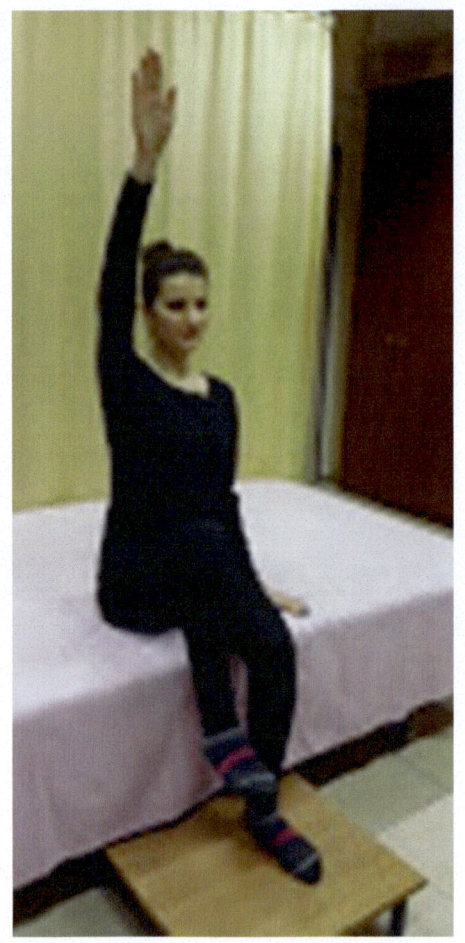

Fig. 8.12 TrA&MF sitting-two point of stable contact

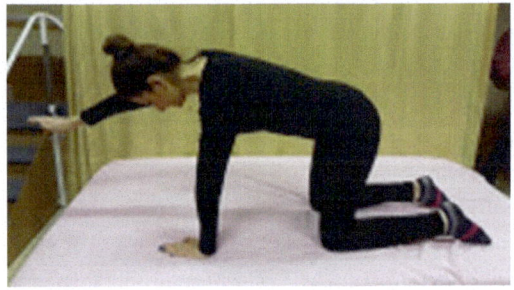

Fig. 8.11 TrA&MF-quadruped—three points of stable contact

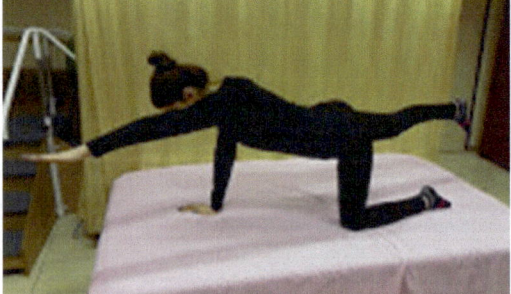

Fig. 8.13 TrA&MF-quadruped-two points of stable contact

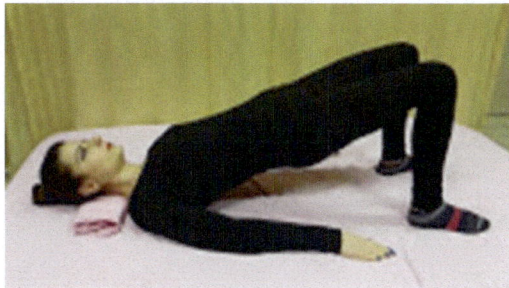

Fig. 8.14 TrA&MF-back bridge

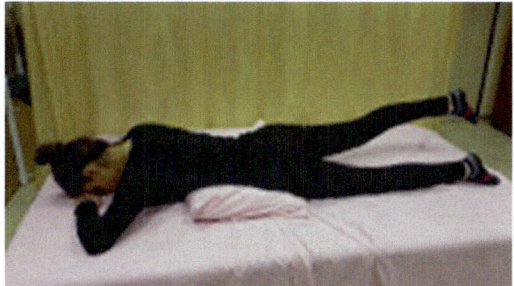

Fig. 8.15 TrA&MF-prone position-leg lift

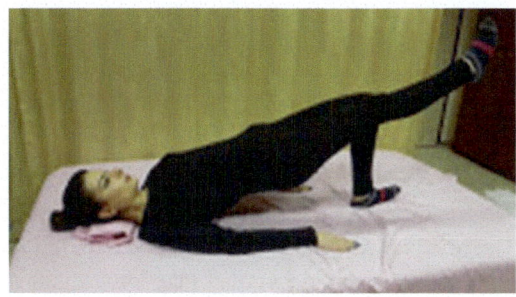

Fig. 8.16 TrA&MF-front bridge-single leg extension

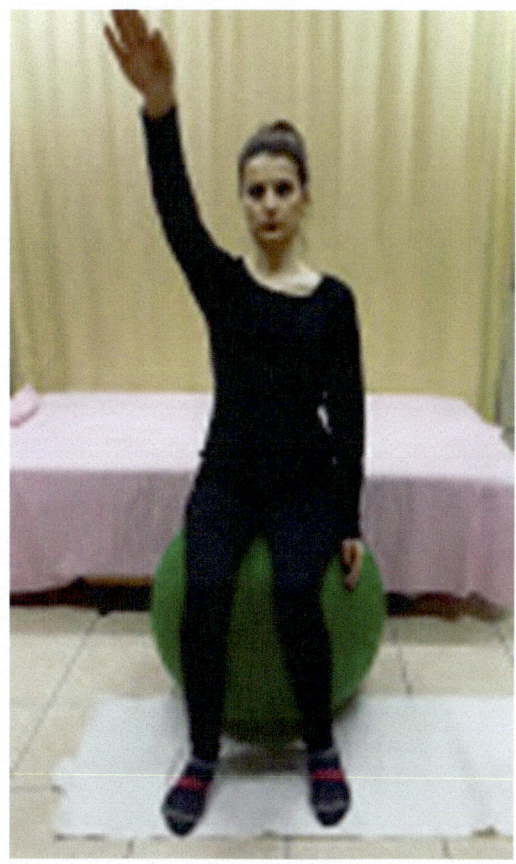

Fig. 8.17 Ball sitting, eyes open and closed arm movement

are very important in supporting cervical lordosis and cervical joints [100].

Cervical stabilization exercise program addresses motor learning and training program comprising three phases [101].

Phase 1: The focus is on low-intensity exercises in order to activate deep cervical and axioscapular muscles and train the basic movement patterns of cervical and axioscapular region.

Phase 2: In the task-oriented exercises, neck and shoulder belt muscle coordination and movement pattern training and muscle reeducation involving deep postural muscles' co-activation are continued. In this phase, loading in exercises is started.

Phase 3: Muscles' strength and endurance are addressed and the training aims for the level that

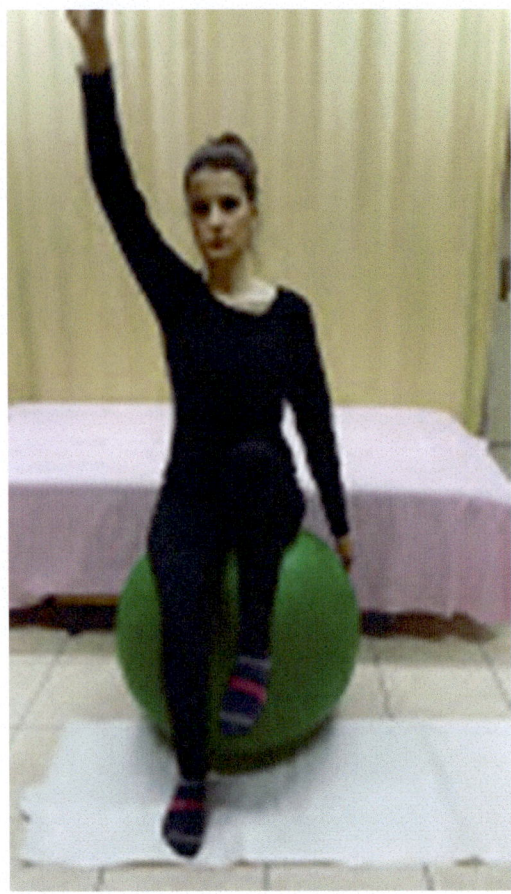

Fig. 8.18 Ball sitting-eyes open, two point of stable contact

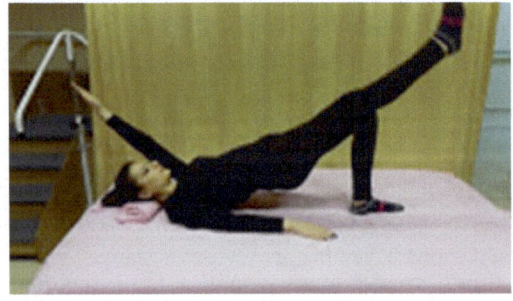

Fig. 8.19 TrA&MF-back bridge-two points of stable contact

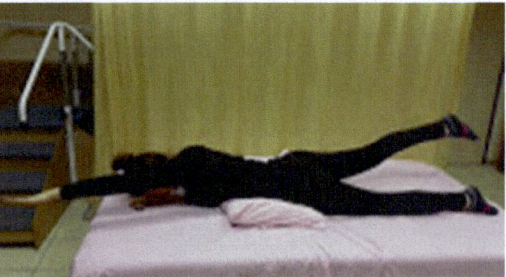

Fig. 8.20 TrA&MF-prone position-contralateral arm and leg lift

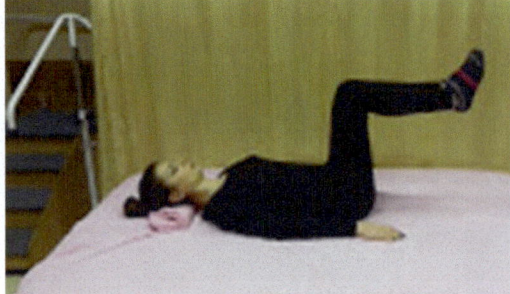

Fig. 8.21 TrA&MF-bilateral knee lift

the patient will return to his/her job, recreational, or sports activities.

8.3.9 Early-Period Post-cervical Surgery

The first phase of the cervical stabilization training includes craniocervical flexion training where muscle activation of deep cervical flexors is increased and low-load endurance exercises for these muscles. It must be begun at the earliest period post-cervical region surgery.

8.3.9.1 Craniocervical Flexion [CCF] Training

During the treatment, "pressurized biofeedback apparatus" is used in order to raise the patients'

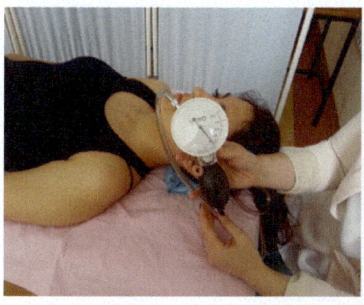 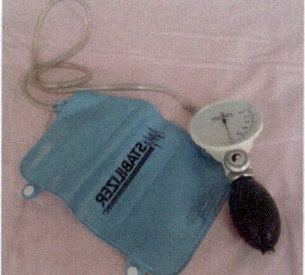 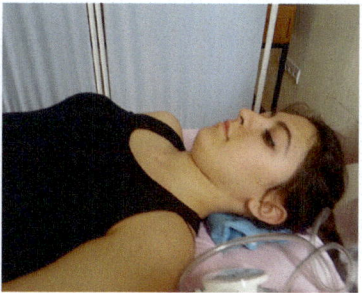

Fig. 8.22 CCF training

awareness and to focus on the desired muscle [102–104]. The patient is positioned in the hook position. Pressurized biofeedback apparatus is placed horizontally between craniocervical and cervical vertebra, in mid-position or in such a way to allow forehead-chin projection. It is inflated to standard 20 mmHg in order to establish contact between the surface and the neck. The patient is asked to gently stare at the midline of the chest (Fig. 8.22) [105, 106].

Since increase in superficial muscle activation is not desired the patient must be reminded that this movement is not a movement that requires force. Again, to reduce the activation of superficial muscles the tongue-palate muscles must be relaxed. For this, the patient is asked to remove his/her tongue from the palate and to slightly open the teeth [107, 108].

It is important that the craniocervical flexion movement is painless. There can be acute pain in patients after cervical surgery, and there might be reservations related with performing the exercises since it is thought that exercise can increase pain. However, the patient should be asked to lightly swing their head to determine the painless movement limits. If any pain occurs during this very light practice, this indicates that either the patient performed the movement in a harsh manner or the movement was performed with the upper cervical regions' pushback movement.

In this case the movement must be taught again. In order to minimize any tension that might occur in the patient, the patient is positioned in hook position, with arms on the abdomen.

- Compensations:
  - If the pressure increases more than 2 mmHg at the beginning
  - If the movement is performed too fast
  - If the activity of superficial muscles is felt
  - If it does not return to starting point when pressure is released
  - If the lordotic angle is lost
  - If the patient lifts his/her head to reach target

If any of the above is true, this means that the "craniocervical flexion" movement is performed incorrectly [109, 110].

8.3.10 Low-Load Endurance Training

Low-level endurance training of deep-neck flexions begins as soon as the patient correctly performs the craniocervical flexion movement. The training begins at a pressure level that the patient can achieve a good movement pattern and hold stable, without using superficial flexor muscles. This is usually the lowest levels of the test [22 or 24 mmHg].

Fig. 8.23 CCF
endurance training

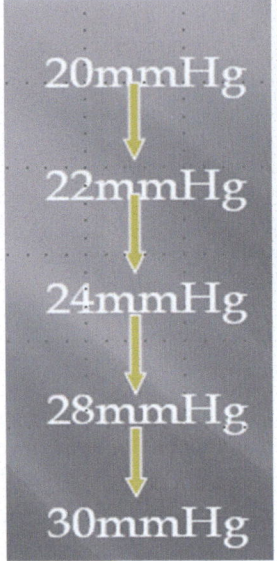
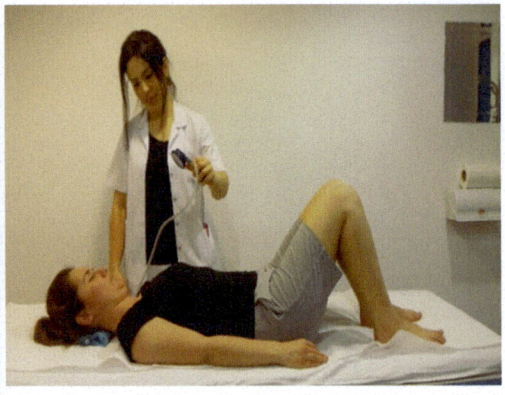

8.3.10.1 Training Protocol

Starting at 20 mmHg and increasing at 2 mmHg steps, the desired level of 30 mmHg is achieved. The movement is maintained for 10 s at each level; ten repetitions are asked with 3–5-s rest intervals. If the level is maintained for 10-s three repetitions then the next level can be started (Fig. 8.23) [111, 112].

Fast and irregular movements are not encouraged since they mask the insufficiencies in deep-neck flexors' activation. The patient follows the superficial muscles' undesired movements by paling the muscles. In this case the patients should first of all focus on the craniocervical flexion movement and later look at the pressure gauge and maintain the pressure level they have achieved. In any case, the training should be performed without any fatigue; otherwise a wrong pattern emerges. The duration required to achieve and maintain the five levels of craniocervical varies; however it is usually achieved within 4–6 weeks.

8.3.11 Reeducation of Neutral Spinal Posture

Preserving the neutral vertical spinal posture at regular intervals during the day has numerous favor-

able benefits and outcomes. Mechanically, vertical neutral posture can eliminate the passive load on cervical structures and the resulting pain. Spinal and pelvic posture control training is the first step of the training. It is a painless exercise that in fact eliminates pain. At the beginning, vertical neutral spinal posture is trained while sitting. Correction begins in the lumbopelvic region. One of the methods that the patient learns in a simple and quick manner is applying pressure on L5 spinous process and facilitating the position (Fig. 8.24). This emphasizes the restoration of normal lordosis through the use of multifidus. Thoracic and cervical postures are usually corrected automatically by correcting the lumbopelvic position. Additional visual feedback through the use of a mirror can also be beneficial to the patient. The patients can be taught the facilitation they perform on their own, for the early periods of the posture training. The patients can repeat the facilitation by placing their thumbs of fingers on the L5 spinous protrusion. Correction continues until an awareness of position and muscles is achieved.

The patients are encouraged to practice the posture correction exercise at 15-min intervals throughout the day and to maintain the position for at least 10 s as they continue their activities. This practice can be performed in sitting or standing position. Scapular correction is in the second phase of the reeducation. This is sometimes postponed until second phase with patients having difficulty in learning the spinal postural position. One last element of posture correction exercise is asking the patient to perform a slight occipital lifting.

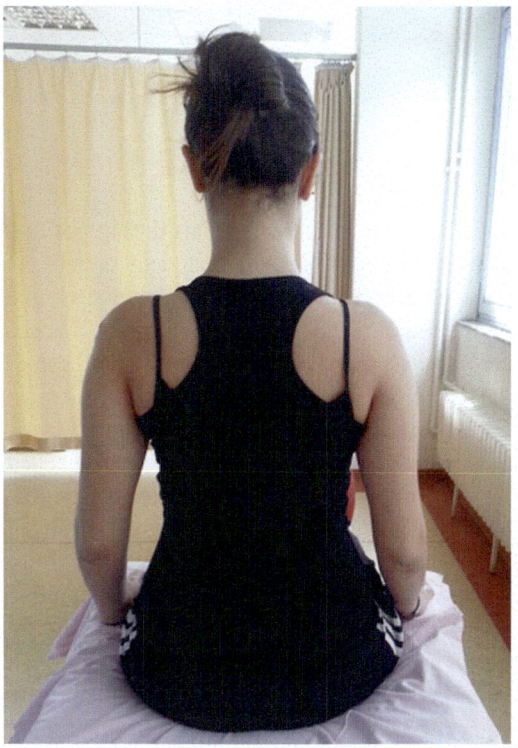

Fig. 8.24 Neutral spine

8.3.12 Late-Period Post-cervical Surgery

The exercise program in this period continues to focus on motor learning; however, the load is increased in exercises. In this phase, a switch is made from the laying-on-back positions, where the gravity is helping, to positions which are against the gravity. Unilateral and bilateral extremity movements are added to the exercise program in order to achieve dynamic stabilization. The patient switches from stationary ground to moving ground and from simple extremity movements to complex movements to help develop position awareness and balance. After gaining control of the movements, weights and elastic bands are added to the exercises (Figs. 8.25, 8.26, 8.27, 8.28, 8.29, 8.30, 8.31, and 8.32).

8.3.13 Vibration and Proprioception

The impact of vibration applications on the sense of position and kinesthesis is a subject frequently researched in the recent years. The sense receptors in the muscles, joints, and skin play an active role in proprioception sense. The most important receptors for proprioception in muscles are in the Golgi tendon organs and muscle fibers. Afferents related with sense of position and movement are found in muscle fibers. These are triggered when the muscle fiber tenses during elongation of the

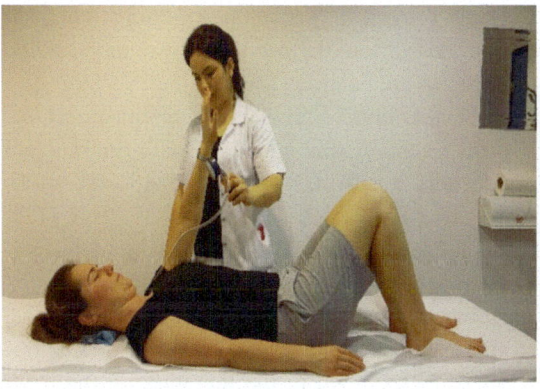
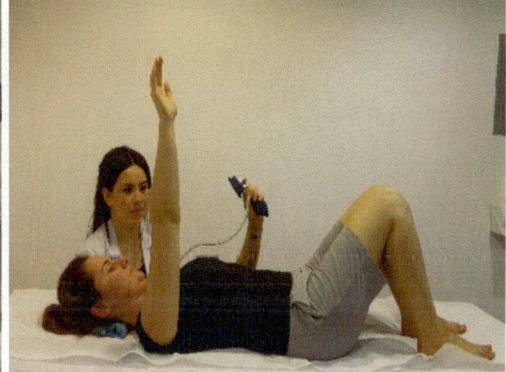

Fig. 8.25 CCF with arm movement

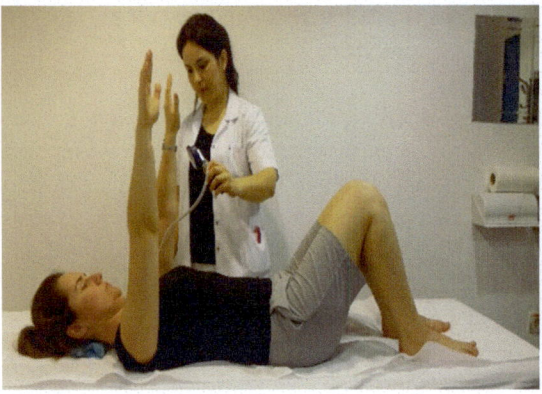 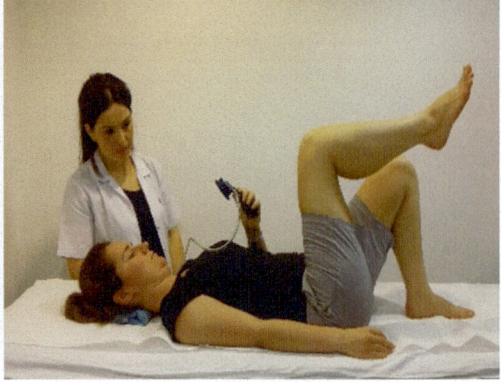

Fig. 8.26 CCF with bilateral arm movement and lift knee

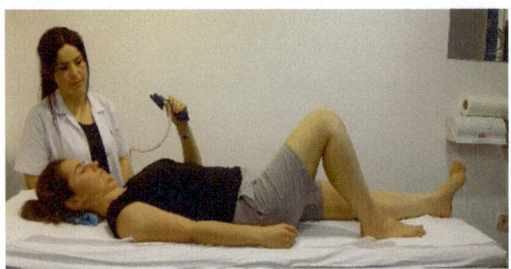

Fig. 8.27 CCF with heel-slide

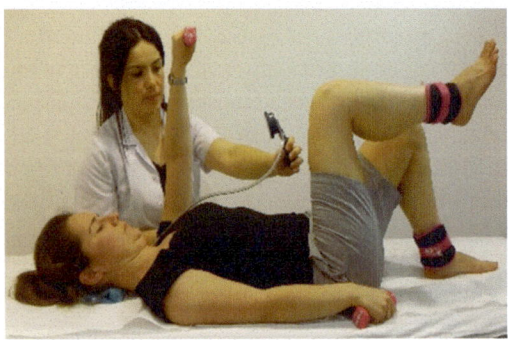

Fig. 8.28 CCF with opposite side arm and leg lift

muscle. While the Ia afferents in the muscle fiber are sensitive to speed variations in the extremities, group II afferents provide information related with position conditions. The activity of muscle fibers increases with the elongation of the muscle. For the sense of position to be picked up, the muscles on both sides of the joint should be able to receive sufficient signals during position and movement. When sufficient activation of the muscle fiber is achieved through vibration applied on the muscle tendon, the joint position changes can be detected. According to the studies conducted, slight variations are seen in skeletal muscle lengths during whole-body vibration. During the application of the vibration, a response called "tonic vibration reflex" arises, which includes the activation of muscle fiber and the activation of muscle fibrils through large alpha motor neurons. Tonic vibration reflex also leads to muscle fiber activation and increasing of the effectiveness of polysynaptic pathways. Vibration applications of 100 Hz and above cause the group Ia fibers to empty and may lead to illusions in position sense and movement perception. Vibration applications below 100 Hz, on the other hand, mostly activate group II fibers. As stated before, since group II fibers provide information regarding the position's condition, the position sense may develop after this application [113–115].

In the literature, vibration applications for proprioception training are usually carried out between 5 and 100 Hz for 30–45-s durations and 15-s rest periods, for a total of 5 min [116, 117]. There are no studies in the literature pertaining vibration application postspinal surgery. However, in the early period post-operation, applications can be done using durations and frequencies specified in the literature on the painful region or slightly away from painful region

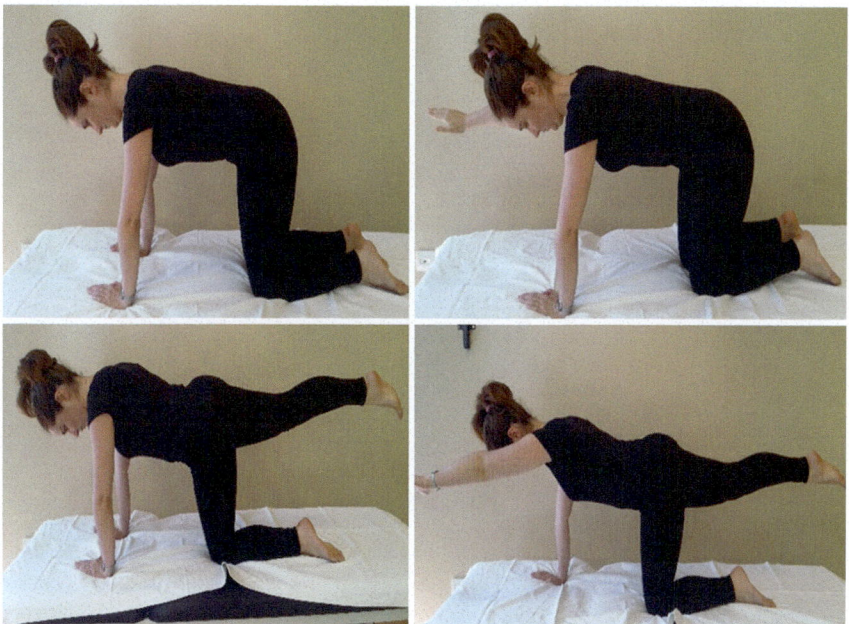

Fig. 8.29 CCF with quadruped position

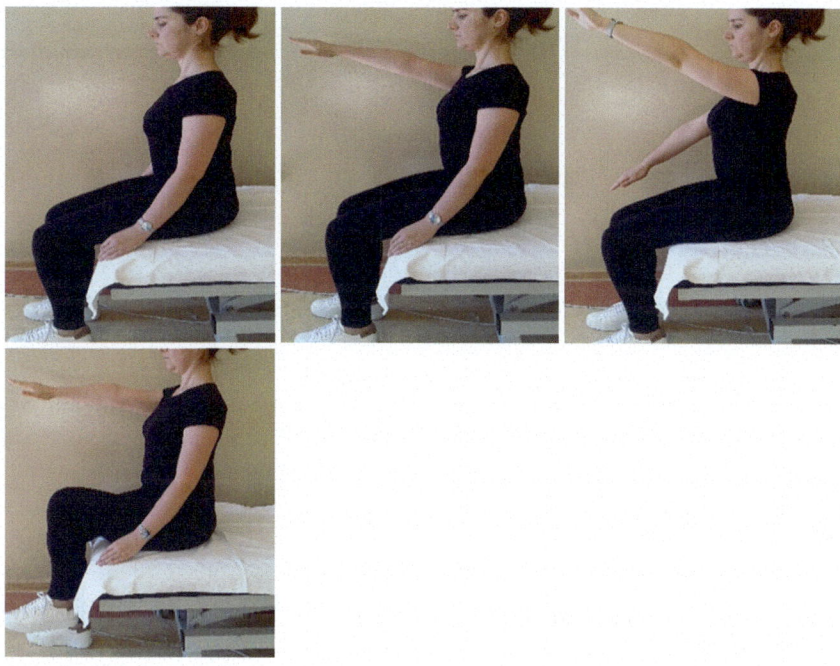

Fig. 8.30 CCF with sitting

Fig. 8.31 CCF with standing

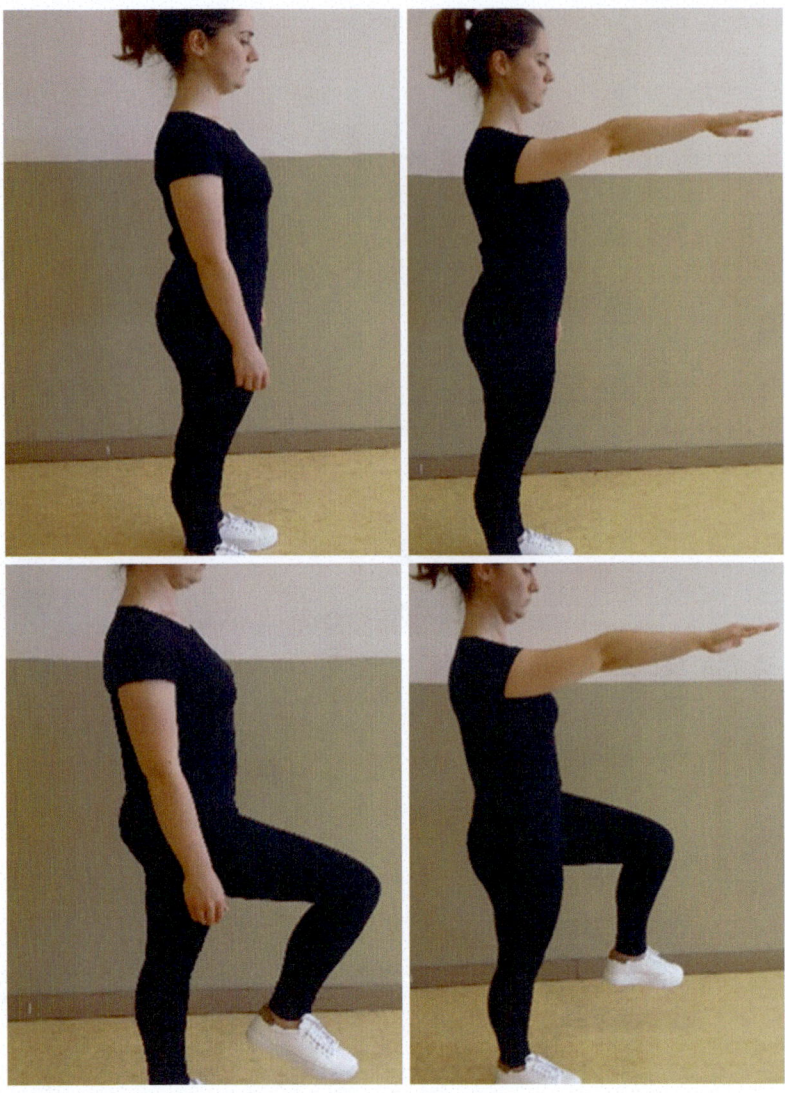

if the pain causes too much discomfort. In the light of all of these developments, even though the effect of vibration applications on proprioception is becoming better known in the recent years, there's definitely a need for more studies to be conducted on the subject.

8.4 Manuel Therapy

8.4.1 Massage Therapy

Massage therapy has local and systemic effects. Local effects are that it helps with the breakdown of tissue adhesions [118] and increases blood flow and oxygenation of muscles [119]. It has been demonstrated that massage alleviates production of inflammatory cytokines TNF-alpha and IL-6 at cellular levels, increasing mitochondrial biogenesis in muscle damages arising from exercises [120]. Increased blood levels of oxytocin and reduced levels of the stress hormone ACTH are among the systemic effects [121]. Depending on the increase in serotonin and endorphins, depression, anxiety, and pain are reduced, which are among the central nervous system effects [118]. It has also been demonstrated that therapeutic massage reduces Hoffman's reflex and alpha-motor

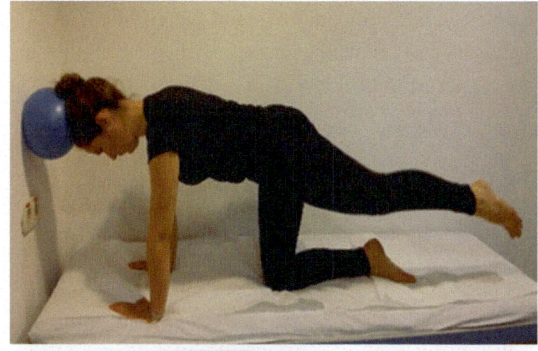

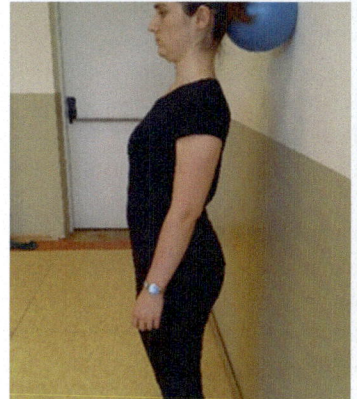 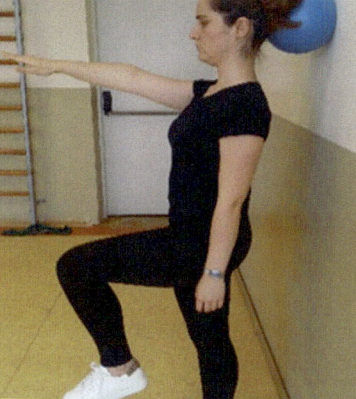 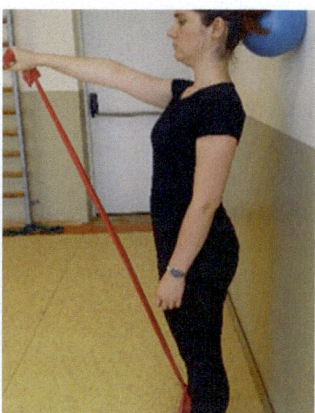

Fig. 8.32 CCF with deep extensor muscle activation

neuron excitability of the flexor carpi radialis muscle [122], and improves cervical range of motion [123, 124].

The term "joint effusion" refers to swelling within a joint capsule, which is commonly seen after acute extremity joint injury, and it may persist for extended periods of time [125]. Skeletal muscle can be inhibited due to joint effusions and it can even impair extremity proprioception even though no pain is felt [126, 127]. A single known event that causes physical injury, or trauma as referred to here [128], is often revealed with musculoskeletal tissue disruption and accompanying damage or destruction mechanoreceptors innervating those tissues [129]. After trauma, and once swelling and pain are resolved, loss of musculoskeletal tissue and its mechanoreceptors is associated with persistent impairment of proprioception [118, 130, 131].

An individual who has had different kinds of surgeries may benefit from the massage therapy as it has been shown by studies. In literature,

effectiveness of massage therapy in the postoperative thoracic surgery setting has been studied. According to one, 160 people completed the pilot study and it was found that patients that had a massage therapy had remarkably reduced pain scores after the massage. Massage therapy reduces reducing muscle hypertonicity and alleviates pain, which is cited as another positive effect [132].

There are however no studies on the effect of massage therapy on proprioception after spinal surgeries. Clinically, the afore-cited local and systemic effects can be employed for improved proprioception after spinal surgical. Also, massage therapy helps to improve proprioception as it stimulates cutaneous receptors.

8.4.2 Soft-Tissue Mobilization

In human body, apart from the bone tissue, all tissues including muscles, tendons, ligaments, and fascia that is a sheet of connective tissue constitute soft tissue of the body. Soft tissues enclose other tissues and organs, attaching, stabilizing, and protecting them. Soft tissues including skin, muscle, and joint capsule contain many mechanosensitive neurons. Mechanoreceptors and mechano-nociceptors, for instance, respond to many mechanical stimuli like compression, stretch, and vibration [133].

Soft-tissue mobilization technique is a form of manual therapy, and it intends to increase soft-tissue mobility by employing methods such as low-load, long-duration forces applied in approximation, traction, and torsional vectors [134]. Contact is often applied to knuckles, knuckle joint, palm, elbow, or forearm.

After an injury, inflammation and proliferation of new cells occur. During such time of inflammation and proliferation, fibrosis and formation of scar tissue in the injured soft tissue may be seen [135]. As a result, often inflammatory pain is felt. When inflammatory occurs in an injured tissue, immune cells step in and phagocytosis occurs. As tissue fragments that are decomposed by phagocytosis or substrates that are secreted by immune cells trigger type III and IV nerve endings pain is induced in the body [136]. It is stated in the literature that soft-tissue mobilization has been effective in reducing inflammation arising from exercise; however a massage technique has been applied in this study here [137].

Soft-tissue mobilization intends to break up the inelastic or fibrous muscle tissue *myofascial adhesions* like scar tissue due to back surgery, hence to move tissue fluids and relax any muscle tensions. This can be applied to all of the muscles that surround the spine, and it is composed of rhythmic stretching and strong pressure. Soft-tissue mobilization techniques may become even more effective with active participation of the patient. At the time of mobilization of restricted tissue, voluntary muscle activation in agonist-antagonist pairs may give more effective results. Relief in soft tissue improves blood and lymph stream, and reduces edema and pain [130].

After a spinal surgery, depending on patient toleration, therapist localizes the area with maximum tissue restriction by employing a layer-by-layer assessment. Soft contacts and longitudinal applications can be used every other day depending on the toleration of the patient and the tissue itself.

8.4.3   Connective Tissue Massage

Connective tissue is richly innervated with mechanosensory and nociceptive neurons. Connective tissue massage is a type of massaging applied by stretching stokes onto connective tissue [138]. There are a few theories relating to mechanism of action of the connective tissue massage. One of them is that strokes applied onto connective tissue result in local mechanical actions on some of the cells (i.e., histamine-releasing mast cells, glycosaminoglycan-producing fibroblasts), diminish sympathetic nervous system activation, and activate reflex mechanisms that lead to vasodilatation. As a result of this, the circulation is stimulated in organs that are associated with parasympathetic ganglion, circulation is improved in the entire body, and pain and muscular spasms are reduced [139]. Most probably connective tissue passage intensely stimulates cutaneous mechanical receptors, which, in turn, triggers the "paingating" mechanism, blocking the sense of pain along small peripheral sensorial fibers that are responsible for carrying the sense of pain towards ascending tracts of spinal cord, hence reducing pain [140]. In addition to this, it is a fact that connective tissue massage can stimulate cutaneovisceral reflex via autonomic nerve system, and lead to improving actions in the internal organs that share the same innervation as dermatomes on skin [141].

It has been demonstrated in literature that connective tissue massage can reduce back pain. In literature, it has been further demonstrated in the case of neck pain that both conventional massage and connective tissue massage can be used for reducing acute pain antispasmoic and quick relief [142].

In early phase of postsurgical immobilization, it has been shown that loss in muscle length is essentially related to shortening of muscular related connective tissue [143, 144]. In clinical applications, after spinal surgeries, despite the damaging role of immobilization and surgical applications on the tissue, dynamically and potentially reversible nature of the connective tissue plasticity can be activated with connective tissue massage applications. Also, connective tissue massage helps to improve proprioception as it stimulates cutaneous receptors.

8.4.4 Kinesio Taping

The Kinesio Taping® technique and Kinesio Tex® tape were developed by Dr. Kenzo Kase, a Japanese chiropractor and acupuncture expert in 1973. According to Dr. Kase, musculoskeletal disorders primarily result from muscular dysfunctions. The technique relies on three concepts, namely space, action, and cooling, indicating that swelling muscles take up the space due to pain, inflammation, and edema. In kinesio taping technique, skin is removed; therefore cutaneous and subcutaneous interstitial area is increased, which, in turn, triggers circulation and action. Increased circulation and action reduces inflammation, which, to some extent, cools it off. This intends to reduce pain, increases performance, triggers reeducation of neuromuscular system, prevents injuries, and accelerates circulation and tissue improvement [145].

In this technique, certain positive impacts can be mentioned depending on the degree of stretching to the tape [145]. These impacts stimulate mechanoreceptor via the skin, transmit signals to the central nervous system creating a positional stimuli in the relevant area, correct array of the fascia tissue, and lift fascia, cutaneous, and subcutaneous soft tissues in painful and inflammatory area for making more space. In addition to this, it creates sensory signals to restrict or otherwise increase the movement, and guides exudate towards the lymph for reduced edema [145].

However, mechanism of actions and effectiveness for kinesio taping techniques suffer from insufficient scientific data in literature—not to mention that literature results are controversial. Some studies defend that periarticular muscular tissue is supported and muscles are strengthened while muscular stability is improved, joint mobility is facilitates, and pressure upon structures such as muscles, ligaments, tendons, and nerves is diminished to a degree of some sort of inhibition that reduces tension and improves proprioception. Some other studies however defend that kinesio taping has no effect on eccentric and concentric muscle force or on proprioception [146–149].

Some researchers have put forth that kinesio taping affects cutaneous mechanoreceptors in a way that is like to adjust proprioception [147, 149]. The kinesio taping, in case of cutaneous and muscular application, alters the skin and superficial fascia length, and muscular fiber stretching, affecting mechanoreceptors that are sensitive to stretching, pressure, and tearing forces [150, 151]. This might lead to specific modifications in muscular motion and tonus. Especially low-pressure stimulation onto connective tissue alters the impact on mechanoreceptors and may even have effect on gamma motor neuron and muscular tonus alignment. The kinesio taping may be influential on increased proprioceptive ability especially in the middle of the action only. At this specific interval, ligament mechanoreceptor is inactive while muscle receptors are active. Responding to joint mobility and position may stimulate sensory afferent transmission, playing on the proprioception improvement. Cutaneous afferent stimuli are in contact with motor cortex, and this is how it affects the central nervous system muscular stimulability [152–154].

The kinesio taping applications on the spine often relate to back pain and postural support purposes. In a study for the impact of kinesio taping application upon lower body joint range of motion, Y-shaped tape recommended to 30 healthy men's and women's sacrospinalis was applied in a way that the base coincides with the center of sacrum, while arms of the shape Y come forward at the time of flexion. Measurements were made for body flexion, extension, and lateral flexion before and after kinesio taping. Researchers have revealed that kinesio taping increased active lower body flexion joint range of motion. Accordingly, it has been indicated that the application could be followed in order to support lower back muscles, provide mechanical support with the body muscles, reduce pain, accelerate tissue healing, and improve body flexion [155–157]. In another study performed in literature, it has been demonstrated that pain, functionality, and body's joint range of motion results gradually improved after kinesio taping applications applied on rectus abdominis, internal oblique, erector spinae, and latissimus dorsi [158].

In case of patients with a neck pain, inhibition occurs in deep-neck flexor and extensor muscles, oil infiltration increases, deformation takes place in type 1 and type 1 fiber ratios, and muscular atrophy is observed. Micro and macro trauma risk increases while support decreases [159–161]. As a result, trapezius group's activation response and exhaustion increase, and neck joint motion and proprioception senses decrease. It is known that scapulothoracic area is also affected in case of neck pain, and especially the response to upper trapezium activation increases while serratus anterior muscular activation response decreases [162, 163]. This shows that scapula orientation and mobility alterations are identical for the patients that suffer from neck pain and shoulder complaints [164, 165]. Alterations in scapula position are classified as down rotation, depression, elevation, addiction, abduction, tilt, and blading [166]. Alterations in scapula position interrupt with the tension of cervicoscapular muscles [upper trapezium, levator scapula], increase stress in the neck area, and are likely to affect the neck functions along the weight transfer from upper extremities [167]. Repeated and extreme stress results in cervical tissue injuries, pain, and restricted neck rotation [168, 169]. Such stress issues also affect cervical inflammation, inhibit proprioceptive sense, and interrupt with motor controls [170, 171]. It has been shown with various studies that kinesio taping, if and once applied with the technique that is supposed to support the scapular position sense, triggers proprioception, and is influential in preventing injuries [172, 173].

8.4.5 Electrotherapy

Both follow-up and rehabilitation are vital after spinal surgery; even a minimal invasive technique entails physical therapy and rehabilitation applications. To ensure maximum recovery and minimum potential troubles in the future, it is vital that muscles function optimally after a spine procedure.

Electrotherapy contains various treatments involving electricity in order to reduce pain, enhance circulation, repair tissues, trigger muscular strengthening, and promote bone growth that leads to better physical functioning. The medical literature on electrotherapy's effectiveness has been mixed, and it has been found that not all electrotherapy treatments are supported by research.

It takes time for the skin, muscle, connective tissues, intervertebral disc, and similar soft tissues to heal in the postspinal surgical period. Cautious and tolerable actions occur in the original surgical area after early period surgery as far as rehabilitation is concerned. To avoid pain and edema in the operated area, action is restricted to minimum for the first week in spine area. Modalities employed for reducing pain are many, such as cold laser therapy, electrotherapy [ultrasound, iontophoresis, transcutaneous electrical nerve stimulation [TENS], pulsed electromagnetic field therapy [PEMF], electrical stimulation and heat/cold has been investigated, and other methods of reducing pain rather than directly addressing the cause of pain [174–180]. Likewise, after minimally invasive surgeries, electrotherapy agents can be useful for controlling the symptoms. As electrotherapy agents used in the postsurgical period alleviate patients' symptoms such as pain and edema and increase mobility in the operated area, it helps to improve proprioception.

References

1. Gray H. Anatomy of the human body. [Online Ed.]. 2000. Bartleby.com.
2. Yaszemski MJ, Augustua AW, Panjabi MM. Biomechanics of the spine. In: Fardon DF, Garfin SR, editors. Orthopaedic knowledge update: spine 2. 2nd ed. Rosemont: American Academy of Orthopaedic Surgeons; 2002. p. 15–23.
3. Kiefer A, Shirazi-Adl A, Parnianpour M. Synergy of the human spine in neutral postures. Eur Spine J. 1998;7:471–9.
4. Oğuz H. Bel Ağrıları. In: Oğuz H, editor. Tıbbi rehabilitasyon. İstanbul: Nobel Kitapevi; 2004. p. 1131–17.

5. Şar C. Lomber Omurganın Anatomik Özellikleri. In: Özcan E, Ketenci A, editors. Bel Ağrısı Tanı ve Tedavi. İstanbul: Nobel Kitapevi; 2002. p. 9–20.

6. Drake RL, Vogl W, Mitchell AWM. Gray's anatomi. Ankara: Güneş Tıp Kitabevleri; 2007.

7. Bland JH, Boushey DR. Anatomy and physiology of the cervical spine. Semin Arthritis Rheum. 1990;20: 1–20.

8. Blakney M, Hertling D. The cervical spine. In: Hertling D, Kesler RM, editors. Management of common musculoskeletal disorders. 3rd ed. Philadelphia: Lippincott-Raven Publisher; 1996. p. 528–58.

9. Cramer GD. The cervical region. In: Cramer GD, Darby SA, editors. Basic and clinical anatomy of the spine spinal cord and ANS. 2nd ed. Missouri: Mosby; 2005. p. 142–209.

10. Gatterman MI. Chiropractic management of neck pain of mechanical origin. In: Giles LGF, Singer KP, editors. Clinical anatomy and management of cervical spine pain, vol. 2. Oxford: Butterworth-Heinemann; 1998. p. 21–5.

11. MacKinnon PCB, Morris JF. Oxford textbook of functional anatomy: head and neck. 2nd ed. New York: Oxford University; 2005. p. 55–62.

12. Waugh A, Grant A. Anatomy and physiology in health and illness. UK: Elsevier Limited; 2011. p. 414–7.

13. Gosselin G, Rassoulian H, Brown I. Effects of neck extensor muscles fatigue on balance. Clin Biomech (Bristol, Avon). 2004;19(5):473–9.

14. Jackson R. The cervical syndrome. Clin Orthop. 1977:138–48.

15. Sedov AS, Raeva SN, Pavlenko VB. Neuronal mechanisms of motor signal transmission in thalamic Voi nucleus in spasmodic torticollis patients. Fiziol Cheloveka. 2014;40(3):28–35.

16. McRae R. Clinical orthopaedic examination. 2nd ed. London: Churchill Livingstone; 1983.

17. Frymoyer JW. The adult spine principles and practice. 2nd ed. Philadelphia: Lippincott; 1996.

18. Field S, Treleaven J, Jull G. Standing balance: a comparison between idiopathic and whiplash-induced neck pain. Man Ther. 2008;13(3):183–91.

19. Mathis JM. Percutaneous vertebroplasty and kyphoplasty. Spine Anal. 2006:10.

20. Dutton M. Dutton's ortopeadic examination evaluation and intervention. McGraw Hill professional; 2012.

21. Neumann DA. Kinesiology of the musculuskeletal system: foundations for rehabilitation. St. Louis: Elsevier Healty Sciences; 2013.

22. Wood KB, Garvey TA, Gundry C, Heithoff KB. Magnetic resonance imaging of the thoracic spine. Evaluation of asymptomatic individuals. J Bone Joint Surg Am. 1995;77(11):1631–8.

23. O'Rahilly R. Basic human anatomy. Philadelphia: Saunders; 1986.

24. Little JP, Adam CJ. Effects of surgical joint destabilization on load sharing between ligamentous structures in the thoracic spine: a finite element investigation. Clin Biomech. 2011;26:895–903.

25. Ibrahim AF, Darwish HH. The costotransverse ligaments in human: a detailed anatomy study. Clin Anat. 2005;18:340–5.

26. Magerl F, Aebi M, Gertzbein SD, Harms J, Nazarian S. A comprehensive classification of thoracic and lumbar injuries. Eur Spine J. 1994;3:184–201.

27. Lenke LG, Sides BA, Koester LA, Hensley M, Blanke KM. Vertebral column resection for the treatment of severe spinal deformity. Clin Orthop Relat Res. 2010;468(3):687–99.

28. Neviaser A, Toro-Arbelaez JB, Lane JM. Is kyphoplasty the standard of care for compression fractures in the spine, especially in the elderly? Am J Orthop. 2005;34:425–9.

29. Haher T, Merola AA. Surgical techniques for the spine. New York: Thieme Medical Publisher; 2003.

30. Lonstein JE. Patient evaluation. MOE'S textbook of scoliosis and other spinal deformities. Philadelphia: W.B. Saunders Company; 1995. p. 45–85.

31. Freeman B, Canale ST. Campbell's operative orthopaedics. Philadelphia: Mosby; 2003. p. 1751–837.

32. Melman C, Al-Sayyad MJ, Crawford AH. Effectiveness of Spinal Release and Halo-Femoral Traction in the Management of Severe Spinal Deformity. 2004;24(6):667–73.

33. Lowe TG, Edgar M, Margulies JY, Miller NH, Raso VJ, Reinker KA, Rivard CH. Etiology of idiopathic scoliosis: current trends in research. J Bone Joint Surg Am. 2000;82-A(8):1157–68.

34. Kindsfater K, Lowe T, Lawellin D, Weinstein D, Akmakjian J. Levels of platelet calmodulin for the prediction of progression and severity of adolescent idiopathic scoliosis. J Bone Joint Surg Am. 1994; 76(8):1186–92.

35. Tsiligiannis T, Grivas T. Pulmonary function in children with idiopathic scoliosis. Scoliosis. 2012;7:7.

36. Weiss HR. Spinal deformities rehabilitation—state of the art review. Scoliosis. 2010;5:28.

37. Cohen SP, Raja SN. Pathogenesis, diagnosis, and treatment of lumbar zygapophysial [facet] joint pain. Anesthesiology. 2007;106(3):591–614.

38. Bogduk N. Clinical anatomy of the lumbal spine and sacrum. New York: Churcill Livingstone; 1997.

39. Adams MA. The biomechanics of back pain. Edinburg, New York: Churchill Livingstone; 2002.

40. Hukins DWL, Kirby MC, Sirkoyn TA, Aspden RM, Cox AJ. Comparison of structure, mechanical properties and functions of lumbar spinal ligaments. Spine. 1990;15(8):787–95.

41. Panjabi M. The stabilising system of the spine. Part II. Neutral zone and stability hypothesis. J Spinal Disord. 1992;5:390 7.

42. Krismer M, Haid C, Ogon M, Behensky H, Wimmer C. Biomechanics of lumbar instability. Orthopade. 1997;26(6):516–20.

43. van Vliet PM, Henegan NR. Motor control and the management of musculoskeletal dysfunction. Man Ther. 2006;11(3):208–13.

44. Mannion AF, Weber BR, Dvorak J, Grob D, Müntener M. Fibre type characteristics of the lumbar

paraspinal muscles in normal healthy subjects and in patients with low back pain. J Orthop Res. 1997; 15(6):881–7.

45. Wu PB, Date ES, Kingery WS. The lumbar multifidus muscle in polysegmentally innervated. Electromyogr Clin Neurophysiol. 2000;40(8):483–5.

46. Chan D, Song Y, Sham P. Genetics of disc herniation. Eur Spine J. 2006;7:586–96.

47. Cholewicki J, McGill SM. Mechanical stability of the in vivo lumbar spine: implications for injury and chronic low back pain. Clin Biomech. 1996;11(1): 1–15.

48. Boerger TO, Limb D, Dickson RA. Does 'canal clearance' affect neurological outcome after thoracolumbar burst fractures? J Bone Joint Surg Br. 2000;82:629–35.

49. Yogandan N, Halliday A, Dicman C. Practical anatomy and fundamental biomecanics spine surgery. Techniques. In: Benzel EC, editor. Complication avoidance and management. 2nd ed. Philadelphia: Livingstone; 1999. p. 113–7.

50. Fagan A, Moore R, Vernon Roberts B, Blumbergs P, Fraser R. ISSLS prize winner the innervation of the intervertebral disc: a quantitative analysis. Spine (Phila Pa 1976). 2003;28:2570–6.

51. Roberts S, Eisenstein SM, Menage J, Evans EH, Ashton IK. Mechanoreceptors in intervertebral discs. Morphology, distribution, and neuropeptides. Spine (Phila Pa 1976). 1995;20:2645–51.

52. Logroscino G, Mazza O, Aulisa A, Pitta L, Pola E, Aulisa L. Spondylolysis and spondylolisthesis in the pediatric and adolescent population. Childs Nerv Syst. 2001;17(11):644–55.

53. Syrmou E, Tsitsopoulos PP, Marinopoulos D, Tsonidis C, Anagnostopoulos I, Tsitsopoulos PD. Spondylolysis: a review and reappraisal. Hippokratia. 2010;14(1):17–21.

54. Standaert CJ. The diagnosis and management of lumbar spondylolysis. Oper Tech Sports Med. 2005;13(2):101–7.

55. Stanitski CL. Spondylolysis and spondylolisthesis in athletes. Oper Tech Sports Med. 2006;14(3):141–6.

56. Fitzgerald JA, Newman PH. Degenerative spondylolisthesis. J Bone Joint Surg Br. 1976;58:184–92.

57. North American Spine Society. Diagnosis and treatment of degenerative lumbar spondylolisthesis. 2nd ed. Burr Ridge, IL: North American Spine Society; 2014. https://www.spine.org/ResearchClinicalCare/QualityImprovement/ClinicalGuidelines.aspx

58. Katz JN, Harris MB. Clinical practice. Lumbar spinal stenosis. N Engl J Med. 2008;358(8):818–25.

59. Binder DK, Schmidt MH, Weinstein PR. Lumbar spinal stenosis. Semin Neurol Jun. 2002;22(2):157–66.

60. Katz JN, Dalgas M, Stucki G, Katz NP, Bayley J, Fossel AH, Chang LC, Lipson SJ. Degenerative lumbar spinal stenosis. Diagnostic value of the history and physical examination. Arthritis Rheum. 1995;38(9):1236–41.

61. Gilman S. Joint position sense and vibration sense: anatomical organisation and assessment. J Neurol Neurosurg Psychiatry. 2002;73:473–7.

62. Proske U. What is the role of muscle receptors in proprioception? Muscle Nerve. 2005;31:780–7.

63. Johnson EO, Babis GC, Soultanis KC, Soucacos PN. Functional neuroanatomy of proprioception. J Surg Orthop Adv. 2008;17:159–64.

64. Malmström E-M. Cervical influence on dizziness and orientation. Lund: Department of Otorhinolaryngology, Head and Neck Surgery, Clinical Sciences, Lund and Department of Health Sciences, Division of Physiotherapy Lund University; 2008. p. 57.

65. Malmström EM, Karlberg M, Melander A, Magnusson M, Moritz U. Cervicogenic dizziness – musculoskeletal findings before and after treatment and long-term outcome. Disabil Rehabil. 2007;29(15):1193–205.

66. Preuss R, Fung J. Can acute low back pain result from segmental spinal buckling during submaximal activities? A review of the current literature. Man Ther. 2005;10:14–20.

67. Swinkels A, Dolan P. Spinal position sense is independent of the magnitude of movement. Spine (Phila Pa 1976). 2000;25:98–104.

68. Gill KP, Callaghan MJ. The measurement of lumbar proprioception in individuals with and without low back pain. JMPT. 1998;21(10):582.

69. Brumagne S, Cordo P, Lysens R, Verschueren S, Swinnen S. The role of paraspinals muscle spindles in lumbosacral position sense in individuals with and without low back pain. Spine. 2000;25(8):989–94.

70. Pettibon B. Spinal biomechanics: detection and correction of the spinal system's subluxation; part 18. Chiropr J. 1997;12(2):30–2.

71. Peterka RJ, Loughlin PJ. Dynamic regulation of sensorimotor integration in human postural control. J Neurophysiol. 2004;91:410–23.

72. Simoneau M, Tinker SW, Hain TC, Lee WA. Effects of predictive mechanisms on head stability during forward trunk perturbation. Exp Brain Res. 2003;148: 338–49.

73. Ghez C. Voluntary movement. In: Kandel E, Schwartz J, Jessell T, editors. Principles of neural science. London: Prentice-Hall International Inc; 1991. p. 609–25.

74. Shumway-Cook A, Woollacott M. Motor control. Theory and practical applications. Philadelphia: Lippincott Williams & Wilkins; 2001.

75. Martin J, Jessell T. Modality coding in the somatic sensory system. In: Kandel E, Schwartz J, Jessell T, editors. Principles of neural science. London: Prentice-Hall International Inc; 1991. p. 341–52.

76. Rothwell J. Control of human voluntary movement. London: Chapman and Hall; 1994.

77. Dhillon MS, Bali K, Prabhakar S. Proprioception in anterior cruciate ligament deficient knees and its relevance in anterior cruciate ligament reconstruction. Indian J Orthop. 2011;45(4):294–300.

78. Janssens L, Brumagne S, Claeys K, Pijnenburg M, Goossens N, Rummens S, Depreitere B. Proprioceptive use and sit-to-stand-to-sit after lumbar microdiscectomy: the effect of surgical approach and early physiotherapy. Clin Biomech. 2016;32:40–8.

79. Haavik H, Murphy B. The role of spinal manipulation in addressing disordered sensorimotor integration and altered motor control. J Electromyogr Kinesiol. 2012;22(5):768–76.

80. Adkins DL, Boychuk J, Remple MS, et al. Motor training induces experience-specific patterns of plasticity across motor cortex and spinal cord. J Appl Physiol. 2006;101(6):1776–82.

81. Tsao H, Galea M, Hodges P. Reorganization of the motor cortex is associated with postural control deficits in recurrent low back pain. Brain. 2008;131(8):2161–71.

82. Tsao H, Galea MP, Hodges PW. Driving plasticity in the motor cortex in recurrent low back pain. Eur J Pain. 2010;14(8):832–9.

83. Chiou S, Shih Y, Chou L, et al. Impaired neural drive in patients with low back pain. Eur J Pain. 2014;18(6):794–802.

84. Bergmark A. Stability of the lumbar spine: a study in mechanical engineering. Acta Orthop Scand. 1989;60(Suppl 230):1–54.

85. Solomonow M, Zhou B, Baratta R, et al. Neuromuscular disorders associated with static lumbar flexion: a feline model. J Electromyogr Kinesiol. 2002;12(2):81–90.

86. Zhu X, Shin G. Kinematics and muscle activities of the lumbar spine during and after working in stooped postures. J Electromyogr Kinesiol. 2013;23(4):801–6.

87. Shin G, D'Souza C. EMG activity of low back extensor muscles during cyclic flexion/extension. J Electromyogr Kinesiol. 2010;20(4):742–9.

88. Storheim K, Berg L, Hellum C, et al. Fat in the lumbar multifidus muscles – predictive value and change following disc prosthesis surgery and multidisciplinary rehabilitation in patients with chronic low back pain and degenerative disc: 2-year follow-up of a randomized trial. BMC Musculoskelet Disord. 2017;18(1):145.

89. Bresnahan LE, Smith JS, Ogden AT, et al. Assessment of Paraspinal muscle cross-sectional area after lumbar decompression: minimally invasive versus open approaches. Clin Spine Surg. 2017;30(3):162–8.

90. Hides J, Stanton W, Mendis MD, et al. The relationship of transversus abdominis and lumbar multifidus clinical muscle tests in patients with chronic low back pain. Man Ther. 2011;16(6):573–7.

91. Lee AS, Cholewicki J, Reeves NP, et al. Comparison of trunk proprioception between patients with low back pain and healthy controls. Arch Phys Med Rehabil. 2010;91:1327–31.

92. O'Sullivan PB, Burnett A, Floyd AN, et al. Lumbar repositioning deficit in a specific low back pain population. Spine (Phila Pa 1976). 2003;28(10):1074–9.

93. Richardson CA, Snijders CJ, Hides JA, et al. The relation between the transversus abdominis muscles, sacroiliac joint mechanics, and low back pain. Spine. 2002;27(4):399–405.

94. Hides J, Wilson S, Stanton W, et al. An MRI İnvestigation İnto the function of the transversus abdominis muscle during "drawing-İn" of the Abdominal Wall. Spine. 2006;31(6):175–8.

95. Hides JA, Miokovic T, Belavý DL, et al. Ultrasound İmaging assessment of abdominal muscle function during drawing-İn of the abdominal wall: an İntrarater reliability study. J Orthop Sports Phys Ther. 2007;37(8):480–6.

96. Shirley D, Hodges P, Eriksson A, et al. Spinal stiffness changes throughout the respiratory cycle. J Appl Physiol. 2003;95(4):1467–75.

97. Bø K, Sherburn M, Allen T. Transabdominal ultrasound measurement of pelvic flor muscle activity when activated directly or via a transversus abdominis muscle contraction. Neurourol Urodyn. 2003;22(6):582–8.

98. Critchley D. Instructing pelvic floor contraction facilitates transversus abdominis thickness increase during low-abdominal hollowing. Physiother Res Int. 2002;7(2):65–75.

99. Boudreau SA, Farina D, Falla D. The role of motor learning and neuroplasticity in designing rehabilitation approaches for musculoskeletal pain disorders. Man Ther. 2010;15(5):410–4.

100. Lluch E, Schomacher J, Gizzi L, et al. Immediate effects of active cranio-cervical flexion exercise versus passive mobilisation of the upper cervical spine on pain and performance on the cranio-cervical flexion test. Man Ther. 2014;19(1):25–31.

101. Jull G, Sterling M, Falla D. Wiplash, headache and neck pain: research-based directions for physical therapies. Edinburg: Elsevier; 2008.

102. Mayoux-Benhamou MA, Revel M, Vallée C, et al. Longus colli has a postural function on cervical curvature. Surg Radiol Anat. 1994;16(4):367–71.

103. Mayoux-Benhamou MA, Revel M, Vallee C, et al. Selective electromyography of dorsal neck muscles in humans. Exp Brain Res. 1997;113(2):353–60.

104. Jun I, Kim K. A comparison of the deep cervical flexor muscle thicknesses in subjects with and without neck pain during craniocervical flexion exercises. J Phys Ther Sci. 2013;25(11):1373–5.

105. Jull G, Kristjansson E, Dall'Alba P. Impairment in the cervical flexors: a comparison of whiplash and insidious onset neck pain patients. Man Ther. 2004;9(2):89–94.

106. Jull GA, O'Leary SP, Falla DL. Clinical assessment of the deep cervical flexor muscles: the craniocervical flexion test. J Manip Physiol Ther. 2008;31(7):525–33.

107. Falla DL, Jull GA, Hodges PW. Patients with neck pain demonstrate reduced electromyographic activ-

ity of the deep cervical flexor muscles during performance of the craniocervical flexion test. Spine.
2004;29(19):2108–014.

108. Iqbal ZA, Rajan R, Khan SA, et al. Effect of deep
cervical flexor muscles training using pressure biofeedback on pain and disability of school teachers
with neck pain. J Phys Ther Sci. 2013;25(6):657–61.

109. Jull GA, Falla D, Vicenzino B, et al. The effect of
therapeutic exercise on activation of the deep cervical flexor muscles in people with chronic neck pain.
Man Ther. 2009;14(6):696–701.

110. James G, Doe T. The craniocervical flexion test:
intra-tester reliability in asymptomatic subjects.
Physiother Res Int. 2010;15(3):144–9.

111. Falla DL, Campbell CD, Fagan AE, et al.
Relationship between cranio-cervical flexion range
of motion and pressure change during the craniocervical flexion test. Man Ther. 2003;8(2):92–6.

112. Falla D, O'Leary S, Farina D, et al. The change in
deep cervical flexor activity after training is associated with the degree of pain reduction in patients
with chronic neck pain. Clin J Pain. 2012;28(7):
628–34.

113. De Gail P, Lance JW, Neilson PD. Differential
effects on tonic and phasic reflex mechanisms produced by vibration of muscles in man. J Neurol
Neurosurg Psychiatry. 1966;29(1):1–11.

114. Aaboe J, Henriksen M, Christensen R, et al. Effect of
whole body vibration exercise on muscle strength
and proprioception in females with knee osteoarthritis. Knee. 2009;16(4):256–61.

115. Gandevia SC, Smith JL, Crawford M, et al. Motor
commands contribute to human position sense. J
Physiol. 2006;571(3):703–10.

116. Beinert K, Preiss S, Huber M, et al. Cervical joint
position sense in neck pain. Immediate effects of
muscle vibration versus mental training interventions: a RCT. Eur J Phys Rehabil Med. 2015;51(6):
825–32.

117. Beinert K, Keller M, Taube W. Neck muscle vibration can improve sensorimotor function in patients
with neck pain. Spine J. 2015;15(3):514–21.

118. Moyer CA, Rounds J, Hannum JW. A meta-analysis
of massage therapy research. Psychol Bull.
2004;130:3–18.

119. Sagar SM, Dryden T, Wong RK. Massage therapy
for cancer patients: a reciprocal relationship between
body and mind. Curr Oncol. 2007;14:45–56.

120. Crane JD, Ogborn DI, Cupido C. Massage therapy
attenuates inflammatory signaling after exercise-
induced muscle damage. Sci Transl Med. 2012;4:119.

121. Morhen V, Beavin LE, Zak PJ. Massage increases
oxytocin and reduces adrenocorticotropin hormone
in humans. Altern Ther Health Med. 2012;18:11018.

122. Sefton JM, Yarar C, Carpenter DM, Berry
JW. Physiologic and clinical changes after therapeutic massage of the neck and shoulders. Man Ther.
2011;16:487–94.

123. Topolska M, Chrzan S, Sapula R. Evaluation of the
effectiveness of therapeutic massage in patients with
neck pain. Ortop Traumatol Rehabil. 2012;14:115–24.

124. Frobell R, Le Graverand M, Buck R, Roos E, Roos
H, Tamez-Pena J. The acutely ACL injured knee
assessed by MRI: changes in joint fluid, bone mar-
row lesions, and cartilage during the first year.
Osteoarthr Cartil. 2009;17(2):161–7.

125. Baxendale R, Ferrell W. Disturbances of proprioception at the human knee resultingfrom acute joint dis-
tension. J Physiol. 1987;392:60.

126. Cho Y, Hong B, Lim S, Kim H, Ko Y, Im S. Effects
of joint effusion on proprioception in patients with
knee osteoarthritis: a single-blind, randomized controlled clinical trial. Osteoarthr Cartil. 2011;19(1):
22–8.

127. van Mechelen W, Hlobil H, Kemper H. Incidence,
severity, aetiology and prevention of sports injuries. A
review of concepts. Sports Med. 1992;14(2):82–99.

128. Dhillon M, Bali K, Vasistha R. Immunohistological
evaluation of proprioceptive potential of the residual
stump of injured anterior cruciate ligaments [ACL].
Int Orthop. 2010;34(5):737–41.

129. Schmidt RA, Lee T. Motor control and learning: a
behavioural emphasis. 5th ed. Champaign, IL:
Human Kinetics; 2011.

130. Borsa P, Lephart S, Irrgang J, Safran M, Fu F. The
effects of joint position and direction of joint motion
on proprioceptive sensibility in anterior cruciate ligament-deficient athletes. Am J Sports Med. 1997;
25(3):336–40.

131. Willems T, Witvrouw E, Verstuyft J, Vaes P, De
Clercq D. Proprioception and muscle strength in
subjects with a history of ankle sprains and chronic
instability. J Athl Train. 2002;37(4):487–93.

132. Ge W, Khalsa PS. Encoding of compressive stress
during indentation by slowly adapting type I mechanoreceptors in rat hairy skin. J Neurophysiol.
2002;87:1686–93.

133. Gerald FG. Mechanoreceptive/mechanosensitive
visceral receptors. Encyclopedia of Pain; 2013.
pp. 1808–10.

134. Sato K, Li Y, Foster W, Fukushima K, Badlani N,
Adachi N, Usas A, FH F, Huard J. Improvement of
muscle healing through enhancement of muscle
regeneration and prevention of fibrosis. Muscle
Nerve. 2003;28:365–72.

135. Graven-Nielsen T, Mense S. The peripheral apparatus of muscle pain: evidence from animal and human
studies. Clin J Pain. 2001;17:2–10.

136. Crane JD, Ogborn D, Cupido C, Melov S, Hubbard
A, Bourgeois JM, Tarnopolsky MA. Massage therapy attenuates inflammatory signaling after exer-
cise-induced muscle damage. Sci Transl Med.
2012;4:119ra13.

137. Holey LA, Dixon J. Connective tissue manipulation:
a review of theory and clinical evidence. J Bodyw
Mov Ther. 2013;18:112–8.

138. Holey LA, Dixon J, Selfe J. An exploratory thermo-graphic investigation of the effects of connective tissue massage on autonomic function. J Manip Physiol Ther. 2011;34:457–62.

139. Gifford J, Gifford L. Chapter 14: Connective tissue massage. In: Wells PE, Frampton V, Bowsher D, editors. Pain: management and control in physiotherapy. London: Heinemann Medical; 1994.

140. Yüksel I, Akbayrak T, Tuğay N, Çıtak-Karakaya I, Demirtürk F, Ekici G. Masaj teknikleri. In: Yüksel I, Akbayrak T, editors. Klasik masaj teknikleri, Konnektif doku masajı. Ankara: Alp Publishers; 2007. [15–50/294–295].

141. Bakar Y, Sertel M, Öztürk A, Tütün Yümin E, Tatarli N, Ankarali H. Short term effects of classic massage compared to connective tissue massage on pressure pain threshold and muscle relaxation response in women with chronic neck pain: a preliminary study. J Manip Physiol Ther. 2014;37(6):415–21.

142. Williams PE, Goldspink G. Connective tissue changes in immobilised muscle. J Anat. 1984; 138(Pt 2):343–50.

143. Langevin HM, Sherman KJ. Pathophysiological model for chronic low back pain integrating connective tissue and nervous system mechanisms. Med Hypotheses. 2007;68:74–80.

144. Kase K, Wallis J, Kase T. Clinical therapeutic application of the kinesio taping method. Tokyo: Ken Ikai Co Ltd; 2003.

145. Cools AM, Witvrouw EE, Danneels LA, Cambier DC. Does taping influence electromyographic muscle activity in the scapular rotators in healthy shoulders? Man Ther. 2002;7:154–62.

146. Slupik A, Dwornik M, Bialoszewski D, Zych E. Effect of Kinesio taping on bioelectrical activity of vastus medialis muscle. Preliminary report. Ortop Traumatol Rehabil. 2007;9:644–51.

147. Chen CY, Lou MY. Effects of the application of Kinesio-tape and traditional tape on motor perception. Br J Sports Med. 2008;42:513–4.

148. Fu TC, Wong AM, Pei YC, Wu KP, Chou SW, Lin YC. Effect of Kinesio taping on muscle strength in athletes-a pilot study. J Sci Med Sport. 2008;11: 198–201.

149. Halseth T, McChesney J, DeBeliso M, Vaughn R, Lien J. The effect of Kinesio taping on proprioception at the ankle. J Sports Sci Med. 2004;3: 1–7.

150. Tobin S, Robinson G. The effect of McConnell's vastus lateralis inhibition taping tecnhique on vastus lateralis and vastus medialis obiquus activity. Physiotherapy. 2000;86:173–83.

151. Winter JA, Allen TJ, Proske U. Muscle spindle signals with the sense of effort to indicate limb position. J Physiol. 2005;568:1035–46.

152. Murray HM, Husk LJ. Effect of Kinesio taping on proprioception in the ankle and in the knee. J Orthop Sports Phys Ther. 2001;31:A-37.

153. Chang HY, Wei SH. The influence of proprioception funciton on shoulder internal and external rotators' fatigue. J Phys Educ Higher Educ. 1999;1:85–96.

154. Sterner RL, Pincivero DM, Lephart SM. The effects of muscular fatigue on shoulder proprioception. Clin J Sport Med. 1998;8:96–101.

155. Chang HY, Chou KY, Lin JJ, Lin CF, Wang CH. Immediate effect of forearm Kinesio taping on maximal grip strength and force sense in healthy collegiate athletes. Phys Ther Sport. 2010;11: 122–7.

156. Yoshida A, Kahanov L. The effect of Kinesio taping on lower trunk range of motion. Res Sports Med. 2007;15:103–12.

157. Paoloni M, Bernetti A, Fratocchi G, Mangone M, Parrinello L, Del Pilar Cooper M. Kinesio taping applied to lumbar muscles influences clinical and electromyographic characteristics in chronic low back pain patients. Eur J Phys Rehabil Med. 2011;47:237–44.

158. Greig AM, Bennell KL, Briggs AM, Hodges PW. Postural taping decreases thoracic kyphosis but does not influence trunk muscle electromyographic activity or balance in women with osteoporosis. Man Ther. 2008;13:249–57.

159. Hwang-Bo G, Lee JH. Effects of Kinesio taping in a physical therapist with acute low back pain due to patient handling: a case report. Int J Occup Med Environ Health. 2011;24:320–3.

160. Schomacher J, Falla D. Function and structure of the deep cervical extensor muscles in patients with neck pain. Man Ther. 2013;18(5):360–6.

161. Elliott JM, Jull G, Noteboom JT, Darnell R, Galloway G, Gibbon WW. Fatty infiltration in the cervical extensor muscles in persistent whiplash-associated disorders: a magnetic resonance imaging analysis. Spine. 2006;31:847–55.

162. Elliott JM, Jull G, Noteboom JT, Galloway G. MRI study of the cross-sectional area for the cervical extensor musculature in patients with persistent whiplash associated disorders [WAD]. Man Ther. 2008;13:258–65.

163. Cools AM, Dewitte V, Lanszweert F, Notebaert D, Roets A, Soetens B. Rehabilitation of scapular muscle balance: which exercises to prescribe? Am J Sports Med. 2007;35:1744–51.

164. Petersen SM, Wyatt SN. Lower trapezius muscle strength in individuals with unilateral neck pain. J Orthop Sports Phys Ther. 2011;41(4):260–5.

165. Kibler WB, McMullen J. Scapular dyskinesis and its relation to shoulder pain. J Am Acad Orthop Surg. 2003;11:142–51.

166. Ludewig PM, Cook TM. Alterations in shoulder kinematics and associated muscle activity in people with symptoms of shoulder impingement. Phys Ther. 2000;80:276–91.

167. Kendall FP, McCreary EK, Provance PG, Rodgers MM, Romani WA. Muscles: testing and function

with posture and pain. Baltimore: Williams & Wilkins; 2005.

168. Van Dillen LR, McDonell MK, Susco TM, Sahrmann SA. The immediate effect of passive scapular elevation on symptoms with active neck rotation in patients with neck pain. Clin J Pain. 2007;23(8): 641–7.

169. McDonnell MK, Sahrmann SA, Van Dillen L. A specific exercise program and modification of postural alignment for treatment of cervicogenic 68 headache: a case report. J Orthop Sports Phys Ther. 2005; 35(1):3–15.

170. Gandevia SC, McCloskey DI, Burke D. Kinesthetic signals and muscle contraction. Trends Neurosci. 1992;15(2):62–5.

171. Hodges PW, Moseley GL. Pain and motor control of the lumbopelvic region: effect and possible mechanisms. J Electromyogr Kinesiol. 2003;13(4): 361–70.

172. Aarseth LM, Suprak DN, Chalmers GR, Lyon L, Dahlquist DT. Kinesio tape and shoulder-joint position sense. J Athl Train. 2015;50(8):785–91.

173. Hsu YH, Chen WY, Lin HC, Wang WT, Shih YF. The effects of taping on scapular kinematics and muscle performance in baseball players with shoulder impingement syndrome. J Electromyogr Kinesiol. 2009;19(6):1092–9.

174. Khadilkar A, Odebiyi DO, Brosseau L. Transcutaneous electrical nerve stimulation [TENS] versus placebo for chronic low-back pain. Cochrane Database Syst Rev. 2008;4:CD003008.

175. Adamczyk A, Kiebzak W, Wilk-Franczuk M. Effectiveness of holistic physiotherapy for low back pain. Ortop Traumatol Rehabil. 2009;11:562–76.

176. Ansari NN, Ebadi S, Talebian S. A randomized, single blind placebo controlled clinical trial on the effect of continuous ultrasound on low back pain. Electromyogr Clin Neurophysiol. 2006;46:329–36.

177. Bunzli S, Gillham D, Esterman A. Physiotherapy-provided operant conditioning in the management of low back pain disability: a systematic review. Physiother Res Int. 2011;16:4–19.

178. French SD, Cameron M, Walker BF. A cochrane review of superficial heat or cold for low back pain. Spine (Phila Pa 1976). 2016;31:998–1006.

179. Kroeling P, Gross A, Graham N. Electrotherapy for neck pain. Cochrane Database Syst Rev. 2013;8: CD004251.

180. Krekoukiasa G, Gelalisa ID, Xenakisa T, Gioftsosb G, Dimitriadisc Z, Sakellarib V. Spinal mobilization vs conventional physiotherapy in the management of chronic low back pain due to spinal disk degeneration: a randomized controlled trial. J Man Manip Ther. 2017;25(2):66–73.

Proprioception After Hip Injury, Surgery, and Rehabilitation

9

John Nyland, Omer Mei-Dan, Kenneth MacKinlay,
Mahmut Calik, Defne Kaya, and Mahmut Nedim Doral

9.1 Hip Anatomy and Pathomechanics

Hip joint health and function is directly related to low back and knee health. The ball and socket morphology of the hip joint and its six degrees of freedom mobility in three planes of motion create an abundance of contractile and noncontractile tissue synergies during functional movements. In many ways, the hip serves as the key linkage between the trunk or lumbo-pelvic regions and the lower extremities [1–4] (Figs. 9.1 and 9.2). The articula-

J. Nyland, D.P.T., S.C.S., Ed.D., A.T.C. (✉)
Kosair Charities College of Health and Natural
Sciences, Spalding University, Louisville, KY, USA
e-mail: jnyland@spalding.edu

O. Mei-Dan, M.D.
Orthopaedic Surgery, University of Colorado
Hospital, University of Colorado, Aurora, CO, USA
e-mail: omermeidan@ucdenver.edu

K. MacKinlay, M.D.
Department of Orthopaedic Surgery, University of
Louisville, Louisville, KY, USA
e-mail: kmack01@louisville.edu

M. Calik, P.T. • D. Kaya, Ph.D., M.Sc., P.T.
Department of Physiotherapy and Rehabilitation,
Faculty of Health Sciences, Uskudar University,
Istanbul, Turkey
e-mail: mahmut.calik@uskudar.edu.tr;
defne.kaya@uskudar.edu.tr

M.N. Doral, M.D.
Department of Orthopedics and Traumatology, Ufuk
University, Faculty of Medicine, Ankara, Turkey
e-mail: mndoral@gmail.com

tion between the femoral head and the acetabulum formed by osseous contributions from the ilium, ischium, and pubic bones is further stabilized by the hip joint labrum, capsular ligaments, and stronger, extracapsular ligaments, including the Iliofemoral ligament ("Y" ligament of Bigelow), the ischiofemoral ligament, and the pubofemoral ligament.

The ligamentum teres represents an interesting intra-articular hip joint structure consisting of two bands that originate on the ischial and pubic sides of the acetabulum notch and blend with the transverse acetabular ligament between these two attachment sites [5]. The two bands insert on the fovea capitis of the femoral head. From its origin, the ligamentum teres begins as a flat, pyramidal ligament transitioning into a more round or tubular morphology at its attachment on the fovea capitis. Anatomically, the ligamentum teres predominantly arises from the transverse acetabular ligament along the inferior margin of the acetabulum. Mechanical testing of the ligamentum teres has shown some similarity in structure and strength to the anterior cruciate ligament (ACL) of the knee [6, 7]. The ligamentum teres is composed of collagen types I, III, and IV and is surrounded by a layer of synovium that contains small arteries (including the artery femoris capitis), veins, and nerve bundles [8] (Fig. 9.3). The mean length of the ligamentum teres is 30–35 mm. At its yield and failure points, the mean length of the ligamentum teres is approximately 38 mm and 53 mm, respectively [9]. Traditionally, there has been no consensus

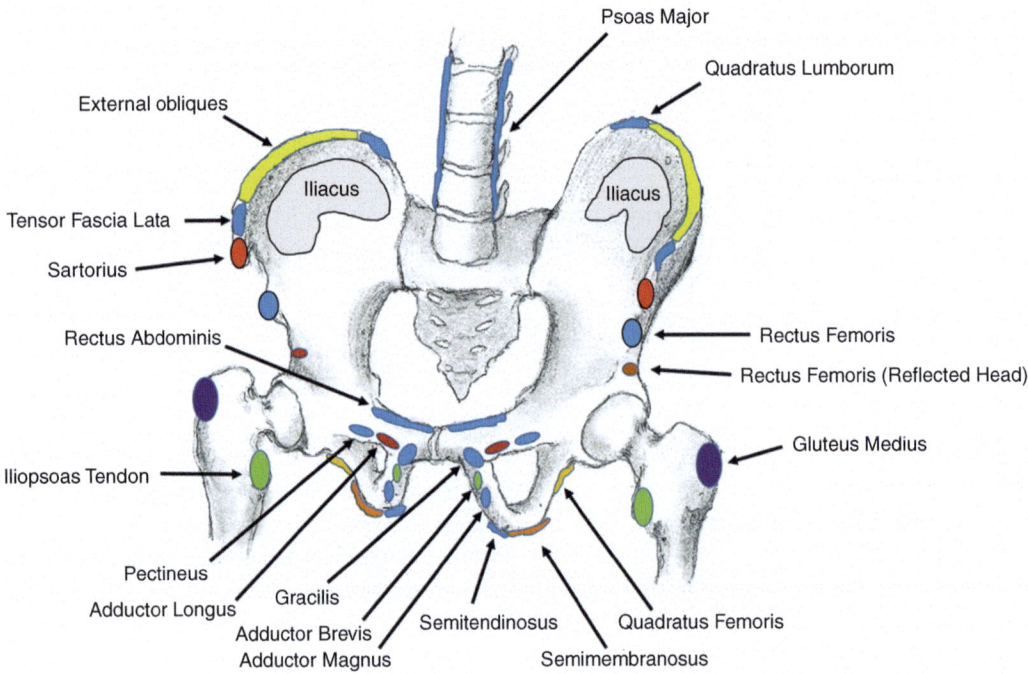

Fig. 9.1 Key tendinous attachments that influence hip, lumbo-pelvic region, and sacroiliac joint function

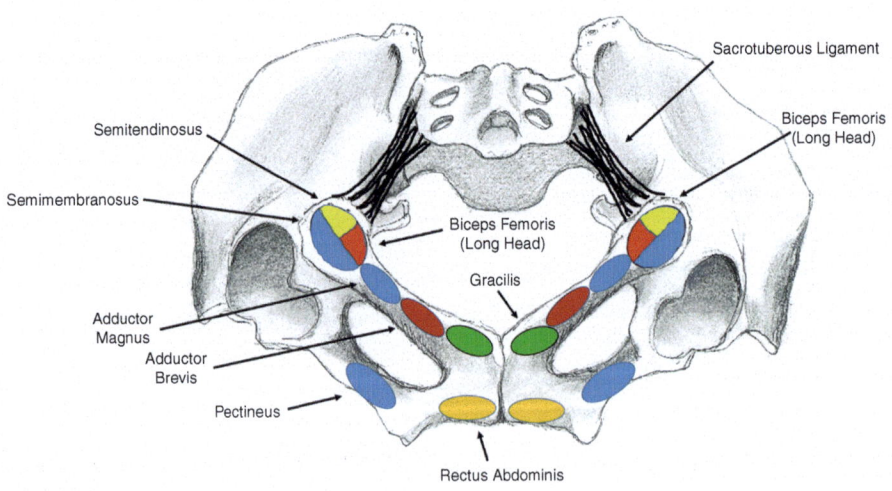

Fig. 9.2 Inferior view of pelvic tendon attachments that influence sacroiliac joint rotation

on the role of the ligamentum teres in providing hip joint stability. Although it has long been considered less than essential for noncontractile hip joint stability purposes, it may have greater importance when hip joint dysplasia or capsuloligamentous deficiency exists [10].

Gray and Villar [6] suggested that by virtue of fovea capitis topography, the ligamentum teres is tightest in a position of hip adduction, flexion, and external rotation. As this is the position in which the joint is least stable, a mechanical, hip stabilizing role of the ligamentum teres was proposed.

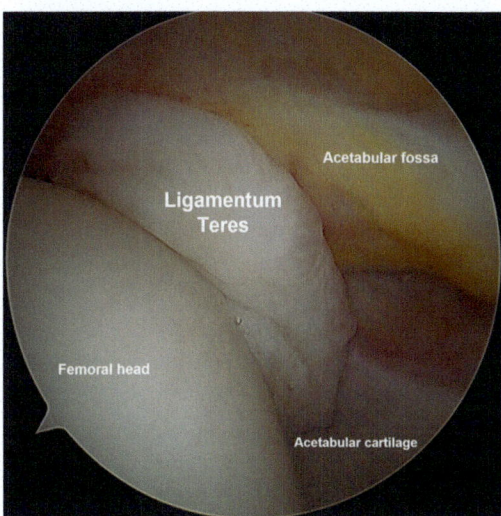

Fig. 9.3 Arthroscopic view of ligamentum teres

Martin et al. [10] used string models to assess the excursion of the ligamentum teres during hip movements. The model found that the ligamentum teres had its greatest excursion when the hip was externally rotated in flexion (ER/FLEX) and internally rotated in extension (IR/EXT). They concluded that the ligamentum teres may contribute to hip stability, particularly when the hip is in ER/FLEX and IR/EXT. In studying 20 patients with ligamentum teres ruptures and an osseous abnormality that appeared to correlate with symptomatic instability, they reported that individuals with osseous risk factors for instability, including inferior acetabular insufficiency, may have instability with squatting (ER/FLEX) and crossing one leg behind the other (IR/EXT). The ligamentum teres serves as an important hip stabilizer when an individual assumes a squatting position (with hips in flexion and external rotation) or when attempting to cross the involved leg behind the other (with hip extension and internal rotation) [10]. These two positions create maximum tension on the ligamentum teres [10]. They argued that the role of ligamentum teres may become more important when the other stabilizers are deficient, such as with deficient bony stability (anteroinferior acetabular deficiency) or deficient capsuloligamentous stability (generalized ligamentous laxity). Kivlan et al. [7] used human cadavers to demonstrate that when

the hip moves into flexion-abduction, the ligamentum teres moves into a position that provides anterior and inferior hip stabilization. The ligamentum teres acts as a "sling-like" structure in supporting the femoral head inferiorly and preventing anterior/inferior hip joint subluxation. The ligamentum teres has been found to be approximately as strong as the ACL and is tightest when the hip is in a position with the least stability (flexion, adduction, external rotation) [11]. It is also known to possess nociceptors and mechanoreceptors [12, 13], further suggesting a direct proprioceptive role far greater than that of a vestigial remnant.

Shoulder and knee arthroscopy has considerably increased in popularity since the mid-1970s. Wide use of hip arthroscopy has developed at a slower pace, with the first textbooks being published in the 1980s [14, 15]. From a joint tissue preservation standpoint, hip joint arthroscopy is a later member to this movement. There is a direct association between acetabular labral tears, developmental hip dysplasia, femoro-acetabular impingement, and early onset hip osteoarthritis [16]. Femoro-acetabular impingement is a general term that encompasses any excessive abutment secondary to repetitive contact between the femoral head–neck junction and the acetabular rim. Over time, irritation from this condition can lead to intra-articular cartilage delamination, regional labral injury, and early osteoarthritis. Femoro-acetabular impingement may involve a lesion on the acetabular side (pincer) (Fig. 9.4) or on the femoral side (cam) (Fig. 9.5) or both. Cam lesions are directly associated with femoral head–neck junction asphericity and are generally located at the anterior-superior aspect of the joint [17]. The cam lesion represents a bony increase in the diameter of the femoral neck at the femoral head–neck junction.

9.2 Proprioceptive and Kinesthetic Considerations of the Hip Region

The proprioceptive system helps preserve neuromuscular hip joint control and dynamic stability. It includes peripheral mechanoreceptors that detect signals and convey proprioceptive information to the sensory cortex of the brain [18, 19]. Afferent-efferent feedback systems help improve movement coordination and postural control, thus helping prevent injuries. A correlation between a decreased number of nerve

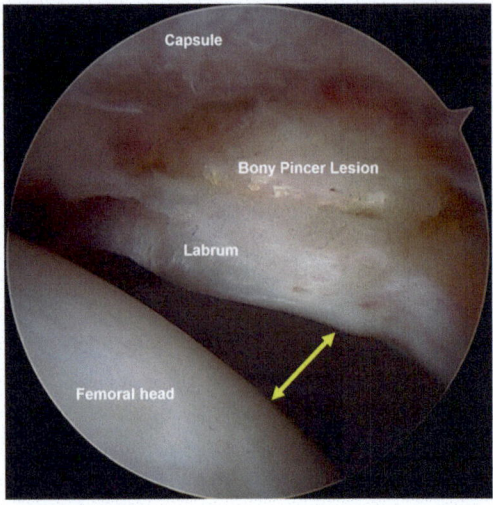

Fig. 9.4 Arthroscopic view of bony pincer lesion at left hip. The yellow arrow depicts the space between the femoral head and acetabulum generated by distraction. A bony pincer lesion can be observed behind the labral tissue after it was exposed using a radio frequency device, prior to its removal using a motorized burr

endings and proprioception deficits has been identified in joint disease [20]. Proprioceptive system performance affects dynamic joint stability and can be a contributing cause of articular cartilage degeneration. In comparing groups with and without hip arthrosis, Moraes et al. [21] reported a significantly greater reduction in the Pacini type ($P < 0.035$) than in the Ruffini type mechanoreceptors among subjects with hip arthrosis and lower overall mechanoreceptor densities. Patients with knee osteoarthritis often have lower extremity sensory deficits described as proprioceptive loss, balance loss, joint position sense loss, and kinesthetic loss [20, 22]. The role of these deficits in the pathophysiology of joint OA is not clear; however, a growing body of evidence suggests that diminished sensory input may impair or reduce protective muscular reflexes around the joint, leading to increased mechanical loading and articular cartilage damage. Shakoor et al. [23] identified significant sensory deficits associated with hip osteoarthritis and these deficits involved both the upper and lower extremities. The mechanism for this remains unclear; however, neurologic feedback mechanisms or an inherent generalized neurologic defect has been proposed [20].

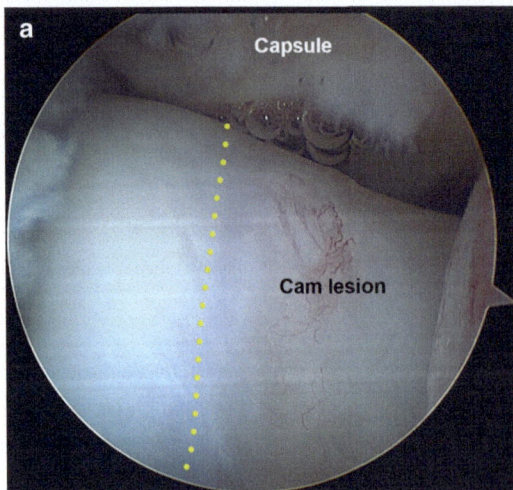
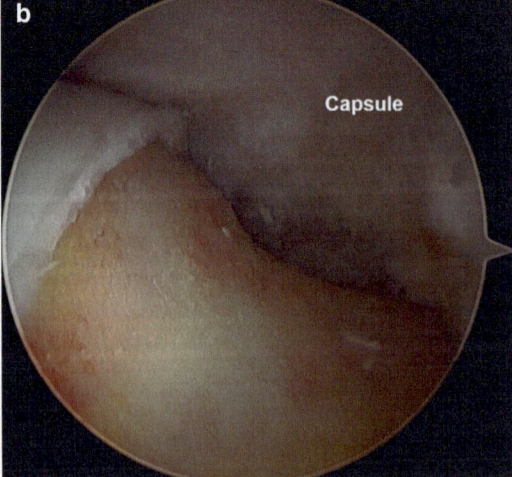
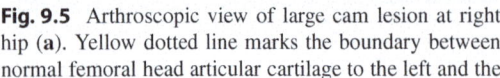

Fig. 9.5 Arthroscopic view of large cam lesion at right hip (**a**). Yellow dotted line marks the boundary between normal femoral head articular cartilage to the left and the osseous bump to the right (**b**). Following lesion decompression, a normal offset normal hip range of motion was restored

Given its generally robust osseous and capsuloligamentous stability compared to the glenohumeral joint (the "other ball and socket joint"), at the hip, concerns related to proprioceptive or kinesthetic function have not received similar attention. However, with growing hip arthroscopy use, the knowledge base of both capsuloligamentous histology and the potential negative influences of hip joint dysplasia on dynamic hip joint stability is increasing [10–13]. Although deeper than the glenoid process of the shoulder, the stability provided by the acetabulum is likewise augmented by a labrum. Mechanoreceptors have been identified in the hip capsule, acetabular labrum, and transverse acetabular ligament. The highest mechanoreceptor density in hip labral tissue is located within its inner zone (tissue closest to the acetabular articular cartilage). The labrum is also only vascularized in the inner third. This, in particular, is an important consideration as surgeons attempt to expand the zone of effective labral repair [24].

The anterior region of the labrum comprised the highest relative contribution of sensory fibers and mechanoreceptors. Alzaharani et al. [25] found the highest level of mechanoreceptors and free nerve endings in the anterosuperior and posterosuperior labral regions between 10 and 2 o'clock around the acetabulum (Fig. 9.6). Haversath et al. [26] found the highest concentration of

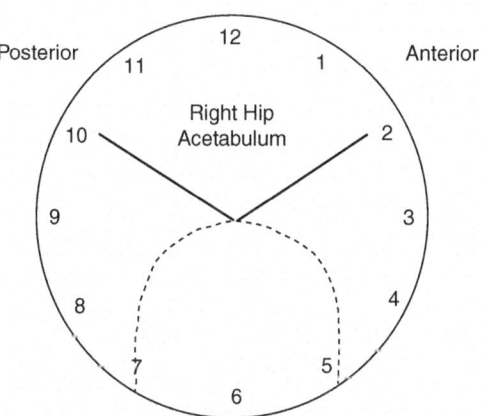

Fig. 9.6 Right hip acetabulum labral clock pattern. Studies report that the greatest concentration of labral mechanoreceptors exists between the 10 and 2 o'clock position

pain receptors in the anterolateral labrum, especially the labral–acetabular junction with fewer pain receptors beyond the 10–2 o'clock position. Labral tissue debridement in these regions may provide pain relief by nociceptive fiber ablation; however, removal of the mechanoreceptors from this area may have deleterious effects on joint proprioception and on dynamic neuromuscular control function. They suggested that labral tears in these zones should be repaired, particularly injuries located at the base of the labrum. In an immunohistological study, Haversath et al. [26] identified a high sensory fiber and mechanoreceptor density in the anterior and superior hip capsule. Kampa et al. [27], however, found a small interneural zone at the anterosuperior capsule that lacked the dense innervation seen in other areas of the capsule. In summary, the highest labral sensory fiber and mechanoreceptor density is located along the anterior and superior capsule, particularly anteromedially.

Physiological studies in the cat hip joint have demonstrated two types of mechanoreceptors: slowly adapting Ruffini mechanoreceptors which are sensitive to capsular stretch or tension, and rapidly adapting Pacinian mechanoreceptors which are sensitive to pressure and vibratory stimuli [19]. Although it has been shown that the most common mechanoreceptor types in hip periarticular tissues are Pacinian and Ruffini mechanoreceptors, others only observed a preponderance of Ruffini mechanoreceptors [28]. Pacinian mechanoreceptors are rapidly adapting receptors that can identify sudden ligament tension changes, but quickly decrease transmitting signals once tension becomes constant. These mechanoreceptors can monitor acceleration and deceleration of a ligament's tension. The fast-adapting Pacinian mechanoreceptors found in abundance in the ACL are not as common in the hip joint. Gerhardt et al. [28] suggested that fast neuro-feedback loops may not be as important in the well-contained, stable hip joint as they are in the knee. Injury to these afferent fibers from hip dislocation, fracture, or surgery may result in decreased proprioceptive acuity, which may lead to decreased coordination, decreased postural control, subsequent re-injury, and/or early onset osteoarthritis.

According to Gerhardt et al. [28], within the hip capsule, the highest areas of innervation were within the superolateral and anterior capsule with 9.6 mechanoreceptors/high powered field and 3.2 free nerve endings/high powered field in the superolateral capsule. In the anterior capsule, there were 4.0 mechanoreceptors/high powered field and 2.2 free nerve endings/high powered field. The anterior hip joint capsule is predominantly supplied by the articular branches of the femoral and obturator nerves, with a frequency of contribution to capsular innervation of 95% and 85%, respectively [27]. Overlap between these two nerves is most apparent on the medial aspect of the hip joint capsule, which may account for the more abundant free nerve endings observed in the anteromedial capsule than elsewhere [18]. In general, the femoral nerve is primarily responsible for innervation of the anterior and anterolateral hip joint capsule, and the obturator nerve supplies the anteromedial and inferior capsule. An accessory obturator nerve contributes to anterior hip joint capsule innervation with a contribution frequency of approximately 5%. Birnbaum et al. [29] identified superior gluteal nerve articular nerve branches that innervated the posterolateral hip joint capsule and articular branches from the nerve to the quadratus femoris muscle that innervated the posteroinferior hip joint capsule. The sciatic nerve supplies the posterosuperior hip joint capsule in a less consistent pattern with a frequency of contribution to capsular innervation of approximately 80% compared to 85% and 100% for the superior gluteal nerve and the nerve to quadratus femoris, respectively [27]. Less consistent is the contribution of the inferior gluteal nerve which contributes to posterior inferior capsular innervations with an approximate 10% frequency. Of considerable interest is that fewer sensory fibers have been identified in the posterior hip joint capsule, suggesting a less robust innervation [28, 30]. Most studies confirm high levels of anterior capsular innervation, while posterior hip joint capsule innervation remains less well understood [31].

9.3 Hip Evaluation and Treatment

The patient with a painful, non-arthritic hip often presents with a diagnostic dilemma, particularly in younger individuals. Hip pain in young adults is often characterized by nonspecific symptoms, normal imaging studies, and vague findings from the history and physical examination [32]. Identification of the exact source and mechanism of the pain can therefore be quite difficult. As our understanding of hip pathology evolves, and arthroscopies and other hip-preserving operative techniques continue to improve, the focus is shifting toward earlier identification of hip pathology. The distinction between differing intra- and extra-articular causes of hip pain is important for treating these patients. Intra-articular sources of hip pain, which are usually addressed arthroscopically, are labral tears, loose bodies, femoro-acetabular impingement, synovitis, ligamentum teres tears, and chondral injury. Extra-articular pain sources that can be managed either surgically or non-operatively include extra-articular bony impingement (trochanteric-pelvic, ischiofemoral, subspine), iliopsoas tendonitis, internal or external snapping hip, abductor tears, and greater trochanteric bursitis, femoral neck stress fracture, myotendinosis injuries (adductors, proximal hamstrings, rectus femoris), piriformis syndrome, deep gluteal syndrome, sacroiliac joint pain, athletic pubalgia, sports hernia, Gilmore's groin, and osteitis pubis [4]. As this formidable list suggests, of all the major joints, the hip remains the most difficult to evaluate for most clinicians who treat patients with musculoskeletal concerns. Especially in the setting of subtle bony abnormalities, such as femoro-acetabular impingement, the clinician's ability to precisely differentiate pain generators in the hip has been ambiguous.

Deciphering the etiology of the pathology versus the pain generators is essential to prescribing proper treatment. A systematic means of determining which hip structures are the source of the pathology, which is the pain generator, and how to best implement treatment has been described [32]. For hip flexion-extension and adduction-abduction, it is important to distinguish pure hip joint motion from compensatory pelvis or lumbar spine motion. When sitting, the pelvis is best stabilized with the hip flexed to 90°. This enables a more accurate assessment of hip internal and external rotation. Total hip internal and external rotation range of motion differences exist in extension and flexion. There should be at least 10° of hip internal rotation for normal function [32]. Decreased hip internal rotation is suggestive of intra-articular hip pathology. Patients with femoro-acetabular impingement or rotational constraint from increased or decreased femoral and/or acetabular anteversion may present with significant side-to-side measurement differences. In adolescent athletes with open growth plates, apophyseal avulsion fracture/injury of the sartorius and rectus femoris of the anterior superior and anterior inferior iliac spines, respectively, are common [32]. Pubic symphysis or ramus tenderness may result from the recurrent stresses generated by the powerful hip adductors and the rectus abdominus/conjointed tendon. It is important that clinicians remember that the loaded pelvis usually rotates over a fixed femur, thus creating anterior and medial forces with instant rotary moments.

9.4 Hip, Core, and Lower Extremity Functional Linkage

The human body uses an effective three-dimensional framework of bones, joints, muscles, and ligaments for posture and movement. In upright posture, the trunk load passes through the sacroiliac joints. The orientation of the sacroiliac joint surfaces, however, is more or less in line with the distribution of loading, which induces high shear forces between the sacrum and the coxal bones. The sacroiliac joints are stabilized by a strong ligamentous system. Having viscoelastic properties during constant trunk load, the sacroiliac ligaments are vulnerable to viscoelastic creep responses and need to be reinforced against high sacroiliac joint shear forces. Biomechanically, an active neuromuscular corset increases compression between the coxal bones and the sacrum, thereby protecting the sacroiliac ligaments and supporting load transfer between the trunk and lower extremities [33, 34]. Sacroiliac joint interlocking may also be assisted by transversely oriented muscles such as the transversus abdominis, piriformis, gluteus maximus, and external and internal obliques. Possession of sufficient sacroiliac joint stability is essential for effectively transferring spinal loads through them to the coxal bones and the lower extremities. Biomechanical modeling of upright standing posture has shown that transversely oriented abdominal transversus abdominis and pelvic floor (coccygeus, pubo- and ilio-coccygeus) muscle activation helps reduce vertical sacroiliac joint shear forces and increases dynamic stability [33]. Within this scenario, force equilibrium is represented by induced iliolumbar and posterior sacroiliac joint ligaments as the transversus abdominus clamps the sacrum between the coxal bones, and as the pelvic floor muscles oppose lateral coxal bone movement.

The sacropelvic parameter of pelvic incidence is a position-independent anatomic parameter that affects lumbar lordosis and pelvic orientation. Pelvic incidence is the angle between the line perpendicular to the sacral endplate at its midpoint and the line connecting this point to the axis of the femoral heads [35] (Fig. 9.7). Pelvic inclination may be associated with femoro-acetabular impingement, as a lower angle may contribute to hip joint cam or pincer lesion development. Proper sagittal plane balance ensures that forces transmitted from the vertebral column to the lower extremities are located posterior to the lumbar spine and the femoral heads [36]. The sacrum and pelvis form a semirigid structure (the sacro-pelvis) that translates and rotates with gait for the necessary compensatory balance around the bicoxofemoral axis [37] which

Fig. 9.7 The pelvic incidence represents the angle between the line perpendicular to the sacral plate and the line connecting the midpoint of the sacral plate to the bicoxofemoral axis. Sacral slope corresponds to the angle between the sacral plate and the horizontal plane. Pelvic tilt is the angle between the lines connecting the midpoint of the sacral plate to the bicoxofemoral axis and the vertical plane

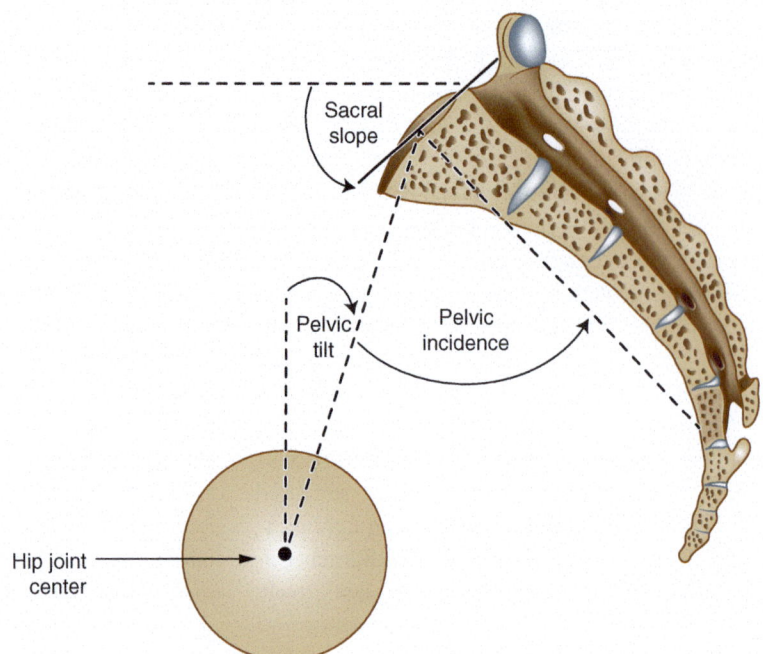

passes through the centers of the left and right femoral heads. Consequently, disruption of this stability often results in a faulty load absorption [38]. Patients with decreased pelvic incidence often attempt to improve sagittal alignment by decreasing lumbar lordosis and tilting the pelvis forward. This increased forward pelvic tilt promotes over-coverage of the femoral head by the anterior acetabulum. This may restrict femoro-acetabular joint movement, and lead to hip joint impingement in addition to possible posterior lumbar spine compression injuries.

Dynamic impingement can be caused by the presence of a cam lesion (decreased femoral head–neck offset), a pincer lesion (acetabular over-coverage of the femoral head), proximal femoral retroversion, or coxa vara. The reduced femoral head-to-neck offset distance that exists with a cam lesion leads to acetabulum contact early in the arc of internal hip rotation. Repetitive contact during sports activity can lead to labral tearing, transition zone articular cartilage delamination, pain, and early onset hip osteoarthritis. Femoro-acetabular impingement decreases physiologic hip internal rotation, placing the labrum and hemi-pelvis at risk for repetitive, abnormal loading when participating in activi-

ties that require greater hip internal rotation than the bony anatomy allows. Femoro-acetabular impingement and athletic pubalgia or sports hernia are being observed with greater frequency as a source of disability among athletically active individuals. A clinical link has been reported between femoro-acetabular impingement and athletic pubalgia [39]. Dynamic cam impingement causes pubic symphysis rotational motion after the point of bony contact. Repetitive loading of the pubic symphysis is a known precursor to athletic pubalgia [40]. This relationship suggests one possible explanation for the clinical observation that patients with femoro-acetabular impingement often also present with athletic pubalgia or osteitis pubis.

Functionally, when a gait disturbance or perturbation causes an initiation or prolongation of the swing phase at one lower extremity, the stance phase of the contralateral lower extremity becomes initiated or prolonged accordingly. Unilateral lower extremity displacements during stance and gait evoke a bilateral response pattern with similar spinal nerve activation onset latencies at both lower extremities [41, 42]. This inter-limb coordination is necessary to keep the body center of gravity over the feet [42, 43].

A major reason for high medical treatment costs in older adults is an increased prevalence of falls and fall-related injuries. Approximately 28–35% of individuals over the age of 65 years experience at least one fall over a 1-year period with 20% of these falls requiring medical attention. Gait instability in terms of greater stride-to-stride variability has been identified as a major intrinsic fall risk factor in old age [44]. There is evidence that gait stride-to-strike variability further increases when two tasks (postural requirement in addition to a secondary cognitive/motor task) are concurrently performed [44, 45]. Granachner et al. [44] identified larger temporal and spatial side-to-side variability in older compared to younger adults when walking during dual task conditions (i.e., walking while verbally reciting serial subtractions by 3 as compared to just walking). Kressig et al. [46] suggested that the degree of stride time variability in dual task walking conditions distinguished fallers from non-fallers in a group of independently walking older inpatients. A systematic review on dual task performance and the prediction of falls indicated that performance changes while dual tasking were significantly associated with an increased risk of falling among older adults [47]. Reduced gait speed may represent a compensatory strategy to enhance dynamic stability during walking to prevent falling.

Postural control is a complex function that involves commands from the central nervous system, peripheral afferents for regulation, and the musculoskeletal system as an effector. Basing their perceptions on the rich innervation of structures situated in and around the joints, several authors since Freeman [48] have hypothesized that a lesion of capsuloligamentous mechanoreceptors, particularly ligaments, could lead to a decrease in proprioception and consequently to joint instability, even in the absence of muscular strength loss or joint surface lesions. While many studies have focused on contributions from the central nervous system and peripheral afferents for postural regulation, fewer studies have envisaged the links between balance and posture in cases of rheumatologic or orthopedic hip disorders. Although the hip articular capsule serves

a proprioceptive role, this role may be less than capsule-ligamentous contributions at the shoulder or knee for example, and has not been instrumentally objectified in coxarthrosis or following total hip arthroplasty [49]. The spinal musculature serves a crucial function in posture and balance as it is both a motor effector and a sensory receptor [50–52]. Proprioception from spine neuromuscular receptors play a fundamental role in static and dynamic postural control, and they contribute to the control of rhythmic gait [53, 54].

Muscle spindles are sensory receptors that provide the central nervous system with information about muscle length, length changes, and joint position sense [52, 55]. Afferent information from muscle spindles is combined with afferent input derived from cutaneous and joint mechanoreceptors. The cervical spine region has an essential role in providing the central nervous system with primary proprioceptive input. This is reflected in the abundance of cervical spine joint mechanoreceptors [50, 56]. Neck muscles are also exceptionally rich in muscle spindles both in animals and in humans, especially in the suboccipital region where there are up to 200 muscle spindles/gram of muscle. In contrast, the first lumbrical in the thumb has only 16 muscle spindles/gram [51, 57, 58]. High muscle spindle concentrations are associated with highly structured, more complex systems [59, 60]. Using differing quantification methods, Voss [61] and Banks [60] each reported greater mean muscle spindle densities more proximally at the trunk muscles, with densities progressively decreasing more distally at the hip and thigh regions (Table 9.1). Studies of peripheral joints in animals and humans suggest that joint mechanoreceptors play a complementary role to muscle receptors in the mediation of postural control, particularly at the extremes of motion or when the joint is specifically distracted or compressed. Muscle spindle receptors take on a greater proprioceptive and dynamic joint stability role during mid-range function.

Sensorimotor control of standing posture and head-neck-eye movements relies on the integrative afferent information processing from the vestibular, visual, and proprioceptive systems which

Table 9.1 Lumbo-pelvic and hip region muscle spindle density region rank comparison

Banks [60]				Voss [61]	
Muscle	Relative muscle spindle abundance	Region rank	Region rank	Muscle	Relative muscle spindle number
Transversus abdominis	2.4			Transversus abdominis	7.3
Iliocostalis	2.0			Longissimus dorsi	4.5
External obliques	2.0			External obliques	3.5
Internal obliques	1.4			Internal obliques	3.0
Rectus abdominus	1.2			Iliocostalis	2.5
	1.8 ± 0.5			Rectus abdominus	2.25
		1	1		3.8 ± 2
Iliopsoas	1.5			Gemellus superior	3.9
Gluteus maximus	1.0			Piriformis	3.5
Gluteus minimus	0.93			Gemellus inferior	3.4
Piriformis	0.87			Gluteus minimus	2.2
Gluteus medius	0.78			Quadratus femoris	1.9
Quadratus femoris	0.47			Iliopsoas	1.8
Gemellus inferior	0.42			Gluteus medius	1.0
Gemellus superior	0.40			Gluteus maximus	0.8
	0.8 ± 0.4	2	2		2.3 ± 1
Adductor magnus	0.88			Gracilis	1.5
Gracilis	0.65			Adductor longus	1.1
Adductor longus	0.58			Adductor magnus	0.9
Adductor brevis	0.51				1.2 ± 0.3
Pectineus	0.44				
	0.6 ± 0.2	4	3		
Vastus lateralis	0.81			Sartorius	1.2
Vastus medialis	0.75			Rectus femoris	0.9
Vastus intermedius	0.69			Vastus intermedius	0.9
Sartorius	0.67			Vastus medialis	0.8
Rectus femoris	0.64			Vastus lateralis	0.7
	0.7 ± 0.1	3	4		0.9 ± 0.2
Semitendinosus	0.79			Semitendinosus	1.4
Biceps femoris	0.63			Biceps femoris	0.8
Semimembranosus	0.37			Semimembranosus	0.6
	0.6 ± 0.2	4	4		0.9 ± 0.4

converge throughout the central nervous system. Eye-head coupling is necessary to modify neck neuromuscular activation depending upon the direction of gaze. The vestibular system provides gaze stability. Rehabilitation attempts to retrain normal cervical kinesthetic performance, largely focusing on improving eye-head coupling. Some researchers recommend kinesthetic retraining protocols in the management of patients who have experienced a cervical spine whiplash injury and in patients presenting with altered head-neck position sense and/or oculomotor control. Research is needed to see if rehabilitation approaches that take full advantage of integrative afferent information processing from the vestibular, visual, and proprioceptive systems can similarly help restore function following musculoskeletal injuries to the upper and lower extremities.

9.5 Therapeutic Considerations that Optimize Hip Function

Lumbar hyperlordosis, anterior pelvic tilt, and sacroiliac joint dysfunction in any combination have been linked to chronic hamstring strain injuries [62]. Lumbar hyperlordosis often correlates with anterior pelvic tilt, placing strain on the origin of the hamstring at the ischial tuberosity, resulting in hamstring musculotendinous pathology [62]. Ideally, when standing or sitting, the innominate bones are in rotational alignment. However, pelvic obliquity often develops with anterior rotation on one side and posterior rotation on the other. Innominate rotational obliquity and sacral torsion may result from any number of forces that are transmitted between the vertebral column, the pelvis, pelvic floor, and the lower extremities. The influence of monthly menstrual cycle hormones in females may further increase this risk as capsuloligamentous tissues become more extensible.

Athletic training errors such as overtraining, excessive unilateral loading as with repetitious or high intensity kicking or throwing, or improper technique can exaggerate normal sacroiliac joint movements [34]. Overtime, unilateral muscle tightness or contractions at the lumbo-pelvic or hip regions can produce innominate rotation. For example, a tight rectus femoris could produce anterior-inferior anterior superior iliac spine rotation, while a tight biceps femoris could produce posteroinferior rotation on the ischial tuberosity [63]. Age-related changes on growth plates largely dictate if injuries in this region represent tendon insertional avulsions, fractures, or primary muscle strains.

Ideally, during hip flexion, the ipsilateral innominate bone rotates posteriorly and inferiorly moving the ischial tuberosity anteriorly and reducing hamstring strains. If however, the innominate is fixed in an anteriorly rotated position, the ischium cannot move anteriorly as the hip flexes. This increases stress at the hamstring origin, particularly during the rapid acceleration associated with sprinting and jumping [64]. Sacroiliac joint dysfunction has also been associated with piriformis spasm on the side of the posteroinferior lateral angle, paravertebral spasm, and gluteal and hamstring muscle spasm [65]. Trunk and pelvic floor muscle activation can assist sacroiliac joint form closure. Muscle activation through the vertebral column and pelvis can also influence sacral positioning, potentially creating sacroiliac joint dysfunction through imbalanced activation or weakness.

The principle of reciprocal inhibition states that during agonist muscle activation, the antagonists do not behave passively, but are actively inhibited by central nervous system mechanisms [66]. This mechanism, long thought to be based in afference from muscles or tendons, can also be mediated by joint mechanoreceptors that may also inhibit or facilitate muscle tone. Failure to appreciate these arthrokinetic circuits may explain the difficulty in achieving neuromuscular re-education or strengthening goals during rehabilitation [67]. In association with this, taking a chronic hamstring strain injury as an example, having a tightened anterior hip joint capsule tends to facilitate iliopsoas muscle activation and stiffness while inhibiting gluteus maximus activation through the arthrokinetic reflex [68]. When this occurs, visible gluteal muscle wasting may be observed. Since the gluteus maximus muscle is the primary hip extensor, its inhibition places undo loads on the hamstring muscles making them more prone to injury [69].

Mobilizing the hip joint to decrease anterior capsuloligamentous tightness and stretching the iliopsoas muscle has been shown to significantly increase gluteus maximus strength [68]. Muscle weakness may therefore be influenced by the inhibition associated with underlying capsuloligamentous joint hypo-mobility. With a tight anterior hip joint capsule and iliopsoas muscle, the gluteus maximus muscle gets inhibited each time the femoral head attempts to translate anteriorly against the tight anterior joint capsule/iliopsoas muscle. Increased anterior femoral head translation can alter mechanoreceptor activation patterns, reducing gluteus maximus muscle neural inhibition while also reciprocally inhibiting iliopsoas muscle activation [68]. Therefore, the therapeutic role of mobilizing joints such as the hip or sacroiliac joints extends beyond normalizing osseous positioning to stimulating joint mechanoreceptors that are directly involved in an arthrokinetic reflex with the hamstring muscle group [62, 70]. Faulty sacroiliac joint positioning can negatively influence joint capsule afferent output. Modified joint capsule afferent signals may also alter the activation of supporting transversus abdominis and multifidus muscles [71]. With capsuloligamentous or musculotendinous restriction of normal joint movement, changes in mechanoreceptor signals to the central nervous system can lead to active weakening (or inhibition) of muscles whose action could take the joint beyond its restrictive barrier. Therefore, trying to strengthen a muscle that is being actively inhibited by the central nervous system may be counterproductive prior to using joint mobilization techniques to evaluate whether or not normal joint play has been re-established. In close accordance with the suggestions of Janda [72], Mahofsky et al. [67] proposed a clinical rule: "stretch what is tight and mobilize what is stiff prior to strengthening what is weak." Joint mechanoreceptors can also be stimulated during tasks that maximize sensory input to the central nervous system, triggering subconscious and automatic neuromuscular responses. Because subcortical regulating systems do not rely on conscious control, they are faster, and with appropriate training, the stabilizing process can become more automatic or "second nature" [73].

Strength deficits may underline "at risk" movement behaviors or maladaptive compensatory movements. Hip muscle performance deficits in particular have been hypothesized to contribute more to increased knee loading [74]. Hip abductor weakness and valgus knee collapse during single-leg landing maneuvers is an example of this relationship [74]. Stearns et al. [75] described a prescriptive hip muscle training program that produced lower extremity biomechanical changes consistent with decreased ACL injury risk. In particular, after participating in a training regimen that focused on hip muscle strengthening, subjects landed

with greater hip flexion and increased hip extensor moments. Furthermore, they had decreased knee/hip moment ratios, suggesting greater use of a different strategy to decelerate the body's center of mass during single-leg landings. The decreased knee/hip extensor moment ratio that was observed was primarily the result of an increase in the hip extensor moments as no significant change in knee extensor moment was observed. During single-leg jump landings, subjects displayed decreased average knee adductor moments, a trend toward decreased peak knee abduction, and improved sagittal and frontal plane lower extremity alignment. As the hip abductors function to control frontal plane lower extremity motion, it is plausible that improved frontal plane knee biomechanics may have been the direct result of the increased hip abductor strength that was observed post-training. These findings suggest that hip muscle strength as opposed to knee extensor strength may be responsible for mitigating biomechanical risk factors associated with ACL injury or re-injury risk [75].

9.6   Hip Surgery and Proprioception

There is no consensus regarding the level of proprioceptive impairment that occurs in association with hip surgical procedures such as internal fixation, labrum repair, and hip arthroplasty. More studies have focused on balance than isolated proprioceptive sense after hip surgery.

9.7   Proprioception After Hip Arthroplasty

Degenerative changes in the hip joint contribute to decreased mobility and significant movement disorders. As in the knee joint, arthroplasty is an effective treatment procedure in the management of degenerative arthritis [21]. In the literature, there are considerably more studies about proprioception post-knee arthroplasty than post-hip arthroplasty. Mechanoreceptors and free nerve endings are known to exist at the hip joint capsule, ligaments around the hip joint, within the femoral head ligament, and in the labrum [21]. The greater volume of these tissues that are surgically resected, the more likely that proprioception will be impaired. However, normalized coxofemoral mechanics with improved hip muscle strength following hip arthroplasty may improve the proprioceptive response [76, 77]. Contrary to expectations, Ishii et al. [77] reported no proprioceptive response differences between patients with total hip arthroplasty, hemiarthroplasty, and healthy age-matched controls group subjects. They emphasized that hip joint proprioception was controlled more by muscle, tendon, and ligament mechanoreceptors than by intracapsular structures following hip arthroplasty.

9.8 Proprioception After the Femoro-acetabular Impingement and Labrum Tear Surgery

Femoro-acetabular impingement (FAI) is characterized by pain due to hip joint shape changes, with or without associated labral and/or chondral pathologies [78]. Additionally, no randomized, controlled study to date has evaluated the effects of differing FAI treatments on hip joint proprioception. Although FAI is seen in young and middle-aged adults, there is a surprisingly lack of investigations regarding its potential influence on hip joint proprioception, particularly among patients who have undergone labral tear resection or repair. In a systematic review, Freke et al. [79] identified involved side dynamic single leg balance impairments among subjects with symptomatic FAI compared to healthy control group subjects.

The increased pain and decreased hip muscle strength associated with FAI decreases patient quality of life [80]. Conservative rehabilitation programs should focus on improving hip function, by decreasing pain, and increasing hip muscle strength and proprioception [80, 81].

Conclusion

The hip joint represents a region of high significance to both surgeons and rehabilitation clinicians. Hip musculotendinous and capsuloligamentous tissues have a considerable influence on trunk, lumbo-pelvic, and composite lower extremity postures, movements and stabilization through neuromuscular control, and kinesthetic and noncontractile proprioceptive properties. Preservation of proprioceptive tissues during arthroscopic procedures and restoration of normalized pain-free range of motion, strength, and proprioception during rehabilitation are essential to optimal function, in addition to core region and composite lower extremity injury prevention.

References

1. Delp SL, Suryanarayanan S, Murray WM, et al. Architecture of the rectus abdominis, quadratus lumborum, and erector spinae. J Biomech. 2001;34:371–5.
2. Gerlach UJ, Lierse W. Functional construction of the superficial and deep fascia system of the lower limb in man. Acta Anat. 1990;139:11–25.
3. Gottschalk F, Kourosh S, Leveau B. The functional anatomy of tensor fasciae latae and gluteus medius and minimus. J Anat. 1989;166:179–89.
4. Nyland J, Kuzemchek S, Parks M, et al. Femoral anteversion influences vastus medialis and gluteus medius EMG amplitude: composite hip abductor EMG amplitude ratios during isometric combined hip abduction-external rotation. J Electromyogr Kinesiol. 2004;14:255–61.
5. Brewster SF. The development of the ligament of the head of the femur. Clin Anat. 1991;4:245–55.
6. Gray AJ, Villar RN. The ligamentum teres of the hip: an arthroscopic classification of its pathology. Arthroscopy. 1997;13:575–8.
7. Kivlan B, Clemente FR, Martin RL, et al. Function of the ligamentum teres during multi-planar movement of the hip joint. Knee Surg Sports Traumatol Arthrosc. 2013;21:1664–8.
8. Dehao BW, Bing TK, Young JL. Understanding the ligamentum teres of the hip: a histological study. Acta Orthop Bras. 2015;23:29–33.
9. Philippon MJ, Rasmussen MT, Turnbull TL, et al. Structural properties of the native ligamentum teres. Orthop J Sports Med. 2014;2:2325967114561962.
10. Martin RL, Kivlan BR, Clemente FR. A cadaveric model for ligamentum teres function: a pilot study. Knee Surg Sports Traumatol Arthrosc. 2012;21:1689–93.

11. Bardakos NV, Villar RN. The ligamentumteres of the adult hip. J Bone Joint Surg Br. 2009;91:8–15.

12. Leunig M, Beck M, Stauffer E, et al. Free nerve endings in the ligamentum capitis femoris. Acta Orthop Scand. 2000;71:452–4.

13. Sarban S, Baba F, Kocabey Y, et al. Free nerve endings and morphological features of the ligamentum capitis femoris in developmental dysplasia of the hip. J Pediatr Orthop. 2007;16:351–6.

14. Byrd T. Overview and history of hip arthroscopy. In: Byrd T, editor. Operative hip arthroscopy. New York: Springer; 2013. p. 1–6.

15. McCarthy JC, Lee JA. History of hip arthroscopy: challenges and opportunities. Clin Sports Med. 2011;30:217–24.

16. Jayasehera N, Aprato A, Villar RN. Hip arthroscopy in the presence of acetabular dysplasia. Open Orthop J. 2015;9:185–7.

17. Gupta A, Redmond JM, Stake CE, et al. Does the femoral cam lesion regrow after osteoplasty for femoroacetabular impingement? Two-year follow-up. Am J Sports Med. 2014;42:2149–55.

18. Gardner E. The innervation of the hip joint. Anat Rec. 1948;101:353–71.

19. Rossi A, Grigg P. Characteristics of hip joint mechanoreceptors in the cat. J Neurophysiol. 1982;47:1029–42.

20. Hurley MV. The role of muscle weakness in the pathogenesis of osteoarthritis. Rheum Dis Clin N Am. 1999;25:283–98.

21. Moraes MRB, Cavalcante MLC, Leite JAD, et al. The characteristics of the mechanoreceptors of the hip with arthrosis. J Orthop Surg Res. 2011;6:58.

22. Nyland J, Wera J, Henzman C, et al. Preserving knee function following osteoarthritis diagnosis: a sustainability theory and social ecology clinical commentary. Phys Ther Sport. 2015;16:3–9.

23. Shakoor N, Lee KJ, Fott LF, et al. Generalized vibratory deficits in osteoarthritis of the hip. Arth Rheum. 2008;59:1237–40.

24. Seides RM, Tan V, Hunt J, et al. Anatomy, histologic features, vascularity of the adult acetabular labrum. Clin Orthop Relat Res. 2001;382:232–40.

25. Alzaharani A, Bali K, Gudena R, et al. The innervation of the human acetabular labrum and hip joint: an anatomic study. BMC Musculoskelet Disord. 2014;15:41. https://doi.org/10.1186/1471-2474-15-41.

26. Haversath M, Hanke J, Landgraeber S, et al. The distribution of nociceptive innervation in the painful hip: a histological investigation. Bone Joint. 2013;J95:770–6.

27. Kampa RJ, Prasthofer A, Lawrence-Watt DJ, et al. The internervous safe zone for incision of the capsule of the hip. J Bone Joint Surg Br. 2007;89:971–6.

28. Gerhardt M, Johnson K, Atkinson R, et al. Characterisation and classification of the neural anatomy in the human hip joint. Hip Int. 2012;22:75–81.

29. Birnbaum K, Prescher A, Hessler S, et al. The sensory innervation of the hip joint—an anatomical study. Surg Radiol Anat. 1997;19:371–5.

30. Dee R. Structure and function of hip joint innervation. Ann R Coll Surg Engl. 1969;45:357–74.

31. Simons MJ, Amin NH, Cushner FD, et al. Characterization of the neural anatomy in the hip joint to optimize periarticular regional anesthesia in total hip arthroplasty. J South Orthop Assoc. 2015;24(4):221–4.

32. Poultsides LA, Bedi A, Kelly BT. An algorithmic approach to mechanical hip pain. HSS J. 2012;8:213–24.

33. Pel JJM, Spoor CW, Pool-Goudzwaard AL, et al. Biomechanical analysis of reducing sacroiliac joint shear load by optimization of pelvic muscle and ligament forces. Ann Biomed Eng. 2008;36:415–24.

34. Ross J. Is the sacroiliac joint mobile and how should it be treated? Br J Sports Med. 2000;34:226.

35. Gebhart JJ, Streit JJ, Bedi A, et al. Correlation of pelvic incidence with cam and pincer lesions. Am J Sports Med. 2014;42:2649–53.

36. Legaye J. Influence of the sagittal balance of the spine on the anterior pelvic plane and on the acetabular orientation. Int Orthop. 2009;33:1695–700.

37. Hack K, Di Primio G, Rakhra K, et al. Prevalence of cam-type femoro-acetabular impingement morphology in asymptomatic volunteers. J Bone Joint Surg Am. 2010;92:2436–44.

38. Yoshimoto H, Sato S, Masuda T, et al. Spinopelvic alignment in patients with osteoarthrosis of the hip: a radiographic comparison to patients with low back pain. Spine. 2005;30:1650–7.

39. Larson CM. Sports hernia/athletic pubalgia: evaluation and management. Sports Health. 2014;6:139–44.

40. Birmingham PM, Kelly BT, Jacobs R, et al. The effect of dynamic femoro-acetabular impingement on pubic symphysis motion. A cadaveric study. Am J Sports Med. 2012;40:1113–8.

41. Dietz V, Berger W. Interlimb coordination of posture in patients with spastic paresis: impaired function of spinal reflexes. Brain. 1984;107:965–78.

42. Dietz V, Muller R, Colombo G. Locomotor activity in spinal man: significance of afferent input form joint and load receptors. Brain. 2002;125:2626–34.

43. Dietz V, Horstmann GA, Berger W. Interlimb coordination of leg muscle activation during perturbation of stance in humans. J Neurophysiol. 1989;62:680–93.

44. Granacher U, Wolf I, Wehrle A, et al. Effects of muscle fatigue on gait characteristics under single and dual-task conditions in young and older adults. J Neuroeng Rehabil. 2010;7:56.

45. Granacher U, Bridenbaugh S, Muehlbauer T, et al. Age-related effects on postural control under multi-task conditions. Gerontology. 2011;57:247–55.

46. Kressig RW, Herrmann FR, Grandjean P, et al. Gait variability while dural-tasking: fall predictor in older inpatients? Aging Clin Exp Res. 2008;20:123–30.

47. Beauchet O, Annweiler C, Dubost V, et al. Stops walking when talking: a predictor of falls in older adults. Eur J Neurol. 2009;16:786–95.

48. Freeman M. Treatment of ruptures of the lateral ligament of the ankle. J Bone Joint Surg Br. 1965;47:661–8.

49. Missaoui B, Portero P, Bendaya S, et al. Posture and equilibrium in orthopedic and rheumatologic diseases. Clin Neurophysiol. 2008;33:447–57.

50. Armstrong B, McNair P, Taylor D. Head and neck position sense. Sports Med. 2008;38:101–17.
51. Boyd-Clark LC, Briggs CA, Galea MP. Muscle spindle distribution, morphology, and density in longus colli and multifidus muscles of the cervical spine. Spine (Phila PA 1976). 2002;27:694–701.
52. McCloskey DI. Kinesthetic sensibility. Physiol Rev. 1978;58:763–820.
53. Haghpanah SA, Farahmand F, Zohoor H. Modular neuromuscular control of human locomotion by central pattern generator. J Biomech. 2017;53:154–62.
54. MacKay-Lyons M. Central pattern generation of locomotion: a review of the evidence. Phys Ther. 2002;82:69–83.
55. Burgess PR, Wei JY, Clark FJ, et al. Signaling of kinesthetic information by peripheral sensory receptors. Annu Rev Neurosci. 1982;5:171–87.
56. Treleaven J. Sensorimotor disturbances in neck disorders affecting postural stability, head and eye movement control. Man Ther. 2008;13:2–11.
57. Kulkarni V, Chandy MJ, Babu KS. Quantitative study of muscle spindles in suboccipital muscles of human fetuses. Neurol India. 2001;49:355–9.
58. Liu JX, Thornell LE, Pedrosa-Domeliof F. Muscle spindles in the deep muscles of the human neck. A morphological and immunocytochemical study. J Histochem Cytochem. 2003;51:175–86.
59. Banks RW. A comparative analysis of the encapsulated end-organs of mammalian skeletal muscles and of their sensory nerve endings. J Anat. 2009;214:859–87.
60. Banks RW. An allometric analysis of the number of muscle spindles in mammalian skeletal muscles. J Anat. 2006;208:753–68.
61. Voss VH. Tabelle der absoluten und relative muskelspindelzahlen der menschlichen skelettmuskulatur. Anat Anz. 1971;129:562–72.
62. Cibulka MT, Rose SJ, Delitto A, et al. Hamstring muscle strain treated by mobilizing the SIJ. Phys Ther. 1986;66:1220–3.
63. Schamberger W. The malalignment syndrome: implications for medicine and sports. Edinburgh: Churchill Livingstone; 2002.
64. Gabbe BJ, Finch CF, Bennell KL, et al. Risk factors for hamstring injuries in community level Australian football. Br J Sports Med. 2005;39:106–10.
65. Dowling DJ. Evaluation of the pelvis. In: DiGiovanna EL, Schiowitz S, Dowling D, editors. An osteopathic approach to diagnosis and treatment. 3rd ed. Philadelphia, PA: Lippincott Williams & Wilkins; 2004. p. 304–22.
66. Day BL, Marsden CD, Obeso JA, et al. Reciprocal inhibition between the muscles of the human forearm. J Physiol. 1984;349:519–34.
67. Makofsky H, Panicker S, Abbruzzese J, et al. Immediate effect of grade IV inferior hip joint mobili

zation on hip abductor torque: a pilot study. J Manual Manipulative Ther. 2007;15:103–11.
68. Yerys S, Makofsky H, Byrd C, et al. Effect of mobilization of the anterior hip capsule on gluteus maximus strength. J Manual Manipulative Ther. 2002;10:218–24.
69. Elphington J. Stability, sport and performance movement: great technique without injury. Berkeley, CA: Lotus Publishing; 2008.
70. Fox M. Effect on hamstring flexibility of hamstring stretching compared to hamstring stretching and sacroiliac joint manipulation. Clin Chiropr. 2006;9:21–32.
71. Pool-Goudzwaard AL, Vleeming A, Stoeckart R, et al. Insufficient lumbopelvic stability: a clinical, anatomical and biomechanical approach to 'a-specific' low back pain. Man Ther. 1998;3:12–20.
72. Janda V. Muscles, central nervous motor regulation and back problems. In: Korr I, editor. The neurobiological mechanisms in manipulative therapy. New York: Plenum Press; 1978.
73. Norris C. Spinal stabilization: an exercise programme to enhance lumbar stabilization. Physiotherapy. 1995;81:31–8.
74. Hewett TE, Myer GD. The mechanistic connection between the trunk, hip, knee, and anterior cruciate ligament injury. Exerc Sport Sci Rev. 2011;39:161–6.
75. Stearns KM, Powers CM. Improvements in hip muscle performance result in increased use of the hip extensors and abductors during a landing task. Am J Sports Med. 2014;42:602–9.
76. Zati A, Degli Esposti S, Spagnoletti C, et al. Does total hip arthroplasty mean sensorial and proprioceptive lesion? A clinical study. Chir Organi Mov. 1997;82:239–47.
77. Ishii Y, Tojo T, Terajima K, et al. Intracapsular components do not change hip proprioception. J Bone Joint Surg Br. 1999;81:345–8.
78. Agricola R, Waarsing J, Arden N, et al. Cam impingement of the hip—a risk factor for hip osteoarthritis. Nat Rev Rheumatol. 2013;9:630–4.
79. Freke MD, Kemp J, Svege I, et al. Physical impairments in symptomatic femoroacetabular impingement: a systematic review of the evidence. Br J Sports Med. 2016;50:1180.
80. Kemp J, Makdissi M, Schache A, et al. Is quality of life following hip arthroscopy in patients with chondrolabral pathology associated with impairments in hip strength or range of motion? Knee Surg Sports Traumatol Arthrosc. 2015;24:3955–61. https://doi.org/10.1007/s00167-015-3679-4.
81. Enseki KR, Kohlrieser D. Rehabilitation following hip arthroscopy: an evolving process. Int J Sports Phys Ther. 2014;9:765–73.

Proprioception After Knee Injury, Surgery and Rehabilitation

10

Defne Kaya, Mahmut Calik, Michael J. Callaghan, Baran Yosmaoglu, and Mahmut Nedim Doral

10.1 Knee Proprioception

The peripheral and central mechanisms underlying proprioceptive control are still unclear. Knee proprioception derives from the integration of afferent signals from proprioceptive receptors in different structures of the knee and is also influenced by signals from outside the knee (e.g. from the vestibular organs, visual system and cutaneous and proprioceptive receptors from other body parts) [1]. About the mechanoreceptors see Table 10.1.

These senses originate from the stimulation of specialized nerve endings or mechanoreceptors in the joint capsule and ligaments. Proprioceptors can convert the mechanical energy of physical deformation into the electrical energy of a nerve action potential and this action potential propagates to the higher centre for motor control [2]. Muscle spindles are thought to be the most important proprioceptive receptors of knee [1]. Reflex contraction of muscles by stimulation of proprioceptors protects joints from mechanical insults. Conscious contractions, in most cases, are too slow to prevent the injury, because their nerve paths are usually longer, therefore slower. Knee proprioception serves to protect against injurious movement and it is critical to the maintenance of joint stability [3]. It is also important for normal joint coordination during movement [4].

In the knee joint, the anterior cruciate ligament (ACL) may have up to 2.5% of neural elements consisting of Ruffini nerve endings, Golgi tendon organs and Pacinian corpuscles [13]. The posterior cruciate ligament (PCL), collateral ligaments (medial and lateral) and menisci also contain similar proprioceptors [11]. Mechanoreceptors of the ACL and PCL carry information about

D. Kaya, Ph.D., M.Sc., P.T. (✉) • M. Calik, P.T.
Department of Physiotherapy and Rehabilitation,
Faculty of Health Sciences, Uskudar University,
Istanbul, Turkey
e-mail: defne.kaya@uskudar.edu.tr;
mahmut.calik@uskudar.edu.tr

M.J. Callaghan, Ph.D., P.T.
Department of Physiotherapy and Rehabilitation,
Manchester Metropolitan University, Manchester, UK

Centre for Musculoskeletal Research, University
of Manchester, Manchester, UK

Department of Physiotherapy and Rehabilitation,
Manchester Royal Infirmary, Manchester, UK
e-mail: Michael.Callaghan@mmu.ac.uk;
michael.callaghan@manchester.ac.uk

B. Yosmaoglu, Ph.D., M.Sc., P.T.
Department of Physiotherapy and Rehabilitation,
Faculty of Health Sciences, Baskent University,
Ankara, Turkey
e-mail: hayribaran@baskent.edu.tr;
baran79@gmail.com

M.N. Doral, M.D.
Department of Orthopaedics and Traumatology,
Ufuk University, Faculty of Medicine,
Ankara, Turkey
e-mail: mndoral@gmail.com

Table 10.1 Mechanoreceptors, location, stimulation and afferent information

Mechanoreceptors	Location	Stimulation	Afferent information
Muscle spindle (Ia, II)	Throughout muscle	All muscle spindles are recruited at just 25% of maximum contraction, making them very sensitive to the stimulus [5]	Muscle tension or length of muscle fibres and the velocity of change in muscle displacement [6]
Golgi tendon organ (Ib)	Musculotendinous junction or within tendons	Golgi tendon organs may not fire during passive movement [7] and hence are thought of as purely active mechanoreceptors	Golgi tendon organs detect differences in tension and force but not length [7], dynamically responding to rapid increases in these two stimuli only. Golgi tendon organs have a protective mechanism near a joint's extreme range of motion, when tension rapidly increases [8]
Pacinian corpuscle (II)	Capsule, ligaments, menisci, skin, fat pad	Pacinian corpuscles rapidly sense acceleration and deceleration and hence changes in movement, but not static or constant joint rotations [8]	Pacinian corpuscles detect the onset or termination of movement, but not constant joint displacement
Ruffini ending (II)	Capsule, ligaments, menisci, skin	Ruffini endings are found in the flexion side of the joint, hence the side that is stretched during extension [9]	Ruffini endings are most sensitive at maximum flexion and extension positions
Free nerve ending (Aδ/C)	Capsule, ligaments, menisci, skin	Free nerve ending is active when damage or injury occurs in the articular tissue [10]	Free nerve ending provides afferent information only once the joint is damaged via nociceptive sensory input [11]
Meissner's corpuscles (Aβ)	Skin	Meissner's corpuscles are responsive to light touch and vibrations	These receptors are secondary or facilitating contributors to proprioceptive sense [12]
Merkel's discs (Aβ)	Skin	Merkel's discs are stimulated by skin pressure and hence contribute to proprioception, when the skin is stretched [12]	

middle-range of knee joint, while mechanoreceptors of the joint capsule carry information about end of the range (full extension and full flexion of knee) to brain [14].

10.2 Proprioception and Patellofemoral Pain Syndrome

Knee joint proprioceptive deficit in patellofemoral joint problems can develop in two ways: (i) abnormal tissue stress with motor control and (ii) inflammation process with pain. The reason for different results in literature can be explained via vast variety in patients' findings (i.e. pain severity, pain duration) and difference among the devices and methods used in measurements. Factors, as many as oedema presence in knee joint, direction and degree of patellar situation disorder, application of test, whether active or passive, can vary sense of joint position. Agreement on the studies in the literature can be observed on the idea for foundation of less error in joint position sense tests without application of any weight on the extremity than application of weight.

The link between patellofemoral pain (PFP) and proprioception deficit was first described as a result of research on histological analyses of the lateral retinacula of subjects with PFP [15]. The discovery of diffuse small nerve damage and neuromata within the retinaculum was thought to originate from the tension and pressure of the malaligned patellofemoral joint; the resultant altered proprioceptive input may cause sudden patellar instability resulting in PFP. Additionally, chronic and atraumatic patellar malignment causes peripatellar plexus dysfunction and it can lead to the loss of proprioception in patients [15].

Sanchis-Alfonso et al. [15] suggested that peripatellar plexus doesn't function properly in chronic patellofemoral pain syndrome due to dislocation of patella, which can be evaluated by means of proprioceptive tests. Researchers mentioned nerve damage and neuromata in peripatellar soft tissue and partly in lateral retinaculum based on their histologic examinations. Also they claimed that changed proprioceptive sense may lead to instability resulting in patellar pain. Finally, the authors concluded that in addition to patellar taping that provides proprioceptive sense input, proprioceptive training is also required in rehabilitation programmes of patients with such findings [15].

Selfe et al. [16] analysed knee joint position sense of patients with patellofemoral pain at 20° and 60° in their study, which examines the effectiveness of number of repetition, joint angle and test type for measurement of knee joint position sense. As a result, they implied that five-time repetition for active joint position sense measurements and six-time repetition for passive joint position sense measurements are required. As knee joint position sense didn't differ at 20° and 60° but it differed in active and passive tests, the authors concluded that it is important whether active or passive test is performed for measurement of joint position sense but not the angle of the joint [16].

Baker et al. [17] examined knee position sense of 20 patients with patellofemoral pain under weight-bearing and non-weight-bearing positions of extremity. The joint position sense test results under non-weight-bearing positions of both affected and asymptomatic extremity revealed that more errors occur at 60° than 20° of knee flexion to achieve tested knee flexion degrees. Patients also made errors achieving the tested knee flexion degree under weight-bearing positions of extremity but not much as it is under non-

weight-bearing positions. Authors emphasized that there is proprioceptive deficit in patients with PFPS compared to healthy people [17].

Hazneci et al. [18] compared 24 patients with patellofemoral pain with 24 healthy people in their study and showed that passive joint position sense at 50° extension and 40° flexion differs between two groups. They also mentioned that 6-week isokinetic exercise training improves passive joint position sense. Authors emphasized that development of joint stability also effects development of proprioception. In addition, it was reported that dynamic factors, such as muscle contraction during active movement, also gets involved in perception of joint position sense, therefore less error may produce, while repeating the determined degree.

Kramer et al. [19] evaluated the active joint position sense under 95% of body weight-bearing and non-weight-bearing positions of extremity at 15°, 30°, 45° and 60° of knee flexion. No difference is found between the measurements of 24 patients with patellofemoral pain and 24 healthy people. Akseki et al. [20] evaluated knee proprioception at four different target angles (15°, 30°, 45°, 60°) by using active joint position sense measurement method in 28 patients with clinically diagnosed unilateral PFPS and 27 healthy controls. It was found that greater error occurs in pathologic knee compared to the opposite knee and both knees of control group at all target degrees. Authors indicated that knee joint proprioception is reduced in patients with PFPS and similarly proprioception of healthy knee is also affected [20].

In one of their studies, Akseki et al. [21] evaluated utility of vibration as a proprioceptive measurement method in patellofemoral pain syndrome. Digital goniometer and 128 Hz frequency standard diapason is used to measure joint position sense and vibration of 19 patients and 10 healthy controls in the study. It was found that patients detect vibration after 7.2 ± 1.3 s in their symptomatic knees at extension position and after 9.1 ± 1.5 s in the opposite knee. Joint position sense measurements have shown that proprioception of symptomatic knee has gone worse in accordance with measurements of vibration feeling duration. While applying 90° flexion measurement, no difference has been detected for feeling the vibration. Authors imply that vibration sense can be used in measurement of proprioception [21].

One aspect of proprioception testing in PFP is the question of clinical relevance and deciding on the cut-off threshold for 'good' and 'poor' proprioception [22]. Decided that if a subject was 5° or more away from their target angle of 45°, this person was declared as having poor proprioception. In an attempt to provide a more reasoned cut-off threshold, Chohan et al. (2014 unpublished data) analysed data from their experiments and through a series of analyses found that different thresholds or cut-off points should be applied to different target angles.

These studies assessed proprioception using active JPS in weight-bearing and non-weight-bearing positions. The results showing significant differences in proprioception status indicated that motor control and proprioception techniques should be considered as a treatment approach for PFP in addition to the existing biomechanical and physiological strategies. Yet it is unclear whether proprioception rehabilitation exercises can prevent PFP. Furthermore, it has been noted in active and passive joint angle reproduction tests that not all patients with PFP have poor proprioception.

It is also known that there are some healthy subjects who have difficulty in accurately reproducing active or passive joint angle [23]. This implies that there may be a subgroup of patients who have both PFP and poor proprioception [24] and whose causes and effects remain uncertain until prospective studies are undertaken. Equally there is a PFP subgroup who has normal proprioception and therefore does not require any treatment or intervention for proprioception training.

10.3 Proprioception and Anterior Cruciate Ligament Injury and Surgery

The anterior cruciate ligament (ACL) is the most commonly injured ligament and is one of the major ligaments providing mechanical stability of knee, controlling the anteroposterior translation and rotation movements, playing a key role in neuromuscular stability, since it is involved in the articular movement sensory feedback, thereby contributing to proprioception [25–27]. Proprioception includes afferent and efferent path of the somatosensory system controlling reflexes and muscle tone of muscles, tendons and articulations [27]. The efferent innervation is given by nerve fibres penetrating the cruciate ligaments and it is based in afferent mechanoreceptors located in peripheral joints, muscles and skin [28]. At the ACL, they represent between 1 and 2% of the volume [26]. The ACL is affected in more than 50% of ligament injuries, and rupture of the fibres of ligament can cause damage of mechanoreceptors present in the joint [29, 30].

After ACL rupture, knee proprioception deficit was displayed. The methods of assessing proprioception in studies after ACL rupture vary. Joint Position Sense (JPS), Threshold to Detection of Passive Motion (TTDPM), balance, EMG muscle timing and delay of muscle contraction are used to assess proprioceptive level after ACL injury [31, 32]. In turn, it is claimed that proprioceptive deficits can adversely affect activity level [33], balance [34], restoring quadriceps strength [35] and increase the risk of further injury [36]. Although rehabilitation regimes are designed to address all these problems, evidence supporting such claims is not readily available as pointed out by Gokeler et al. [32]. Such a wide variation in assessment methods inevitably hinders arrival at a consensus of association between proprioception deficit and ACL injury. Nevertheless, even with the variety of assessment methods, studies have consistently showed proprioceptive deficits in the subjects with ACL deficiency. The increase in female participation in sports that have a high risk of ACL injury has led some researchers to investigate the reasons why the incidence of ACL injury is at least four times greater in females [37]. Among the reasons cited is poorer neuromuscular control, which contributes to proprioception deficit. This has been termed 'dynamic neuromuscular imbalance' and may consist of three parts [37]. The first is the tendency for females to be ligament dominant, which refers to the absence of muscle control of mediolateral knee motion resulting in high valgus knee torques and high ground reaction forces. The second imbalance is quadriceps dominance, in which sportswomen activate their knee extensors preferentially over their knee flexors to stabilize their knee, which accentuates and perpetuates strength and recruitment imbalances between these muscles. The third is dominant leg dominance, which is the imbalance between muscular strength and recruitment on opposite limbs, with the non-dominant limb often having weaker and less coordinated hamstring muscles. In a similar scenario to PFP, an essential aspect is addressing the question of the clinical relevance of these findings. In other words, how much proprioception deficit signifies poor proprioception? The recent systematic review [32] suggests that proprioception testing to date has, in general, only a low-to-moderate correlation with function after ACL injury.

Despite the well-accepted link between ACL rupture and instability, there are an approximately one-third of people who do not have recurrent instability when they perform sporting activity despite their ACL rupture [38]. One reason for their ability to 'cope' with the lack of ACL was proposed by Kapreli et al. [39]. These researchers considered the fact that the ACL contains mechanoreceptors, which inform the central nervous system about joint sense position and kinaesthesia and suggested that ACL injury might be regarded as a neurophysiological dysfunction, not being a simple musculoskeletal injury. Further evidence for this theory was gained using fMRI techniques of patients with ACL rupture, who were classified at either 'copers' or 'non-copers'.

10.4 Surgery of the Anterior Cruciate Ligament and Proprioception

Surgery of the anterior cruciate ligament (ACL) is among the most studied issues in the field of orthopaedics and sports physiology today [40]. This operation aims at restoring the function of the injured dysfunctional ACL and the stabilization of the knee joint [41]. Various autografts

and allografts have been used for ACL reconstruction. Patellar tendon and hamstring tendon autografts are the most commonly preferred autografts. Various fixation techniques and materials are used for inserting the hamstring or patellar tendon grafts harvested from the injured knee as ACL. However, a gold standard is not available for graft selection and fixation techniques [42]. Efforts continue to find out the optimal graft of the operation technique.

The success of ACL reconstruction depends on both mechanic and neuromuscular stability of the knee. Neuromuscular stability certainly depends on achieving the proprioception of the knee. Nerve fibres in the proximal of ACL are activated when ligament deformation occurs and influences the motor activity of the muscles around the knee [43]. ACL's ability to perform proprioception is directly proportional with the number of mechanoreceptors in ACL [41]. ACL injury leads to the injury or destruction of the mechanoreceptors [44]. Denti et al. have reported that number of mechanoreceptors gradually decreases beginning from 3rd month after the injury and only a few free nerve ends remain after 9th month [44]. Biopsy examinations have revealed that free nerve ends disappear after 1 year [44].

The critical question is whether ACL reconstruction would provide an improvement in proprioception of the knee. Results of proprioception studies are conflicting. While some studies have revealed that knee joint position is not restored after ACL reconstruction [42, 45–47], some others have reported an improvement [48]. One of the most important determinants is the time after reconstruction. While mechanic stabilization of the graft may occur in a very short time, ligamentization may take years. Hence, proprioceptive sufficiency-related performance would also be associated with the time after surgery. The most important time for proprioceptive recovery is expected to be between 3 and 6 months after surgery [28]. In ACL reconstruction, use of hamstring or patellar tendon graft or inserting the same graft using different surgical techniques do not influence proprioception loss in post-operative period [42, 48]. It should be emphasized that none of the currently available proprioception tests can discriminate the proprioception from mechanoreceptors on ACL and the proprioception from the soft tissues around the knee and joint capsule. Therefore, none of the tests can provide a certain opinion about the mechanoreceptors in ACL [49]. It is essential to evaluate the joint under dynamic conditions in order to understand the normal control pattern. Although it may be possible to provide mechanic stability through ACL, it should not be neglected that restoring neuromuscular stability completely would be a much more difficult process.

10.5 Meniscus and Proprioception

Functions of menisci could not be understood for long years. Although the most main functions of menisci have been known until the beginning of 2000s, how they are vital for the knee joint has been overlooked. Radical procedures which are performed to remove menisci completely or incompletely have been performed frequently when a traumatic or degenerative tear occurs in menisci. However, cartilage degenerations developing much faster in cartilage tissues of the knee joint after surgery in vast majority of the patients whose menisci have been surgically removed has led to understand the important and indispensable role of menisci for functional movements of the knee. That tibiofibular osteoarthritis risk increases independently from the tear type and meniscus region included in surgery in subjects whose meniscus has been removed although partial has been shown with long-term studies [50]. Today, meniscus is accepted to be a very important structure for functional sufficiency of the knee joint. The role of menisci during sportive and functional activities should be known well to better understand this importance. The most important role of menisci arises when compression load occurs on the joint during functional activities. Menisci reduce the load when transferring to the bones through absorbing the load as they are located

within the joint just like a cushion. Therefore, they prevent the injury of the cartilages in joint surfaces of femoral and tibial joints. They are also seen to be placed to reduce the incompatibility between femur and tibia bones. They prevent joint cartilage degeneration through equally distributing the load beside shock-absorbing effect when there is a load on the joint [51]. The amount of load transferred over menisci is known to vary depending on flexion, rotation angle and translation amount of tibia. Menisci facilitate to distribute joint fluid equally onto all joint surfaces and enable to increase the lifespan of the cartilage through contributing to joint nourishment [51, 52]. The main functional stability of the knee is known to be provided by strong ligaments like anterior and posterior cruciate ligaments and internal and external lateral ligaments. Torn ligaments lead to significant dysfunction of the knee [53–56]; however, critical location of menisci between femur and tibia has great importance for providing functional stabilization of the knee. Although a tear in meniscus usually leads to pain and function loss, no symptoms may develop when degeneration or tear occurs.

The influence of menisci on proprioception is not a focused issue. However, even the close association of particularly medial meniscus and joint capsule where mechanoreceptors are intense is enough to suggest the close relationship with proprioception. While mechanoreceptors in medial meniscus are located in outer rim which has a connection with joint capsule, number of mechanoreceptors is small in lateral meniscus where a connection with joint capsule is not present [57, 58]. Therefore, particularly medial meniscus injury may lead to proprioception loss in knee joint. A study conducted with 105 osteoarthritis patients in order to investigate the relationship between reduced proprioception and medial meniscus injury also verifies this possibility. While the threshold for detection of knee joint movement has been found to be related with the number and magnitude of injured regions on medial meniscus, it was not found to be related with muscle power, joint laxity, pain, age, gender and body mass index [59]. Similarly, a study conducted with 23 subjects with meniscus abnormality has shown that proprioception which is tested with knee angle reproduction capability significantly reduces in subjects with medial meniscus injury compared to healthy controls [10]. These studies clearly indicate the importance of meniscus tissue with regard to proprioception besides its many other important functions.

Arthroscopic repair, menisectomy and meniscus implants are frequently performed for reducing tissue loss-related symptoms arising from meniscus injury. However, application and philosophy of these operations largely vary. Arthroscopic meniscus repair seems as a more advantageous operation with regard to proprioception as it aims at keeping the maximum possible meniscus tissue within the joint. Partial menisectomy is the excision of the torn meniscus tissue and thereby it has the likelihood of reducing mechanoreceptor number. Limited number of studies conducted with the patients who underwent these operations verify the influenced proprioception. A reduction was reported in the control of the operated knee muscles and in proprioception even 1–2 years after partial menisectomy [60]. Similarly, a study conducted with 50 patients with partial menisectomy injury has revealed that the lack in single leg postural stability scores continues after menisectomy despite the absence of an impairment in clinical outcomes [61]. Isolated proprioception tests conducted in arthroscopic partial menisectomy have revealed similar results. A significant reduction develops in angle reproduction performance at 60° and 75° of flexion in operated knee compared to healthy controls [62].

Meniscus transplantation is a surgery type which has increased in treatment of meniscus abnormalities in recent years; however, it has not become widespread due to complications. Allograft meniscus implant has shown to reveal positive effects on position sense of the knee independently from pain and functional performance. The results of this study suggest that although no significant improvement of pain and functionality of the operated knee occurred at this short-term follow-up period, a meniscal allograft transplantation seems to have a significant positive effect on the joint position sense of the previously meniscectomized knee [63]. However, further scientific evidence is needed to indicate how successfully meniscus implants can improve proprioception, function and symptoms of the knee in meniscus injury.

10.6 Proprioception and Knee Rehabilitation Approaches

Under the present heading, the effects of the rehabilitation approaches such as taping, brace and exercises on knee proprioceptive sense for patellofemoral pain syndrome, ACL injury/surgery and meniscal injury/surgery have been discussed.

10.6.1 Effects of Taping on Knee Proprioceptive Sense in Rehabilitation

Taping is commonly used for knee problems, especially for PFPS, partly after ACL injury/surgery, and other knee ligament injuries. Aims of taping are: to decrease the oedema, to support the soft tissue around the knee joint and to improve proprioceptive input. Consequently, there have been a number of studies, which have focused on taping's role in proprioception enhancement.

10.6.1.1 Taping for Patellofemoral Pain Syndrome

Patellar taping is a simple and cost-effective technique introduced in the mid-1980s to alleviate the symptoms of patellofemoral pain syndrome (PFPS) or anterior knee pain [64]. Since then, several reviews have confirmed the efficacy of the technique, yet all have concluded that the mechanism, by which this efficacy is achieved, is open for debate [65–67]. The effect of taping or bandages on the position and congruence of the patellofemoral joint are uncertain. Some results suggest that rather than physically repositioning the joint, there may be other more subtle sensory mechanisms at work through skin, tendon and muscle stimulation that may account for the improvement of a joint position sense (JPS) task and for the success of patellar taping. All proprioception studies so far have measured variables along the efferent and afferent pathways or have assessed the final outcome of skeletal muscle activation and joint movement with techniques such as JPS.

An improvement in JPS with the application of patellar taping has been shown with asymptomatic, healthy people and symptomatic subjects with patellofemoral pain syndrome (PFPS) [23, 24]. However, it seems that the improvement is not uniform, with some people benefiting more than others. Initial results of a study on healthy subjects showed that patellar taping in the form of a simple strip of tape applied across the patella and anterior knee did not significantly change the JPS of 56 healthy subjects. Using a threshold of 5° from the target angle of 45°, those with 'good' proprioception (less than 5° from the target angle) derived little improvement in their ability to be closer to the target angle. On the other hand, those with 'poor' proprioception (5° or more from the target angle) were significantly closer as a result of the tape intervention [23]. These findings may occur because people with good JPS could not be 'improved' any further, whereas the tape would have its greatest 'treatment effect' on those with poor JPS, who could be improved more.

A later study was conducted on subjects with clinically diagnosed PFPS [24]. Here the researchers found that taping significantly improved JPS in these subjects, when similar thresholds were applied. These results confirmed that sub-classification of PFPS patients in the domain of proprioception is a consideration, when applying treatment. There appeared to be some PFPS patients with poorer JPS proprioceptive status than others and treatment of these patients may be more appropriately applied, if they could be easily identified and appropriately categorized. There was the intriguing possibility that the subgroup helped by tape is comprised of patients with neural damage within the lateral retinaculum or nerve sensitization due to pain.

A three-way comparison of malalignment, proprioception and histological findings would be an intricate but useful area of further research.

Why does taping improve proprioception as measured by JPS? A possible explanation may be either in chemical sensitizing of small and large diameter nerve fibres, as a response to pain [68] or microscopic small nerve damage in the lateral retinaculum [69–71]. The application of some form of knee support is thought to augment afferent input via the enhancement of cutaneous stimulation [72].

These results suggest that taping has a subtle, non-mechanical effect on the knee by affecting the areas of brain concerned with coordination, decision-making and motor control. In order to provide proof of these subtle mechanisms, functional magnetic resonance imaging (fMRI) provided an opportunity to examine brain activity in areas associated with proprioception, coordination and motor control [73]. fMRI uses the blood oxygenation level-dependent (BOLD) contrast technique, which reflects the loss of oxygen from haemoglobin causing its iron to become paramagnetic. When a task is performed, there is consequent neuronal activity and an increase in oxygen usage. These changes are followed within a few seconds by a larger fractional increase in blood flow and an increase in blood volume, resulting in a decrease in the amount of deoxygenated blood present. It is this change that the BOLD contrast technique detects. The fMRI technique has been used to show that a simple non-weight-bearing JPS task of knee extension and flexion increases brain activation in the cerebellum and decreases activation in the supplementary motor cortex.

Tape applied across the patellar without any intended patellar displacement or realignment during the same task causes primary sensorimotor and supplementary motor cortices to have significantly increased bilateral activity whereas the primary sensorimotor cortex has decreased activity.

Kinesiotaping can be applied at 50–85% tensions on the skin to restrict partial or full joint motion, but the taping tension was insufficient to correct the patellar alignment. The effects of Kinesiotape in patients with patellofemoral pain are still unclear [74]. Studies showed that Kinesiotaping can relive pain in patients with patellofemoral pain [75, 76]. The results of several studies showed that Kinesio- and McConnell taping can reduce pain in patients with patellofemoral pain [74–81] and they speculate that Kinesio- and/or McConnell taping should stimulate cutaneous mechanoreceptors and improve knee proprioception [78, 79]. Kinesiotaping is effective in controlling patellar tracking through increased muscle force sense and that might be the mechanism of pain relief in PFPS patients. McConnell taping to correct patellar alignment also cause pain relief in PFPS patients [77, 81].

10.6.1.2 Taping for ACL Injury/Surgery

A few studies focused on the effects of Kinesiotaping after ACL reconstruction, while there is no study for ACL injury. All studies showed no significant difference in the reduction of swelling or improvement of knee score and total range of motion except the pain relief [82–85]. Engrossingly, there is no study in the literature to investigate the effects of the taping on proprioception in patients with ACL injured/reconstructed.

10.6.1.3 Taping for Meniscal Injury/ Surgery

There is unique study to investigate the effects of the patellar taping on during a slow step descent task in patients with meniscal lesions [86] while the present study did not assess the proprioception of knee.

10.6.2 Effects of Bracing on Knee Proprioceptive Sense in Rehabilitation

Braces are commonly used for chronic problems such as PFPS and after traumatic ACL and other ligament injuries. Although one of the aims of bracing is to provide mechanical stability to

the joint, there has been speculation that proprioception enhancement also plays a role in the positive effects seen in military recruits [87]. Consequently, there have been a number of studies, which have focused on bracing's role in proprioception enhancement. Although there is a myriad of brace designs, JPS has been assessed in the knee by applying a sleeve type brace, often made of neoprene. In terms of proprioception, there is no consensus that one brace is better than another. It is possible therefore that, in terms of effecting JPS, an expensive brace is no more efficacious than an inexpensive one or even the simple elasticated bandages.

10.6.2.1 Bracing for Patellofemoral Pain Syndrome

Studies on healthy subjects have shown that a neoprene sleeve brace and similar styles of braces can improve knee proprioception using a variety of tests [88–90]. Other types of braces specially designed for the patellar can also compensate for JPS impairment brought on by a fatigued state after exercise in healthy subjects [91]. Interestingly, like Callaghan et al. [23] these researchers also applied the criterion of a cut-off to distinguish between good and poor proprioception; those who had 'poor' proprioception had a greater enhancement of their JPS, when they wore a brace compared to those who had 'good' proprioception. In a similar experiment to that done with patella taping, fMRI has also been used to assess the effects of a neoprene knee sleeve brace on centres of the brain [92]. Using the BOLD technique this study showed that different proprioceptive inputs to the knee joint by the neoprene brace had a direct influence on brain activity during knee movement. An increased level of brain activation was seen with the application of a brace and sleeve, respectively, compared to the condition, when no brace or sleeve was present at the knee. However, as the movements of the knee were active movements from $0°$ to $90°$ of knee flexion rather than angle active reproduction to assess JPS, the true effect on JPS and therefore proprioception is unknown.

10.6.2.2 Bracing for ACL Injury/ Surgery

After ACL injury/surgery and/or during rehabilitation, some clinicians prefer to use functional knee braces. Rigid shell or sleeve braces can provide mechanical stabilization and proprioceptive input. Elastic knee braces increase postural control by approximately 22% in patients with ACL rupture, while there is no difference in postural stability between uninjured and injured legs in the braced condition [93]. As known, braces help to improve proprioceptive sense and postural control in patients with ACL injury. Sleeve braces help to improve dynamic balance after perturbation and dynamic lower limb peak rate of force development compared to the non-braced condition [92]. Authors indicated that the effects might be caused by the flexible area of support and the incorporated mechanisms to address proprioceptive aspects.

In light of the new studies, there is no doubt about that braces do not protect against postoperative injury, decrease pain, improve range of knee motion or improve knee stability in patient with ACL reconstruction [94].

10.6.2.3 Bracing for Meniscal Injury/ Surgery

After arthroscopic meniscectomy (especially partial), risk of knee osteoarthritis development increases because of increased medial compartment loading. Knee valgus braces should be used to support the medial side of the knee during forward lunge and one-leg rise condition, which increased peak knee flexion [95]. After arthroscopic isolated meniscus repair, hinged braces should be used to control knee range of motion during the activities and exercises. Conservatively, after arthroscopic isolated meniscus repair, hinged brace use with a gradual increase ROM to 90° and only touch weight bearing during the 6 weeks [96].

It is unfortunate that we have to inform, there is no study to investigate the effects of bracing on proprioceptive sense in patients with meniscal lesions/surgery in the literature.

10.6.3 Effects of Exercises on Knee Proprioceptive Sense in Rehabilitation

Exercise is commonly used for treatment of musculoskeletal problems. Aims of exercises are: to increase the muscle strength and endurance, to provide high functional performance, to improve mechanical stability and/or control and to provide proprioceptive input. Consequently, there have only been a limited number of studies, which have focused on exercises role in proprioception enhancement.

10.6.3.1 Effects of Exercise on Knee Proprioceptive Sense in Patellofemoral Pain Syndrome

Exercises for patients with patellofemoral pain syndrome are effective, regardless of the type of exercise (e.g. in weight bearing or not; targeting hip or knee). In 2016, International Patellofemoral Pain Research Retreat published their recommendation for patellofemoral pain syndrome treatment [97]. They estipulated that: (1) Exercise is recommended to reduce pain in short, medium and long term and improve function in medium and long term. (2) Combining hip and knee exercises is recommended to reduce pain and improve function in short, medium and long term, and this combination should be used in preference to knee exercises alone.

Although it is known that muscle strength is highly correlated with the joint position sense [98], there are a few studies to investigate the effects of the exercise therapy on the joint position sense in patients with patellofemoral pain syndrome. For instance, Guney et al. showed that quadriceps eccentric strength is correlated more to joint position sense than concentric strength. JPS results are poorer on the painful knee, when compared to uninvolved side. While eccentric strength correlated with both JPS target angles, concentric strength is correlated only with 20°.

In light of our literature research, there are only two studies to investigate the effects of the exercises therapy on the knee joint position sense [18, 99]. Hazneci et al. investigate the effects of isokinetic exercise on knee joint position sense and muscle strength [18]. Isokinetic exercise protocol was carried out at angular velocities of 60°/s and 180°/s three times per week during the 6 weeks. Passive knee joint position sense, quadriceps and hamstring muscle strength and pain assessments were collected: After the isokinetic exercise therapy, passive reproduction of knee joint position sense for 40° of flexion and 50° of extension, in addition to flexion peak torque, extension peak torque, flexion total work, extension total work and pain score, has improved significantly in the patellofemoral pain syndrome group. Authors concluded that isokinetic exercises have positive effects on passive position sense of knee joints, increasing the muscular strength and work capacity. These findings show that using the present isokinetic exercise in rehabilitation protocols of patients with patellofemoral pain syndrome not only improves the knee joint stabilization but also the proprioceptive acuity [18]. Balci et al. [99] investigated the effects of two different closed kinetic chain exercises in patients with patellofemoral pain syndrome. Forty female patients with unilateral PFPS were randomly divided into two groups, to receive exercises with the hip internally rotated or externally rotated with the use of the Monitored Rehab Functional Squat (MRFS) System. The duration of exercises was 4 weeks with a total of 20 sessions. Both groups were evaluated before exercises therapy, after 4 weeks of exercises and after 6 weeks of home exercise programme with the MRFS System for muscle strength and proprioception, with a visual analogue scale for pain and with the Kujala questionnaire for functional assessment. Their results showed that concentric proprioceptive deficit improved significantly in both groups after treatment. Eccentric proprioceptive deficit, however, did not change significantly both after treatment and home exercises. Authors emphasized that functional knee squat

exercises with internally and externally rotated hip positions provide similar improvements in muscle strength and proprioception in patients with patellofemoral pain syndrome [99].

10.6.3.2 Effects of Exercise on Knee Proprioceptive Sense in ACL Injury/Surgery

Exercises after ACL rupture or ACL surgery (reconstruction/repair) are effective and critical part of the rehabilitation programme. Pinczewski et al. [100] reported that one in four patients undergoing an ACL reconstruction will suffer a second tear within 10 years of their first. Paterno et al. [101] also reported that an incidence rate of a second ACL injury within 2 years after returning to sports was six times greater than healthy. Paterno et al. also demonstrated deficits in muscular strength, kinaesthetic sense, balance, and force attenuation for 6 months to 2 years following reconstruction [101]. Taking into account all of these, efficient exercise programme should take lead to return to sports, safely and successfully. As known, anterior cruciate ligament (ACL) rupture and surgery leads to a proprioceptive deficit and therefore joint position sense [102, 103]. Efficient exercises, which improve knee proprioception, make its way into rehabilitation programme and return to sports. Proprioceptive exercises should take place from early phases of the rehabilitation programme and to further during all steps of rehabilitation. There are a lot of studies to investigate the effects of exercises on balance in patients with ACL injury/reconstruction, while this chapter and the book focus on only proprioceptive sense. Therefore, we will not mention those studies which focus on balance, in this chapter.

Friemert et al. [104] compared the effects of continuous active motion and continuous passive motion on knee joint position sense before and after ACL surgery. Significantly better results were, however, obtained in the continuous active motion group. During the first post-operative week, a continuous active motion exercise produced a significantly greater reduction in the proprioceptive deficit. Authors emphasized that active exercises should be the first choice in immediately post-operative rehabilitation after ACL replacement [104].

Cooper et al. investigated the effect of proprioceptive and balance exercises on people with an injured or reconstructed anterior cruciate ligament. Authors received some evidence regarding that proprioceptive and balance exercises improve outcomes. Improvements have been found in joint position sense and proprioception, in addition to muscle strength, knee functions and hop test [24].

Ordahan et al. [105] evaluated knee proprioception in patients with anterior cruciate ligament (ACL) injuries and to assess the effectiveness of an exercise programme consisting mainly of proprioception exercises addressing pain, proprioception and functional status following ACL reconstruction. A significant improvement in pain severity, proprioception and functional capacity after the post-operative 6-month rehabilitation programme with intensive proprioceptive exercises was shown. Authors' emphasized rehabilitation programme predominantly consisting of proprioception exercises provided considerable improvement on knee proprioception and functional status [105].

Cho et al. examined the effect of closed kinetic chain exercises performed by an unstable exercise group and a stable exercise group on the knee joint proprioception and functional scores of patients, who underwent anterior cruciate ligament reconstruction [106]. A 60-min exercise programme, three times a week for 6 weeks was performed in both groups. The results of the clinical evaluation at 45° proprioception showed statistically significant differences between the two groups. The results of the clinical evaluation at 15° proprioception showed no statistically significant differences between the two groups. The proprioception and functional scores of the patients in the unstable exercise group, who underwent ACL reconstruction, were superior to those in the stable exercises group.

10.6.3.3 Effects of Exercise on Knee Proprioceptive Sense in Meniscus Injury/Surgery

The partial meniscectomy and/or meniscal repair leads to proprioceptive knee deficits in a short period after the arthroscopic procedure [107], however, to our knowledge, there is no study to focus on the effect of the exercises on knee proprioception in patients with meniscus lesion and/or undergo surgery such as meniscectomy or partial meniscal repair.

Conclusion

Large prospective longitudinal studies are needed to evaluate therapeutic interventions designed to improve proprioception in the knee joint. Rehabilitation programme predominantly consisting of proprioceptive exercises, plyometrics, strengthening, functional full body exercises such as Tai Chi-yoga-pilates etc., weight-bearing exercises, neuromuscular training, and sports-specific exercises provided considerable improvement on knee proprioception and functional status (see Figs. 10.1 and 10.2).

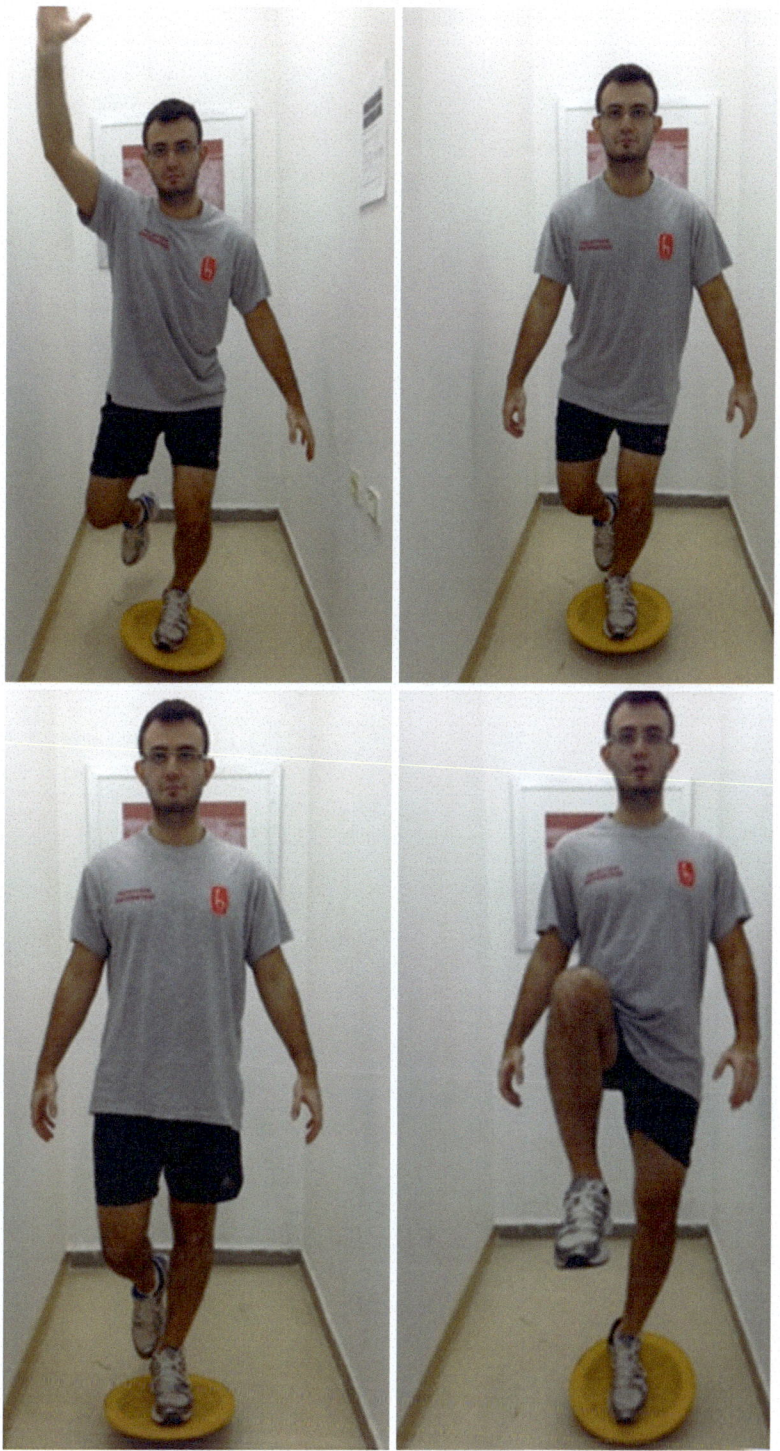

Fig. 10.1 Examples for functional proprioceptive exercises for patients with knee lesions

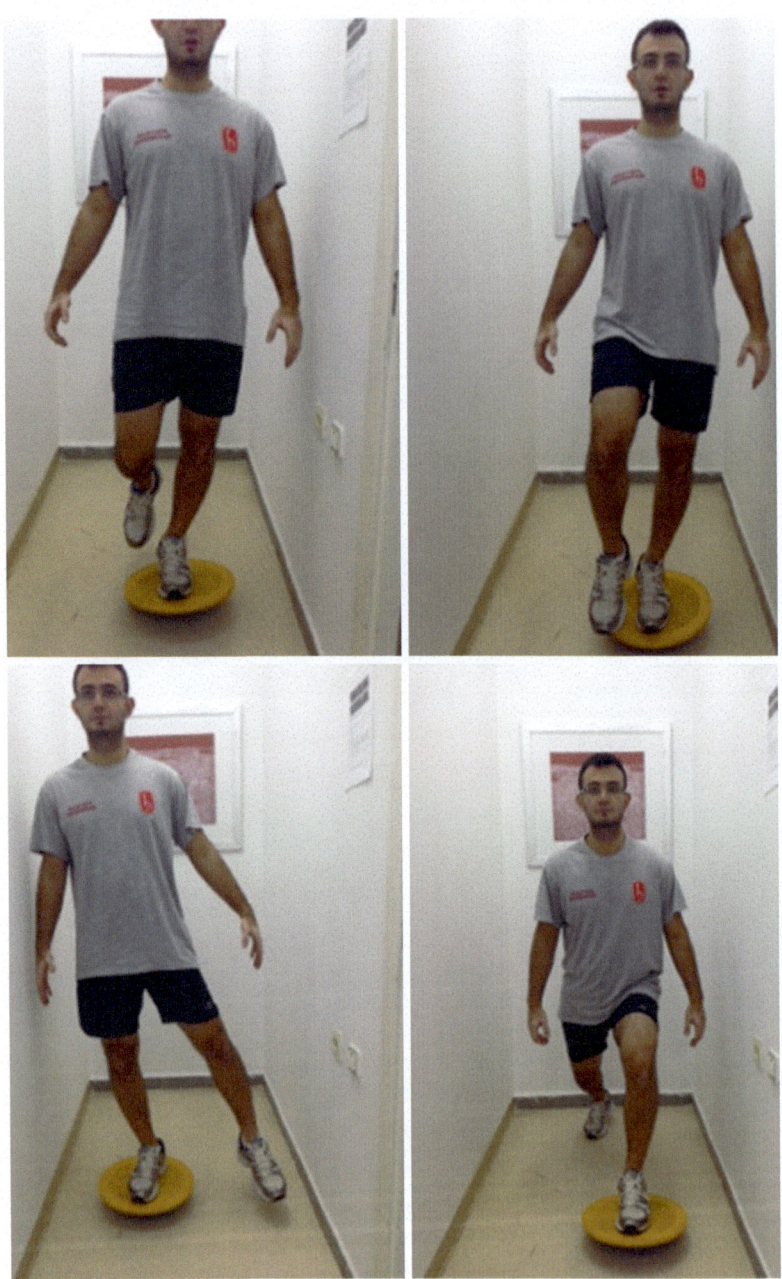

Fig. 10.1 (continued)

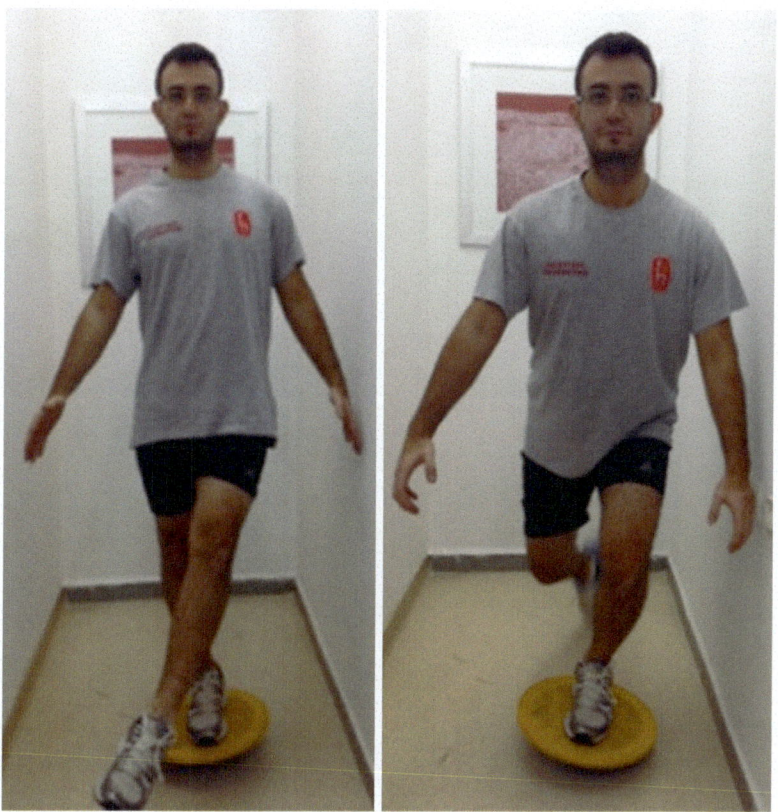

Fig. 10.1 (continued)

Fig. 10.2 Examples of
Tai Chi exercises for
patients with knee
lesions. (**a**) Pubu, (**b**)
Lochiaobu (brush the
knee), (**c**) Liu (flat
stance), (**d**) Liu, (**e**) Jade
lady before shuttles, (**f**)
Blocking before punch
(With permission:
Photos: Ozge Cakır, PT,
PhD, Assist Prof.)

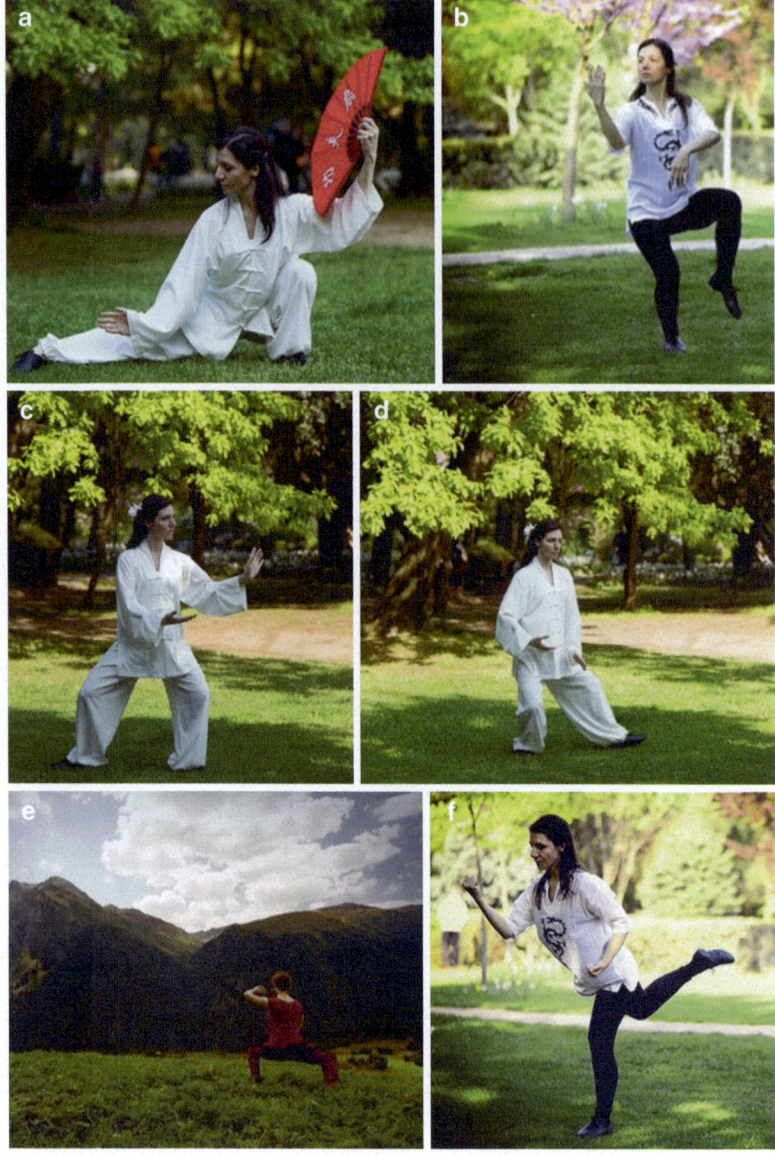

References

1. Sharma L. Proprioceptive impairment in knee osteo-arthritis. Rheum Dis Clin N Am. 1999;25:299–314.
2. Gardner EP, Martin JH. Coding of sensory information. In: Kandel ER, Schwartz JH, Jessell TM, editors. Principles of neuroscience. 4th ed. New York, NY: McGraw-Hill; 2000. p. 411–28.
3. Pai YC, Rymer WZ, Chang RW, et al. Effect of age and osteoarthritis on knee proprioception. Arthritis Rheum. 1997;40:2260–5.
4. Abelew TA, Miller MD, Cope TC, et al. Local loss of proprioception results in disruption of inter-joint coordination during locomotion in the cat. J Neurophysiol. 2000;84:2704–14.
5. Proske U. Kinesthesia: the role of muscle receptors. Muscle Nerve. 2006;34:545–58.
6. Lundy-Ekman L. Neuroscience: fundamentals for rehabilitation. Philadelphia, PA: Elsevier Health Science Division; 2012.
7. Riemann BL, Lephart SM. The sensorimotor system. Part I. The physiologic basis of functional joint stability. J Athlc Train. 2002;37:71–9.
8. Johansson H, Pederson J, Bergenheim M, et al. Peripheral afferents of the knee: their effects on central mechanisms regulating muscle stiffness, joint stability and proprioception and coordination.

In: Lephart SM, Fu FH, editors. Proprioception and neuromuscular control in joint stability. Champaign, IL: Human Kinetics; 2000. p. 5–22.

9. Grigg P. Peripheral neural mechanisms in proprioception. J Sport Rehabil. 1994;3:2–17.

10. Jerosch J, Prymka M, Castro WH. Proprioception of knee joints with a lesion of the medial meniscus. Acta Orthop Belg. 1996;62:41–5.

11. Solomonow M, Krogsgaard M. Sensorimotor control of knee stability. A review. Scand J Med Sci Sports. 2001;11:64–80.

12. Burgess PR, Wei JY, Clark FJ, et al. Signaling of kinesthetic information by peripheral sensory receptors. Annu Rev Neurosci. 1982;5:171–87.

13. Jennings AG. A proprioceptive role for the anterior cruciate ligament: a review of the literature. J Orthop Rheumatol. 1994;7:3–13.

14. Lephart SM, Riemann BL, Fu FH. Introduction to the sensorimotor system. In: Lephart SM, Fu FH, editors. Proprioception and neuromuscular control in joint stability. Champaign, IL: Human Kinetics; 2000.

15. Sanchis-Alfonso V, Rosello-Sastre E, Martinez-Sanjuan V. Pathogenesis of anterior knee pain syndrome and functional patellofemoral instability in the active young. Am J Knee Surg. 1999;12:29–40.

16. Selfe J, Callaghan M, McHenry A, et al. An investigation into the effect of number of trials during proprioceptive testing in patients with patellofemoral pain syndrome. J Orthop Res. 2006;24:1218–24.

17. Baker V, Bennell K, Stillman B, et al. Abnormal knee joint position sense in individuals with patellofemoral pain syndrome. J Orthop Res. 2002;20:208–14.

18. Hazneci B, Yildiz Y, Sekir U, et al. Efficacy of isokinetic exercise on joint position sense and muscle strength in patellofemoral pain syndrome. Am J Phys Med Rehabil. 2005;84:521–7.

19. Kramer J, Handfield T, Kiefer G, et al. Comparisons of weight-bearing and non-weight-bearing tests of knee proprioception performed by patients with patello-femoral pain syndrome and asymptomatic individuals. Clin J Sport Med. 1997;7:113–8.

20. Akseki D, Akkaya G, Erduran M, et al. Proprioception of the knee joint in patellofemoral pain syndrome. Acta Orthop Traumatol Turc. 2008;42:316–21.

21. Akseki D, Erduran M, Ozarslan S, et al. Parallelism of vibration sense with proprioception sense in patients with patellofemoral pain syndrome: a pilot study. Eklem Hastalik Cerrahisi. 2010;21:23–30.

22. Perlau R, Frank C. The effect of elastic bandages on human knee proprioception on the uninjured population. Am J Sports Med, 1995;23:251–5.

23. Callaghan MJ, Selfe J, Bagley P, et al. The effect of patellar taping on knee joint proprioception. J Athl Train. 2002;37:19–24.

24. Callaghan MJ, Selfe J, McHenry A, et al. Effects of patellar taping on knee joint proprioception in patients with patellofemoral pain syndrome. Man Ther. 2008;13:192–9.

25. Adachi N, Ochi M, Uchio Y, et al. Reconstruction of the anterior cruciate ligament. Single- versus double-bundle multistranded hamstring tendons. J Bone Joint Surg Br. 2004;86:515–20.

26. Anders JO, Venbrocks RA, Weinberg M. Proprioceptive skills and functional outcome after anterior cruciate ligament reconstruction with a bone-tendon-bone graft. Int Orthop. 2008;32:627–33.

27. Angoules AG, Mavrogenis AF, Dimitriou R, et al. Knee proprioception following ACL reconstruction: a prospective trial comparing hamstrings with bone-patellar tendon-bone autograft. Knee. 2011;18:76–82.

28. Fremerey RW, Lobenhoffer P, Zeichen J, et al. Proprioception after rehabilitation and reconstruction in knees with deficiency of the anterior cruciate ligament: a prospective, longitudinal study. J Bone Joint Surg Br. 2000;82:801–6.

29. Machotka Z, Scarborough I, Duncan W, et al. Anterior cruciate ligament repair with LARS (ligament advanced reinforcement system): a systematic review. Sports Med Arthrosc Rehabil Ther Technol. 2010;2:29.

30. Madhavan S, Shields RK. Neuromuscular responses in individuals with anterior cruciate ligament repair. Clin Neurophysiol. 2011;122:997–1004.

31. Beard DJ, Dodd CA, Trundle HR, et al. Proprioceptive enhancement for anterior cruciate ligament deficiency: a prospective randomised trial for two physiotherapy regimes. J Bone Joint Surg Br. 1994;76:654–9.

32. Gokeler A, Benjaminse A, Hewett TE, et al. Proprioceptive deficits after ACL injury: are they clinically relevant? Br J Sports Med. 2012;46:180–92.

33. Roberts D, Fridén T, Zätterström R, et al. Proprioception in people with anterior cruciate ligament-deficient knees: comparison of symptomatic and asymptomatic patients. J Orthop Sports Phys Ther. 1999;29:587–94.

34. Bonfim TR, Jansen Paccola CA, Barela JA. Proprioceptive and behavior impairments in individuals with anterior cruciate ligament reconstructed knees. Arch Phys Med Rehabil. 2003;84:1217–23.

35. Fridén T, Roberts D, Ageberg E, et al. Review of knee proprioception and the relation to extremity function after an anterior cruciate ligament rupture. J Orthop Sports Phys Ther. 2001;31:567–76.

36. Cooper RL, Taylor NF, Feller JA. A randomised controlled trial of proprioceptive and balance training after surgical reconstruction of the anterior cruciate ligament. Res Sports Med. 2005;13:217–30.

37. Hewett TE, Myer GD, Ford KR, et al. Dynamic neuromuscular analysis training for preventing anterior cruciate ligament injury in female athletes. Instr Course Lect. 2007;56:397–406.

38. Noyes FR, McGinniss GH, Mooar LA. Functional disability in the anterior cruciate insufficient knee syndrome. Review of knee rating systems and

projected risk factors in determining treatment. Sports Med. 1984;1:278–302.

39. Kapreli E, Athanasopoulos S. The anterior cruciate ligament deficiency as a model of brain plasticity. Med Hypotheses. 2006;67:645–50.

40. Gottlob CA, Baker CL, Pellissier JM, et al. Cost effectiveness of anterior crucite ligament reconstruction in young adults. Clin Orthop Relat Res. 1999;367:272–82.

41. Adachi N, Ochi M, Uchio Y, et al. Mechanoreceptors in the anterior cruciate ligament contribute to the joint position sense. Acta Orthop Scand. 2002;73:330–4.

42. Yosmaoglu HB, Baltacı G, Kaya D, et al. Comparison of functional outcomes of two anterior cruciate ligament reconstruction methods with hamstring tendon graft. Acta Orthop Traumatol Turc. 2011;45:240–7.

43. Krogsgaard MR, Dyhre-Poulsen P, Fischer-Rasmussen T. Cruciate ligament reflexes. J Electromyogr Kinesiol. 2002;12:177–82.

44. Denti M, Monteleone M, Berardi A, et al. Anterior cruciate ligament mechanoreceptors. Histologic studies on lesions and reconstruction. Clin Orthop Relat Res. 1994;308:29–32.

45. MacDonald PB, Hedden D, Pacin O, et al. Proprioception in anterior cruciate ligament-deficient and reconstructed knees. Am J Sports Med. 1996;24:774–8.

46. Yosmaoglu HB, Baltacı G, Kaya D, et al. Tracking ability, motor coordination, and functional determinants after anterior cruciate ligament reconstruction. J Sport Rehabil. 2011;20:207–18.

47. Yosmaoglu HB, Baltacı G, Ozer H, et al. Effects of additional gracilis tendon harvest on muscle torque, motor coordination, and knee laxity in ACL reconstruction. Knee Surg Sports Traumatol Arthrosc. 2011;19:1287–92.

48. Reider B, Arcand MA, Diehl LH, et al. Proprioception of the knee before and after anterior cruciate ligament reconstruction. Arthroscopy. 2003;19:2–12.

49. Hogervorst T, Brand R. Mechanoreceptors in joint function. J Bone Joint Surg Am. 1998;80:1365–78.

50. Englund M, Lohmander LS. Risk factors for symptomatic knee osteoarthritis fifteen to twenty-two years after meniscectomy. Arthritis Rheum. 2004;50:2811–9.

51. Makris EA, Hadidi P, Athanasiou KA. The knee meniscus: structure–function, pathophysiology, current repair techniques, and prospects for regeneration. Biomaterials. 2011;32:7411–31.

52. Hauger O, Frank LR, Boutin RD, et al. Characterization of the "red zone" of knee meniscus: MR imaging and histologic correlation. Radiology. 2000;217:193–200.

53. Aglietti P, Buzzi R, Zaccherotti G, et al. Patellar tendon versus doubled semitendinosus and gracilis tendons for anterior cruciate ligament reconstruction. Am J Sports Med. 1994;22:211–7.

54. Amiel D, Kleiner JB, Roux RD, et al. The phenomenon of "ligamentization": anterior cruciate ligament reconstruction with autogenous patellar tendon. J Orthop Res. 1986;4:162–72.

55. Amis AA, Dawkins GP. Functional anatomy of the anterior cruciate ligament. Fibre bundle actions related to ligament replacements and injuries. J Bone Joint Surg Br. 1991;3:260–7.

56. Anderson AF, Dome DC, Gautam S, et al. Correlation of anthropometric measurements, strength, anterior cruciate ligament size, and intercondylar notch characteristics to sex differences in anterior cruciate ligament tears. Am J Sports Med. 2001;29:58–63.

57. Assimakopoulos AP, Katonis PG, Agapitos MV, et al. The innervation of the human meniscus. Clin Orthrop Relat Res. 1992;275:232–6.

58. Messner K, Gao J. The menisci of the knee joint. Anatomical and functional characteristics, and a rationale for clinical treatment. J Anat. 1998;193:161–78.

59. Van der Esch M, Knoop J, Hunter DJ, et al. The association between reduced knee joint proprioception and medial meniscal abnormalities using MRI in knee osteoarthritis: results from the Amsterdam osteoarthritis cohort. Osteoarthr Cartil. 2013;21:676–81.

60. Malliou P, Gioftsidou A, Pafis G, et al. Proprioception and functional deficits of partial meniscectomized knees. Eur J Phys Rehabil Med. 2012;48:231–6.

61. Al-Dadah O, Shepstone L, Donell ST. Proprioception following partial meniscectomy in stable knees. Knee Surg Sports Traumatol Arthrosc. 2011;19:207–13.

62. Karahan M, Kocaoglu B, Cabukoglu C, et al. Effect of partial medial meniscectomy on the proprioceptive function of the knee. Arch Orthop Trauma Surg. 2010;130:427–31.

63. Thijs Y, Witvrouw E, Evens B, et al. A prospective study on knee proprioception after meniscal allograft transplantation. Scand J Med Sci Sports. 2007;17:223–9.

64. McConnell J. The management of chondromalacia patellae: a long term solution. Aust J Physiother. 1986;32:215–23.

65. Barton C, Balachandar V, Lack S, et al. Patellar taping for patellofemoral pain: a systematic review and metaanalysis to evaluate clinical outcomes and biomechanical mechanisms. Br J Sports Med. 2014;48:417–24.

66. Callaghan MJ. Patellar taping, the theory versus the evidence: a review. Phys Ther Rev. 1997;2:181–3.

67. Crossley K, Cowan SM, Bennell KL, et al. Patellar taping: is clinical success supported by scientific evidence? Man Ther. 2000;5:142–50.

68. Capra NF, Ro JY. Experimental muscle pain produces central modulation of proprioceptive signals arising from jaw muscle spindles. Pain. 2000;86:151–62.

69. Fulkerson JP. Disorders of the patellofemoral joint. 4th ed. Baltimore, MD: Williams & Wilkins; 2004.

70. Sanchis-Alfonso V, Roselló-Sastre E. Immunohistochemical analysis for neural markers of the lateral retinaculum in patients with isolated symptomatic

patellofemoral malalignment. A neuroanatomic basis for anterior knee pain in the active young patient. Am J Sports Med. 2000;28:725–31.

71. Sanchis-Alfonso V, Roselló-Sastre E, Revert F. Neural growth factor expression in the lateral retinaculum in painful patellofemoral malalignment. Acta Orthop Scand. 2001;72:146–9.

72. Lephart SM, Kocher MS, FH F, et al. Proprioception following anterior cruciate ligament reconstruction. J Sport Rehabil. 1992;1:188–96.

73. Callaghan MJ, McKie S, Richardson P, et al. Effects of patellar taping on brain activity during knee joint proprioception tests using functional magnetic resonance imaging. Phys Ther. 2012;92:821–30.

74. Lan TY, Lin WP, Jiang CC, et al. Immediate effect and predictors of effectiveness of taping for patellofemoral pain syndrome: a prospective cohort study. Am J Sports Med. 2010;38:1626–30.

75. Akbas E, Atay AO, Yuksel I. The effects of additional kinesio taping over exercise in the treatment of patellofemoral pain syndrome. Acta Orthop Traumatol Turc. 2011;45:335–41.

76. Kuru T, Yaliman A, Dereli EE. Comparison of efficiency of kinesio taping and electrical stimulation in patients with patellofemoral pain syndrome. Acta Orthop Traumatol Turc. 2012;46:385–92.

77. Aminaka N, Gribble PA. Patellar taping, patellofemoral pain syndrome, lower extremity kinematics, and dynamic postural control. J Athl Train. 2008;43:21–8.

78. Aytar A, Ozunlu N, Surenkok O. Initial effects of kinesio taping in patients with patellofemoral pain syndrome: a randomized, double-blind study. Isokinet Exerc Sci. 2011;19:135–42.

79. Campolo M, Babu J, Dmochowska K, et al. A comparison of two taping techniques (kinesio and mcconnell) and their effect on anterior knee pain during functional activities. Int J Sports Phys Ther. 2013;8:105–10.

80. Derasari A, Brindle TJ, Alter KE, et al. McConnell taping shifts the patella inferiorly in patients with patellofemoral pain: a dynamic magnetic resonance imaging study. Phys Ther. 2010;90:411–9.

81. Kaya D, Callaghan MJ, Ozkan H, et al. The effect of an exercise program in conjunction with short-period patellar taping on pain, electromyogram activity, and muscle strength in patellofemoral pain syndrome. Sports Health. 2010;2:410–6.

82. Balki S, Göktaş HE, Öztemur Z. Kinesio taping as a treatment method in the acute phase of ACL reconstruction: a double-blind, placebo-controlled study. Acta Orthop Traumatol Turc. 2016;50:628–34.

83. Boguszewski D, Tomaszewska I, Adamczyk JG, et al. Evaluation of effectiveness of kinesiology taping as an adjunct to rehabilitation following anterior cruciate ligament reconstruction. Preliminary report. Ortop Traumatol Rehabil. 2013;15:469–78.

84. Chan MC, Wee JW, Lim MH. Does kinesiology taping improve the early postoperative outcomes

in anterior cruciate ligament reconstruction? A randomized controlled study. Clin J Sport Med. 2017;27:260–5.

85. Laborie M, Klouche S, Herman S, et al. Inefficacy of Kinesio-Taping® on early postoperative pain after ACL reconstruction: prospective comparative study. Orthop Traumatol Surg Res. 2015;101:963–7.

86. Roy N, Gaudreault N, Tousignant M, et al. Patellar taping alters knee kinematics during step descent in individuals with a meniscalinjury: an exploratory study. Clin Biomech (Bristol, Avon). 2016;31:74–8.

87. Van Tiggelen D, Witvrouw E, Roget P, et al. Effect of bracing on the prevention of anterior knee pain—a prospective randomized study. Knee Surg Sports Traumatol Arthrosc. 2004;12:434–9.

88. Baltaci G, Aktas G, Camci E, et al. The effect of prophylactic knee bracing on performance: balance, proprioception, coordination, and muscular power. Knee Surg Sports Traumatol Arthrosc. 2011;19:1722–8.

89. Birmingham TB, Kramer JF, Inglis JT, et al. Effect of a neoprene sleeve on knee joint position sense during sitting open kinetic chain and supine closed kinetic chain tests. Am J Sports Med. 1998;26:562–6.

90. McNair PJ, Stanley SN, Strauss GR. Knee bracing: effects of proprioception. Arch Phys Med Rehabil. 1996;77:287–9.

91. Tiggelen DV, Coorevits P, Witvrouw E. The effects of a neoprene knee sleeve on subjects with a poor versus good joint position sense subjected to an isokinetic fatigue protocol. Clin J Sport Med. 2008;18:259–65.

92. Strutzenberger G, Braig M, Sell S, et al. Effect of brace design on patients with ACL-ruptures. Int J Sports Med. 2012;33:934–9.

93. Palm HG, Brattinger F, Stegmueller B, et al. Effects of knee bracing on postural control after anterior cruciate ligament rupture. Knee. 2012;19:664–71.

94. Kruse LM, Gray B, Wright RW. Rehabilitation after anterior cruciate ligament reconstruction: a systematic review. J Bone Joint Surg Am. 2012;94:1737–48.

95. Thorning M, Thorlund JB, Roos EM, et al. Immediate effect of valgus bracing on knee joint moments in meniscectomised patients: an exploratory study. J Sci Med Sport. 2016;19:964–9.

96. Lind M, Nielsen T, Faunø P, et al. Free rehabilitation is safe after isolated meniscus repair: a prospective randomized trial comparing free with restricted rehabilitation regimens. Am J Sports Med. 2013;41:2753–8.

97. Crossley KM, van Middelkoop M, Callaghan MJ, et al. 2016 Patellofemoral pain consensus statement from the 4th International Patellofemoral Pain Research Retreat, Manchester. Part 2: recommended physical interventions (exercise, taping, bracing, foot orthoses and combined interventions). Br J Sports Med. 2016;50:844–52.

98. Guney H, Yuksel I, Kaya D, et al. The relationship between quadriceps strength and joint position

sense, functional outcome and painful activities in patellofemoral pain syndrome. Knee Surg Sports Traumatol Arthrosc. 2016;24:2966–72.

99. Balci P, Tunay VB, Baltaci G, et al. The effects of two different closed kinetic chain exercises on muscle strength and proprioception in patients with patellofemoral pain syndrome. Acta Orthop Traumatol Turc. 2009;43:419–25.

100. Pinczewski LA, Lyman J, Salmaon LJ, et al. A 10-year study comparison of anterior cruciate ligament reconstruction with hamstring tendon and patellar tendon autograft: a controlled, prospective trial. Am J Sports Med. 2007;35:564–74.

101. Paterno MV, Rauth MJ, Schmitt LC, et al. Incidence of second ACL injuries 2 years after primary ACL reconstruction and return to sport. Am J Sports Med. 2014;42:1567–73.

102. Kim HJ, Lee JH, Lee DH. Proprioception in patients with anterior cruciate ligament tears. Am J Sports Med. 2016. https://doi.org/10.1177/0363546516682231.

103. Relph N, Herrington L, Tyson S. The effects of ACL injury on knee proprioception: a meta-analysis. Physiotherapy. 2014;100:187–95.

104. Friemert B, Bach C, Schwarz W, et al. Benefits of active motion for joint position sense. Knee Surg Sports Traumatol Arthrosc. 2006;14:564–70.

105. Ordahan B, Küçükşen S, Tuncay İ, et al. The effect of proprioception exercises on functional status in patients with anterior cruciate ligament reconstruction. J Back Musculoskelet Rehabil. 2015;28: 531–7.

106. Cho SH, Bae CH, Gak HB. Effects of closed kinetic chain exercises on proprioception and functional scores of the knee after anterior cruciate ligament reconstruction. J Phys Ther Sci. 2013;25: 1239–41.

107. Thijs Y, Vingerhoets G, Pattyn E, et al. Does bracing influence brain activity during knee movement: an fMRI study. Knee Surg Sports Traumatol Arthrosc. 2010;18:1145–9.

Proprioception After Ankle Injury, Surgery, and Rehabilitation

11

Tekin Kerem Ulku, Baris Kocaoglu,
Menderes Murat Caglar, and Jon Karlsson

11.1 Introduction

Ankle injuries are among the most common sports-related injuries. Lateral ankle sprains constitute the vast majority of these injuries, estimated at approximately two million injuries per year [1]. This constitutes nearly 20% of all sports injuries. Studies have shown that 10–40% of these acute injuries may eventually progress to chronic ankle instability (CAI) [2–4].

The underlying cause of the progression to CAI still remains controversial. Mechanical effects induced by ligamentous laxity are believed to be one factor. However, several patients with torn ligaments have been shown to have a stable ankle joint and vice versa, patients without clearly increased laxity can have CAI [5]. This phenomenon is referred as functional instability.

Patients with functional instability are thought to have impaired neuromuscular control of ankle

joint caused by damaged receptors and soft tissues during initial trauma [6–8]. Since the ankle–foot complex is the only part of the body contacting the ground in most activities, this may hamper the total body balance ability.

Especially for high competitive levels in sports, superior balance ability is essential. To control balance, central nervous system integrates data from visual, vestibular, and proprioceptive systems and produces efferent commands to all muscle groups. However, especially during contact sports visual pathway is preoccupied with visual inputs from the environment, which causes the proprioceptive information to be more important.

Ankle proprioception can be influenced by training, fatigue, and ankle injuries [9, 10]. There are systems that can be used to measure ankle proprioception before and after injury or surgical trauma; joint position sense, peroneal reaction time, EMG evaluation of peroneal muscles, and balance tests are some of them. These balance tests can be static (single leg stance) or dynamic (single leg hop test).

There are still some questions that need an answer. Which are the exact anatomical structures that are responsible for proprioception? What happens to proprioception after injury or surgery? How is the balance maintained after surgery? What kind of intervention is useful to improve proprioception?

T.K. Ulku, M.D. (✉) • B. Kocaoglu, M.D.
Department of Orthopedics and Traumatology,
Faculty of Medicine, Acıbadem University,
Istanbul, Turkey
e-mail: tekin.ulku@acibadem.edu.tr

M.M. Caglar, P.T., MSc.
Clinical Sports Physiotherapy Center, Sportomed,
Istanbul, Turkey

J. Karlsson, M.D.
Department of Orthopedics, University of
Gothenburg, Goteborg, Sweden

© Springer International Publishing AG, part of Springer Nature 2018
D. Kaya et al. (eds.), *Proprioception in Orthopaedics, Sports Medicine and Rehabilitation*,
https://doi.org/10.1007/978-3-319-66640-2_11

Muscle spindles are considered to be the primary proprioceptors of the foot and ankle complex. The muscles around the ankle joint act as two groups. The extrinsic group is primarily responsible for detection of foot orientation relative to the body and the intrinsic muscle group sends information about the feet relative position to earth. Muscle spindles are known to be primarily responsible for this phenomenon, but exact mechanism still needs to be investigated.

Two anatomical structures around the foot and ankle have importance in terms of proprioception. One is the superior and inferior extensor ankle retinaculum. Vesalio described that ankle retinacula are simply pulleys preserving tendons close to bony structures [11]. However, in histological studies, Viladot in 1984 [12] and Pisani in 2004 [13] showed that the retinacula are more than just a mechanical stabilizer. Stecco et al. also showed that their histological features resemble network of receptors rather than a pulley [14]. It is also suggested that the peroneal retinaculum is stretched during inversion maneuver, thus inducing peroneal stretch reflex [14].

The lateral ankle ligament complex is the second important anatomical structure for proprioceptive function. Freeman stated that injured lateral ligament complex and capsule causes deafferentiation due to damaged mechanoreceptors [15]. More recent studies have shown that individuals with CAI have depressed levels of alpha motor neuron activity in quadriceps and hamstring muscles [16, 17]. However, more studies are needed to understand exact anatomical structures responsible for proprioception and how they work as one unit.

Surgical versus nonsurgical treatment for acute lateral ankle ligament sprain is still controversial. Surgery is more favorable than nonsurgical treatment in terms of return to sports, pain, and functional instability according to Kerkhoffs et al. [3]. After surgery, the ankle should be immobilized using a soft ankle brace for no more than 2 weeks. Normal range of motion and strength exercises should be started to restore normal ankle motion within 2 days after the surgery (Fig. 11.1). Endurance training using treadmill, sports-specific drills, and balance improving on a balance board should be started at 2–3 weeks after surgery [3, 17, 18] (Fig. 11.2).

Functional treatment includes a short period of immobilization followed by an early active range of motion exercises and early weight bearing (Fig. 11.3). However, there are only few studies reporting that early functional rehabilitation is superior to immobilization after ankle surgery. Karlsson et al. showed earlier return to sports when patients began an early ankle range of motion exercises as compared with those who were treated with 6 weeks of

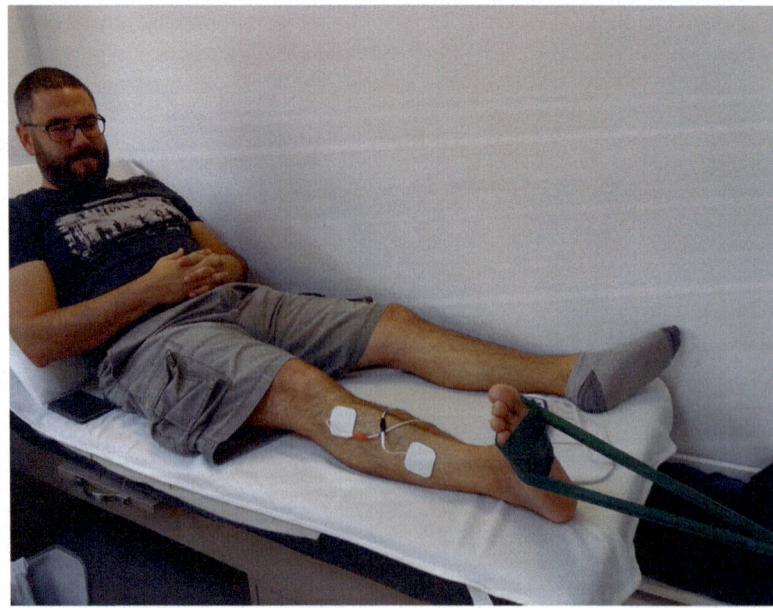

Fig. 11.1 Normal range of motion and strength exercises should be started to restore normal ankle motion within 2 days after the surgery

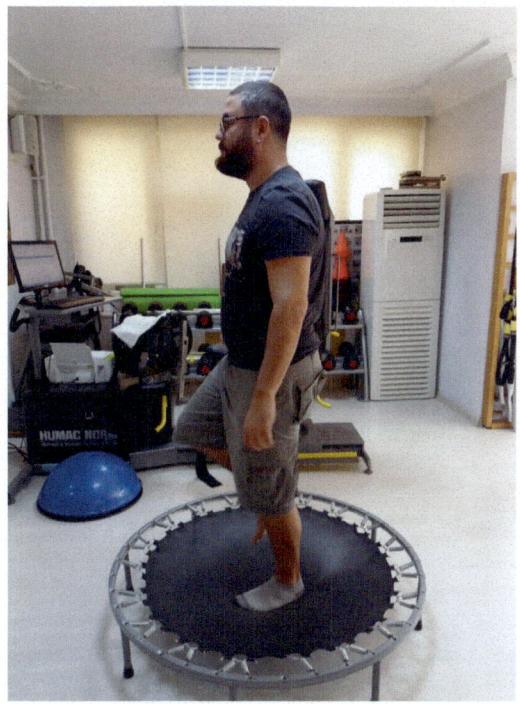

Fig. 11.2 Balance training could be started at 2–3 weeks after surgery

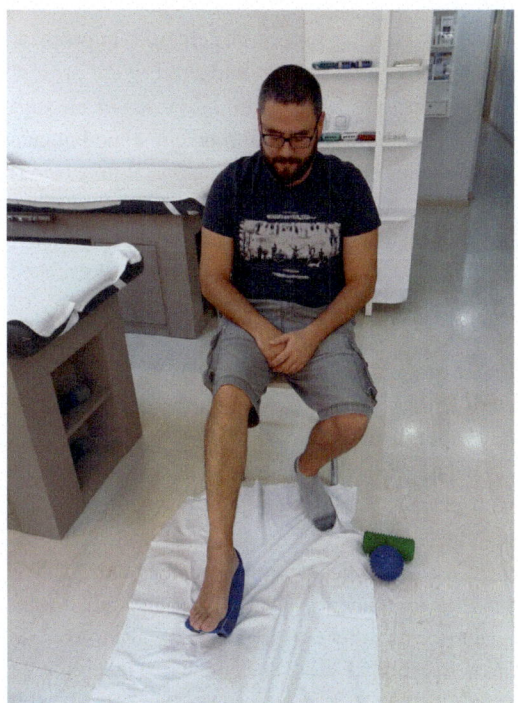

Fig. 11.3 Functional treatment has been developed mainly for nonsurgical treatment of ankle ligament injuries. It includes a short period of immobilization followed by an early active range of motion exercise and early weight-bearing

cast immobilization after surgery for chronic ankle instability [19].

The aim of functional rehabilitation is to prepare the patient for return to the pre-injury level of activity/sports as quickly as possible without affecting the surgical and functional outcome. Functional rehabilitation and sports-specific activity programs should include well-designed exercises that stress the tendons, ligaments, and muscles of the ankle. It should be born in mind that functional exercises should be individualized according to the specific needs of the patient.

Functional rehabilitation is a criterion-oriented program, which aims to improve range of motion, strength, proprioception, and sports-specific activities. During the first and second weeks after ankle surgery, rest and immobilization are important in order to reduce swelling and pain. However, patients should be encouraged to perform activities of daily living and weight-bearing as soon as possible. Unloading and immobilization have been shown to be deleterious to the healing of articular cartilage [19, 20]. At the end of functional rehabilitation, eccentric training should be started.

Eccentric training could be performed after a period of concentric exercises without pain. Eccentric exercises are always easier for patients who have pain while performing concentric exercises. Moreover, it has been stated that eccentric training creates greater force due to the "decreased rate of cross-bridge muscle detachments." It is possible to generate more muscle force for forceful activities with eccentric than concentric training [21].

Eccentric training for the calf muscles and ankle joint was first described in 1998 in the treatment of patients with Achilles tendinopathies. The treatment model with heavy-load eccentric calf muscle training had a good short-term effect on athletes [18].

Proprioception is another issue to be discussed. It is the sensory feedback that contributes to muscle sense, total posture, and joint stability. Proprioceptors are located within the muscles, tendons, ligaments, and other soft tissues in the body. They are sensors, which relay information to the brain about joint position, pressure, and muscle stretch. The proprioceptors of the ankle joint can be affected after ankle injury.

Proprioceptive deficits can predispose to both acute and chronic injury [22].

Strong proprioceptive sense allows for neuromuscular control of dynamic actions contributing to overall joint stability. Maintenance and improvements in neuromuscular control through proprioceptive training contribute greatly to increasing ankle stability. The proprioception can be improved by using functional and proprioceptive exercises. Isolated proprioceptive exercises are composed of three parts: proprioception of joints, balance capacity, and neuromuscular control [23].

Proprioceptive exercise programs vary in methodology, including duration, intensity, and protocols, but they all have effect on decreased reoccurrence of ankle sprains, increased muscular response time, and proprioception. With proprioceptive training, patients pass from the cognitive to the associative phase of learning. After months or years, they pass to the autonomous learning phase [24].

Clinicians have commonly used proprioceptive training as a part of their rehabilitation protocols. Progression of the proprioceptive training should be non-weight-bearing to weight-bearing (with/without external load), static to dynamic (such as running, lateral movements, backward movements, jumping, cutting, twisting, and pivoting), from slow speed to faster speed with balance and control, from two legs to one leg, and with visual control to no visual control (Fig. 11.4).

Wester et al. showed a 12-week proprioceptive training program that can improve the ankle joint position sense, while Riemann et al. did not find any significant improvement after a 4-week with proprioceptive training program [25, 26]. On the other hand, the effectiveness of 4–8 weeks of wobble board training on postural control and perceived stability has been well documented, and residual symptoms following ankle sprains can be reduced by a 12-week wobble board training program [27]. Potential explanations for these discrepancies might be the setting of the training programs (intensity, duration, and frequency) or the assessment techniques.

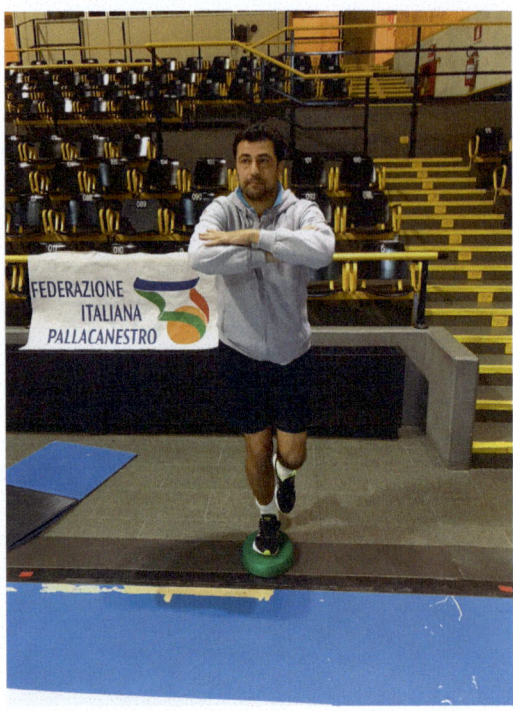

Fig. 11.4 Balance and control, two legs to one leg, and with visual or no visual control

Several studies in terms of changes in proprioception after ankle injury and surgery are present in the literature [28]. Although Vries et al. suggested that there is no difference in static balance tests in patients with chronic ankle injury (CAI) acute trauma and healthy controls, many studies have shown that after an acute inversion trauma and in CAI proprioceptive control is decreased [6, 7, 29–31]. After ankle stabilization surgery Li et al. studied postural sway [11]. They concluded that postural control is increased in patients operated with a modified Broström technique after 6 months of surgery.

Halasi studied joint position sense in patients with chronic ankle instability surgery [28]. After treatment using the Karlsson's surgical technique there was a significant improvement in joint position sense in ten patients. Kynsburg et al. studied joint position sense after nonsurgical treatment of chronic ankle instability [32]. They concluded that physical therapy is an effective way of treating patients with CAI and increases joint position sense.

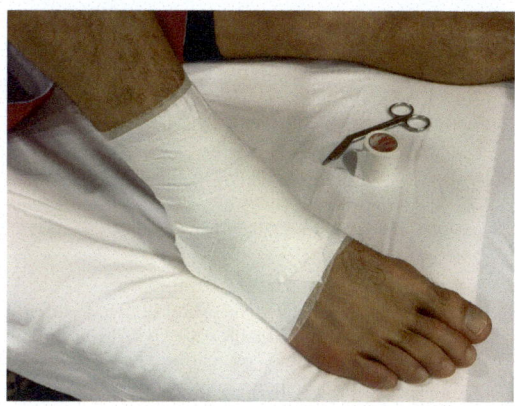

Fig. 11.5 Taping and ankle bracing improve proprioception

Physical therapists use active and passive interventions to improve proprioception and balance after injury. Taping, bracing, compression, and insoles are commonly studied passive intervention methods (Fig. 11.5). Most evidence shows that passive methods are mainly ineffective except insoles [33]. Studies in soccer players have shown positive effects. They probably increase perception capacity in the central nervous system (CNS) by creating an increased essential noise [34]. Since the time is too short to increase the number of mechanoreceptors, the CNS is probably learning faster to provide balance. Another issue is whether training should cover only the injured side or the non-injured as well? Some evidence shows that motor skills are transferrable between the hemispheres, indicating that only training uninjured side can also be beneficial [35].

Conclusion

Ankle proprioception plays an essential role in balance control. Proprioception is negatively affected in patients after an acute inversion trauma and in CAI. Although the exact mechanisms and anatomical structures responsible are unknown, surgery, insoles, and active intervention methods such as physical therapy appear to increase the proprioceptive control. Thus, rehabilitation programs should include proprioceptive training, balance, strengthening

exercises, functional movement, and endurance training after ankle surgery. Balance, functional exercises, and coordination training should continue to be an integral part of rehabilitation protocols.

References

1. Janssen KW, Kamper SJ. Ankle taping and bracing for proprioception. Br J Sports Med. 2013;47:527–8.
2. Karlsson J, Lansinger O. Lateral instability of the ankle joint. Clin Orthop Relat Res. 1992;276:253–61.
3. Kerkhoffs GM, Handoll HH, de Bie R, Rowe BH, Struijs PA. Surgical versus conservative treatment for acute injuries of the lateral ligament complex of the ankle in adults. Cochrane Database Syst Rev. 2007;(2):CD000380.
4. Valderrabano V, Wiewiorski M, Frigg A, Hintermann B, Leumann A. Chronic ankle instability. Unfallchirurg. 2007;110:691–700.
5. Tropp H, Odenrick P, Gillquist J. Stabilometry recordings in functional and mechanical instability of the ankle joint. Int J Sports Med. 1985;6:180–2.
6. Becker HP, Rosenbaum D. Chronic recurrent ligament instability on the lateral ankle. Orthopade. 1999;28:483–92.
7. Hertel J. Functional anatomy, pathomechanics, and pathophysiology of lateral ankle instability. J Athl Train. 2002;37:364–75.
8. Richie DH. Functional instability of the ankle and the role of neuromuscular control: a comprehensive review. J Foot Ankle Surg. 2001;40:240–51.
9. Winter T, Beck H, Walther A, Zwipp H, Rein S. Influence of a proprioceptive training on functional ankle stability in young speed skaters: a prospective randomized study. J Sports Sci. 2015;33(8):831–40.
10. Kynsburg A, Panics G, Halasi T. Long-term neuromus- cular training and ankle joint position sense. Acta Physiol Hung. 2010;97(2):183–91.
11. Li HY, Zheng JJ, Zhang J, Cai YH, Hua YH, Chen SY. The improvement of postural control in patients with mechanical ankle instability after lateral ankle-ligaments reconstruction. Knee Surg Sports Traumatol Arthrosc. 2016;24(4):1081–5.
12. Viladot A, Lorenzo JC, Salazar J, Rodríguez A. The subtalar joint: embryology and morphology. Foot Ankle Int. 1984;5:54–66.
13. Pisani G. Trattato di chirurgia del piede. 3rd ed. Torino: Minerva Medica; 2004.
14. Stecco C, Macchi V, Porzionato A, Morra A, Parenti A. The ankle retinacula: morphological evidence of the proprioceptive role of the facial system. Cells Tissues Organs. 2010;192:200–10.
15. Hertel J. Sensorimotor deficits with ankle sprains and chronic ankle instability. Clin Sports Med. 2008;27:353–70.

16. McVey ED, Palmieri RM, Docherty CL, Zinder SM, Ingersoll CD. Arthrogenic muscle inhibition in the leg muscles of subjects exhibiting functional ankle instability. Foot Ankle Int. 2005;26:1055–61.

17. Sedory EJ, McVey ED, Cross KM, Ingersoll CD, Hertel J. Arthrogenic muscle response of the quadriceps and hamstrings with chronic ankle instability. J Athl Train. 2007;42:355–60.

18. Alfredson H, Pietila T, Jonsson P, Lorentzon R. Heavy-load eccentric calf muscle training for the treatment of chronic Achilles tendinosis. Am J Sports Med. 1998;26:360–6.

19. Karlsson J, Lundin O, Lind K, Styf J. Early mobilization versus immobilization after ankle ligament stabilization. Scand J Med Sci Sports. 1999;9:299–303.

20. Behrens F, Kraft EL, Oegema TR. Biochemical changes in articular cartilage after joint immobilization by casting or external fixation. J Orthop Res. 1989;7:335–43.

21. Clark VM, Burden AM. A 4-week wobble board exercise programme improved muscle onset latency and perceived stability in individuals with a functionally unstable ankle. Phys Ther Sport. 2005;6:181–7.

22. Feuerbach JW, Grabiner MD, Koh TJ, Weiker GG. Effect of an ankle orthosis and ankle anesthesia on ankle joint proprioception. Am J Sports Med. 1994;22:223–9.

23. Eils E, Rosenbaum D. A multi-station proprioceptive exercise program in patients with ankle instability. Med Sci Sports Exerc. 2001;33:1991–8.

24. Fitzgerald GK, Axe MJ, Snyder-Mackler L. The efficacy of perturbation training in nonoperative anterior cruciate ligament rehabilitation programs for physically active individuals. Phys Ther. 2000;80:128–40.

25. Wester JU, Jespersen SM, Nielsen KD, Neumann L. Wobble board training after partial sprains of the lateral ligaments of the ankle: a prospective randomized study. J Orthop Sports Phys Ther. 1996;23:332–6.

26. Riemann BL, Tray NC, Lephart SM. Unilateral multiaxial coordination training and ankle kinesthesia, muscle strength, and postural control. J Sport Rehabil. 2003;12:13–30.

27. Hertel J. Functional instability following lateral ankle sprain. Sports Med. 2000;29:361–71.

28. Halasi T, Kynsburg A, Tállay A, Berkes I. Changes in joint position sense after surgically treated chronic lateral ankle instability. Br J Sports Med. 2005;39(11):818–24.

29. Vries S, Kingma I, Blankevoort L, van Dijk CN. Difference in balance measures between patients with chronic ankle instability and patients after an acute ankle inversion trauma. Knee Surg Sports Traumatol Arthrosc. 2010;18(5):601–6.

30. Docherty CL, Valovich McLeod TC, Shultz SJ. Postural control deficits in participants with functional ankle instability as measured by the balance error scoring system. Clin J Sport Med. 2006;16:203–8.

31. Jerosch J, Hoffstetter I, Bork H, Bischof M. The influence of orthoses on the proprioception of the ankle joint. Knee Surg Sports Traumatol Arthrosc. 1995;3:39–46.

32. Kynsburg A, Halasi T, Tállay A, Berkes I. Changes in joint position sense after conservatively treated chronic lateral ankle instability. Knee Surg Sports Traumatol Arthrosc. 2006;14(12):1299–306.

33. Han J, Anson J, Waddington G, Adams R, Liu Y. The role of ankle proprioception for balance control in relation to sports performance and injury. Biomed Res Int. 2015;2015:842–04.

34. You SH, Granata KP, Bunker LK. Effects of circumferential ankle pressure on ankle proprioception, stiffness, and postural stability: a preliminary investigation. J Orthop Sports Phys Ther. 2004;34(8):449–60.

35. Kaya D, Yuksel I, Turhan E, Asik M, Doral M. Proprioceptive and functional exercises after ankle surgery. Sports Injuries. 2015;4:1779–91.

Proprioception After the Arthroplasty

12

Hande Guney-Deniz and Michael Callaghan

12.1 Proprioception

Proprioception is defined as the ability to be aware of the conscious and unconscious level of the body parts and its positions and movements in space. Proprioception connects the stimuli derived from somatosensory, vestibular, and visual systems to regulate periarticular muscle activity, which provides joint stabilization by the central nervous system [1, 2]. The ability to sense motion, speed, and direction is defined as "kinesthesia" and is considered a part of the proprioceptive system. In other words, kinesthesia is a conscious awareness of joint position and movement with proprioceptive stimulation reaching the central nervous system [1, 2]. Another major component of proprioception is "joint position sense," which can be examined by active or passive reproduction testing of

H. Guney-Deniz, Ph.D., M.Sc., P.T. (✉)
Physiotherapy and Rehabilitation Department,
Faculty of Health Sciences, Hacettepe University,
Ankara, Turkey
e-mail: hande.guney@hacettepe.edu.tr

M. Callaghan, Ph.D., M.Sc., P.T.
Clinical Physiotherapy, Manchester Metropolitan
University, Manchester, UK

Centre for Musculoskeletal Research, University of
Manchester, Manchester, UK

Department of Physiotherapy, Manchester Royal
Infirmary, Manchester, UK
e-mail: michael.callaghan@mmu.ac.uk

a limb or joint without visual or vestibular input. A commonly used method is for subjects to move their extremity to the target angle, and then return to the neutral position before asking them to recreate the angle [3].

The somatosensory and sensorimotor systems are responsible for the harmonious and smooth movement of body parts and the proprioceptive sense controls the rhythmic organization of these two systems. Therefore, the proprioceptive system is considered as a preventive mechanism for the musculoskeletal injuries [4, 5].

12.2 Proprioception and Mechanoreceptors

Mechanoreceptors are specialized sensory receptors, which are responsible for converting stimuli into sensory impulses. These impulses are then interpreted by the central nervous system (CNS) to generate a response that regulates muscle tone and coordination [4–6]. The CNS incorporates the visual and vestibular inputs with the sensory impulses to produce the sense of position, kinesthesia, and coordinated movement [4].

The primary proprioceptive receptors are defined as length sensing muscle spindles in skeletal muscle, stretch receptors in the joint capsule, and Golgi tendon organs (GTOs) in tendons and ligaments. Those located in the deep skin and facial layers are considered to be supplementary receptors [5, 7]. The muscle spindles are able to provide afferent information across the entire range of motion, while the cutaneous and joint receptors are stimulated mainly at the end ranges of the joint movement [1, 8]. Tension-sensitive GTOs located in the tendinous segment of muscles provide afferent feedback when a muscle contraction causes tension on the tendon. As a protective mechanism, GTOs cause contraction of the antagonist muscle and facilitate the relaxation of the agonist muscle [1, 5, 7, 8].

The operative approach for implantation of a total joint arthroplasty or hemi-arthroplasty includes the cutting and subsequent repair of the muscles and usually releasing and sacrificing of ligaments, menisci, capsule, and other soft tissues around the joint which directly provide the proprioceptive input. Therefore, arthroplasty itself is likely to deteriorate proprioceptive sense [7, 9].

12.3 Proprioception and Balance and Falling

An integration of proprioceptive, visual, and vestibular inputs is required to maintain balance. Aging plays a certain role in decreased proprioceptive sense as well as impairments in vestibular and visual inputs, resulting in an overall reduction in sensory input required for balance [9–11]. It has been showed that impairment of just one of these three inputs does not directly affect balance as the other two are able to compensate for the other. However, disturbance of more than one input of the three is likely to adversely affect the balance in the elderly population [12].

Postural control is defined as achieving or restoring a state of balance during any posture or activity and is directly associated with balance. Anticipatory postural adjustments (APA) and compensatory postural adjustments (CPA) are the main mechanisms to retain postural control and balance. The muscle mass decreases up to 20–40% with aging [13, 14], resulting in a loss in postural musculature strength and impairment of postural control. In the elderly, the delay of the APA results with increase in CPA, suggesting decreased postural control and increased risk of falling [13, 14].

Depending on aging, joint replacement surgery is considered a permanent solution for degenerative joints, which are anatomically deformed, painful, and unable to execute motor and functional activities. Consequently, in the elderly, lower extremity joint replacement surgery might negatively affect a patient's balance by disrupting the natural proprioceptive system of the joint. Therefore, it is important to determine the risk factors of falling before the surgery due to the positive correlation between the preoperative risk factors and postoperative falling rate [15].

12.4 Proprioception After Knee Arthroplasty

Late stage knee osteoarthritis is the main cause of knee pain and functional limitations during daily activities and also is a primary reason for having total knee arthroplasty (TKA). The soft tissue adaptations during aging and long-term impaired kinematics affect proprioception in patients with knee arthritis [16]. Both dynamic and static stabilizers can be impaired with aging, which contribute to proprioceptive and functional damage. Combination of these morphological and biomechanical changes with knee arthroplasty might have an adverse effect on proprioceptive sensation [17, 18]. On the other hand, it is stated that tissues around the knee that remain after TKA contribute to proprioception and that the influence of proper gap balancing during the surgical procedure plays a large role in preserving proprioception and may influence patient outcomes after TKA [19].

Intraoperative MRI studies showed that anterior cruciate ligament is intact in 60% of osteoarthritis patients who are scheduled for knee arthroplasty [20]. Knee arthroplasty procedures other than TKA, such as uni-compartmental replacement, usually preserve the anterior or posterior cruciate ligaments. Retaining the anterior cruciate ligament in the knee arthroplasty is as critical as the posterior cruciate ligament. It is well known that the anterior cruciate ligament carries direct proprioceptive sensation to the central nervous system [21].

The importance of the surgical procedure itself in maintaining proprioception cannot be overstated. Numerous papers have assessed certain factors regarding the surgical procedure and their effect on postoperative proprioception (Table 12.1).

Another surgical factor is the presence of bilateral knee OA. Performing bilateral TKA may be beneficial to balance. One study found improved balance after the postoperative period. The authors interpreted that the position of the center of gravity became more centralized in

Table 12.1 Alterations in proprioception after total knee arthroplasty

Paper	Operation and no. of patients	Procedure	Main outcome measure	Results
Barrett et al. (1991) [22]	Unilateral TKA, $n = 45$ OA knees, $n = 21$ replacements, $n = 81$ healthy controls	Semi-constrained ($n = 10$), hinged joint replacement ($n = 11$)	JPS	Patients with semi-constrained TKA showed more improvement in proprioception than those with hinge replacements
Warren et al. (1993) [23]	Unilateral TKA, $n = 40$	PCL retaining ($n = 20$), PCL substituting ($n = 20$)	JPS	PCL retained TKA had better JPS results compared to sacrificed PCL
Simmons et al. [16]	Unilateral TKA, $n = 28$, UKA, $n = 10$	ACL and PCL retained in UKA ACL substituted and PCL retained ($n = 15$) and ACL and PCL substituted ($n = 13$) in TKA	Kinesthesia (threshold of perception) JPS	No difference in kinesthesia and JPS among any of the three groups Maintaining the ACL and PCL did not reveal improved proprioception in UKA nor did maintaining the PCL reveal improved proprioception in TKA
Cash et al. (1996) [24]	Unilateral TKA, $n = 60$	PCL retaining $n = 30$, PCL substituting $n = 30$	Threshold of perception	No differences between groups in proprioception
Ishii et al. (1997) [25]	Unilateral TKA, $n = 55$ knees	Semi-constrained, With and without; PCL retention, patellar resurfacing, cement for fixation	JPS	No difference among all the arthroplasty groups
Fuchs and Thorwesten (1999) [26]	Unilateral TKA, $n = 28$, 25 healthy controls	Non-constrained, PCL retaining	JPS	Significant proprioceptive deficit both in the operated and non-operated extremity, particularly marked at 60° of knee flexion
Swanik et al. (2004) [27]	Unilateral TKA, $n = 20$	PCL retaining ($n = 10$) Posterior stabilized prosthesis ($n = 10$)	Kinesthesia JPS Balance	Posterior stabilized prosthesis reproduced more accurate JPS when the knee was extended from a flexed position No significant improvement detected between groups when preoperative and postoperative 6th months results were compared
Bathis et al. (2005) [28]	Unilateral TKA $n = 50$	Surgical approach; midvastus versus parapatellar	JPS	Midvastus approach had better JPS results compared to parapatellar approach

(continued)

Table 12.1 (continued)

Paper	Operation and no. of patients	Procedure	Main outcome measure	Results
Isaac et al. (2007) [29]	Unilateral TKA (n = 17) and UKA (17)		JPS Postural sway	Improvement in JPS was similar in both groups between preoperatively and at 6th months postoperatively Postural sway improvement was found better in UKA compared to TKA Dynamic aspects of proprioception improve more after UKA than TKA
Gauchard et al. [30]	Unilateral TKA, n = 10, controls, n = 20		Sensory organization test with posturography	No significant difference between controls and patients at 6th week after surgery
Vandekerckhove et al. (2015) [31]	Unilateral TKA, n = 45	PCL substituting (n = 27) PCL retaining (n = 18)	Balance and postural control	Retaining the PCL in TKA does not result in an improved proprioception
Baumann et al. (2016) [32]	Unilateral arthroplasty, n = 60	Bicruciate-retaining knee arthroplasty, UKA, Posterior stabilized total knee arthroplasty	Single leg balance testing	Superior static balance ability after preservation of both cruciate ligaments in arthroplasty of the knee, indicating superior proprioceptive function

those with bilateral TKAs, whereas in the unilateral TKA group it remained on the operative extremity [33].

The critical time for proprioceptive loss in the early postoperative period is described as 6 weeks. It has been suggested that this time may be a transition point between proprioceptive loss and early adaptations to new, learned motor patterns. It has been recommended that postoperative rehabilitation protocols include motor re-learning principles in an attempt to train the patient to recognize a new pattern of knee load distribution [34].

12.5 Proprioception After Hip Arthroplasty

As in the knee joint, degenerative changes in the hip are related to decreased mobility and impairments in the daily living. Total hip arthroplasty (THA) is a gold standard operative technique for pain relief and improving functional capacity [35].

The hip joint receives the proprioceptive inputs from the Pacini, Ruffini, and Golgi corpuscles around joint capsule, ligaments, and labrum [36]. Ishii et al. showed no decrease in the joint proprioception between THA patients and hemiarthroplasty and control groups despite capsulotomy being performed in all patients. The authors suggested that factors like tension receptors in the adjacent tendons and muscles might have greater effects than the capsular component on hip proprioception [37]. Karanjia et al. reported that in THA patients with capsulotomy, there were minimal influences on passive hip joint position sense. They specified that the velocity of the passive movement during testing was the major component for the joint position detection [38].

All the previous findings indicated that proprioceptive sense does not only depend on capsular receptors but also depends on afferents in muscles, tendons, and ligaments.

Studies also showed proprioceptive sense did not decrease after surgery, although, the joint capsule and the mechanoreceptors were sacrificed during the arthroplasty. A possible explanation for this improvement is that improved joint biomechanics allow for a better proprioceptive response. Also, it is suggested that muscle receptors are the prominent determinants of joint position sense and the capsular receptors might play a secondary role [39].

Different surgery procedures such as total hip arthroplasty and hemi-arthroplasty have no influence on hip joint proprioception [37], suggesting that joint and bone receptors play a smaller role than the periarticular tendon receptors [37, 40]. On the other hand, a decrease of receptor activity was reported in patients with THA at 1 week postoperatively with a significant increase in proprioception after 40 days [41].

12.6   Proprioception and Ankle Arthroplasty

Proprioception and maintaining the balance are important topics for improvement of the functional outcomes after total ankle arthroplasty [42]. Several studies investigated proprioceptive sense differences after total ankle arthroplasty. Conti et al. [43] evaluated joint position sense in 13 total ankle arthroplasty patients in a 2-year follow-up study and demonstrated that there were no differences in proprioception between a total ankle arthroplasty and the unaffected side. Lee et al. [44] compared static and dynamic postural balance in patients with unilateral total ankle arthroplasty and age-matched controls. They detected a higher degree of dynamic postural imbalance in patients and concluded that these changes might be due to the damaged proprioceptive receptors caused by capsular excision, weakness of ankle plantar flexors, restricted range of motion, and altered weight bearing.

In general, joint arthroplasty in the lower extremity is a successful procedure that significantly relieves the pain associated with end-stage osteoarthritis. The alleviating of pain following surgery is associated with functional improvement.

Improvement in proprioceptive sense is one the major aims for maintaining the balance and function after lower extremity arthroplasty. In general, patients following total hip and knee arthroplasty exhibit better unilateral proprioception and balance in comparison with total ankle arthroplasty patients. It may be beneficial to include a rigorous proprioception and balance-training program in total ankle arthroplasty patients to optimize functional outcomes [45].

12.7   Proprioception and Shoulder Arthroplasty

Chronic rotator cuff deficiency, degenerative disease, previous trauma, or surgery may lead to glenohumeral osteoarthritis which is associated with pain and loss of range of motion in the shoulder joint. Shoulder arthroplasty is a frequently used treatment modality in glenohumeral osteoarthritis and may enhance the shoulder function [35, 46, 47].

The perception of joint position and motion in the shoulder is essential for the placement of the hand in upper limb function. A feedback mechanism exists for control of shoulder muscular action, which serves as a protective mechanism against excessive strain in the capsule and ligamentous structures. Patients with shoulder problems, especially with end-stage osteoarthritis, have a loss of cartilage and mechanoreceptors, joint laxity, and significant inflammation resulting in reduced proprioception. On the other hand, the cutting (and subsequent repair) of the subscapularis muscle and release of all glenohumeral ligaments during shoulder arthroplasty surgery may contribute to proprioceptive deficits [46, 47].

There are a few studies, which investigated changes in proprioception after total shoulder arthroplasty. In one study, a passive and guided angle reproduction test was performed in 20 patients with shoulder osteoarthritis before and 6 months after total shoulder arthroplasty. The authors reported significant improvements in the joint position sense and perception of movement at the 6th month postoperatively [46]. Conversely, another study found no difference in proprioception at 6 months after surgery [47]. Authors also indicated that active joint reproduction did not change with different types of shoulder arthroplasty such as total shoulder arthroplasty, hemiarthroplasty, and reverse shoulder arthroplasty [47]. In addition, Maier et al. found no differences in a shoulder active angle reproduction test in total shoulder arthroplasty and hemi-arthroplasty 6 months and 3 years after surgery. The authors also indicated that the postoperative deterioration of proprioception was more distinctive in hemi-arthroplasty than in total arthroplasty group [47]. These results implied that arthroplasty in the shoulder joint might adversely affect shoulder proprioception and this was mainly associated with the surgical approach that contained dissection of the subscapularis muscle and the glenohumeral ligaments. In order to be able to reduce the negative impacts on postoperative proprioceptive sense, further studies are needed on the effectiveness of preoperative and postoperative proprioceptive exercises after shoulder arthroplasty.

12.8 Proprioception and Elbow Arthroplasty

Total elbow arthroplasty is a reliable surgical option for patients with painful arthritis, segmental and comminuted distal humeral fractures [48, 49]. Arthroplasty in the elbow joint is traumatic surgery and the soft tissue damage is significant. The triceps is reflected along with the forearm fascia. Both flexor and extensor origins are released from the epicondyles. Collateral ligaments are also released, and the capsule is excised. This means that significant damage to the main tissue sources of proprioceptive afferents, including skin, capsule, muscle, and tendon, can be expected.

In one study, proprioception in the total elbow arthroplasty patients was found significantly inferior compared with the contralateral side and with healthy controls. The authors interpreted these results that the extensive surgery damaged the tissues that were the main sources of proprioceptive input (skin, muscle, tendon, capsule, and ligaments). The role of proprioception in patients' disability and elbow stability after total elbow arthroplasty is still unknown and caution is suggested when using an approach on the extensor aspect, preservation of muscle attachment when possible, and avoidance of large elevation of skin flaps from over the muscle [49].

12.9 Development of Proprioception After Arthroplasty

The primary aim of the rehabilitation is to restore functional outcomes while protecting the mechanical stability of the arthroplasty. Therefore, proprioceptive exercises and balance must be included in rehabilitation programs especially before and after surgery for functional recovery. These exercises should be designed to stimulate the neuromotor programming, which leads to increased proprioceptive afferent input to the central nervous system. By this way, the stimulus-response-recognition circuits, which are already compromised by the pathology and surgery, would be activated, and improve functional stability [50].

It is commonplace to prescribe several sessions of physiotherapy in an attempt to maintain range of motion and prevent postoperative arthrofibrosis. Rehabilitation in the immediate and early (3–6 months) postoperative periods results in a measurable improvement in motor coordination in especially lower limb arthroplasty [30, 51]. As mentioned before, proprioceptive loss can be seen in the early postoperative period; therefore, it is recommended to begin proprioceptive exercises as soon as possible [9, 47]. The postoperative rehabilitation protocols should include motor re-learning principles in an attempt to train the body to recognize the new pattern of joint load distributions.

In addition, the preoperative training programs on proprioception has also been recommended and was found to result in improved balance and gait speed after lower limb arthroplasty, as well as subjective function scores [19].

12.10 Strategies for Maintaining or Improving Proprioception After Arthroplasty

12.10.1 Strengthening Exercises

As the main proprioceptive receptors are located in the muscles, the muscle strengthening is essential for the improvement of proprioceptive sense before and after surgery. It is reported that hip muscle strength is the most important factor for maintaining the postural control and balance in patients with lower limb arthroplasty [52]. It is well known that gluteus medius weakness is disturbing the postural control [52, 53]. It is found that, the quick stair climbing and single leg stance is strongly correlated with the strength of the quadriceps and hip abductor muscles in total knee arthroplasty patients [52–54].

Strengthening of the muscles before and in the early period after surgery would improve joint stability, mobility, and postural control. In this manner, isometric strengthening, range of motion exercises, and core stability exercises can be applied to the patients with arthroplasty.

12.10.2 Closed and Open Kinetic Chain Exercises

Closed kinetic chain (CKC) exercises are the form of exercises in which the distal portion of the extremity is fixed and remains in constant contact with the ground. CKC exercises result in decreased shear forces, increased joint stability, increased proprioceptive inputs, and enhanced dynamic stability. Therefore after surgery, CKC exercises can be easily and securely applicable. The open kinetic chain (OKC) exercises can be applied after CKC exercises in the postoperative period because CKC exercises are proposed to be safer than the OKC exercises. Both OKC and CKC exercises can be performed as aquatic exercises, when gradual weight bearing can be introduced, resistance exercises gradually progressed, and proprioceptive tasks practiced [55, 56].

12.10.3 Passive and Active Joint Repositioning

Joint positioning exercises, when performed at the end rage of joint motion would stimulate motor programming from conscious to unconscious levels [1]. On the other hand, passive repositioning would stimulate mechanoreceptors around joint capsule and ligaments, while active repositioning relies on input from both articular and muscle receptors [1, 7, 38].

12.10.4 Proprioceptive Neuromuscular Facilitation (PNF)

PNF techniques are designed to improve the neuromuscular response by stimulating the stretch receptors in the musculo-tendinous unit [57]. Rhythmic stabilization (RS) is one of the form of PNF techniques that stimulates the articular and muscular mechanoreceptors resulting with the improvement of dynamic joint stabilization. RS exercises can be performed in the functional position of each joint as well as in OKC with manual perturbations or assistance or in CKC with the use of Swiss balls, wobble boards, Bosu balls, or other unstable surfaces [57].

12.10.5 Aquatherapy

Aquatherapy is widely used in the rehabilitation of total joint replacement and is an effective way to reduce pain, to improve range of motion, and to strengthen muscles. The buoyancy of the water allows assisted, active, and resisted exercises while hydrostatic pressure supports and stabilizes the joints, allowing patients to perform exercises without a fear of falling, decreasing pain and improving cardiovascular functions. In addition, tactile stimulation from the turbulence generated during movements provides feedback that supports the proprioceptive inputs and maintains the balance [58, 59].

12.10.6 Balance Training and Proprioception

It is well known that in the lower limb arthroplasty patients a possible reason of balance deficit would be the loss of proprioception [53, 60]. Therefore, the rehabilitation programs should include weight bearing and balance exercises [61]. Balance training, including static stabilization of stance (such as foam activity) and dynamic stabilization of stance (such as tilt board activity or an ankle platform system), activates the hip and ankle proprioceptors and may help improve a patient's proprioception, balance, and postural control strategies [53]. Side steps, tandem walk, cross-over steps, stepping over obstacle, slope ascend and descend, and stair climbing exercises should also be incorporated into balance exercises [53, 62].

Recently, virtual reality and video game systems are commonly implemented in rehabilitation programs. The balance board included in these gaming systems is similar in concept to a force plate. This board measures and interprets the pressure distribution of weight applied by the user and provides feedback on exercises performed. Thus, these kinds of systems are potentially acceptable as an adjunct to rehabilitation programs following arthroplasty surgery. Provided the game is carefully chosen by a knowledgeable physiotherapist, it should simulate the desired activities to encourage lower extremity movement, challenge balance, and require the patient to remain in a standing position during the game. The preliminary research findings are quite promising although further research is required to establish the effects on proprioception after arthroplasties [63, 64].

Conclusion

Documenting the alterations in proprioceptive sense after arthroplasty is important for improving postural control, joint position, and smooth movement. However, there are controversies on the effects of different type of arthroplasty and surgical procedures on proprioception as well as the appropriate pre- and postoperative rehabilitation protocols. Further research is required to establish the effects of both surgical techniques and different rehabilitation protocols on proprioception and functional outcomes after arthroplasty surgery.

References

1. Lephart SM, Riemann BL, Fu FH. Introduction to the sensorimotor system. In: Lephart SM, Fu FH, editors. Proprioception and neuromuscular control in joint stability. Champaign, IL: Human Kinetics; 2000.
2. Riemann BL, Lephart SM. The sensorimotor system. Part I: The physiologic basis of functional joint stability. J Athl Train. 2002;37(1):71.
3. Goble DJ. Proprioceptive acuity assessment via joint position matching: from basic science to general practice. Phys Ther. 2010;90(8):1176.
4. Myers JB, Lephart SM. The role of the sensorimotor system in the athletic shoulder. J Athl Train. 2000;35(3):351.
5. Proske U, Gandevia SC. The kinaesthetic senses. J Physiol. 2009;587(17):4139–46.
6. Stillman BC. Making sense of proprioception: the meaning of proprioception, kinaesthesia and related terms. Physiotherapy. 2002;88(11):667–76.
7. Karakaya IC, Karakaya MG. Proprioception and gender. In: Kaya D, editor. Proprioception: the forgotten sixth sense. Foster City: OMICS Group eBooks; 2014.
8. Ribeiro F, Oliveira J. Factors influencing proprioception: what do they reveal? INTECH Open Access Publisher; 2011.
9. Wodowski AJ, Swigler CW, Liu H, Nord KM, Toy PC, Mihalko WM. Proprioception and knee arthroplasty: a literature review. Orthop Clin North Am. 2016;47(2):301–9.
10. Baloh RW, Jacobson KM, Socotch TM. The effect of aging on visual-vestibuloocular responses. Exp Brain Res. 1993;95(3):509–16.
11. Paige GD. Senescence of human visual-vestibular interactions. 1. Vestibulo-ocular reflex and adaptive plasticity with aging. J Vestib Res. 1991;2(2):133–51.
12. Teasdale N, Stelmach GE, Breunig A. Postural sway characteristics of the elderly under normal and altered visual and support surface conditions. J Gerontol. 1991;46(6):B238–B44.
13. Doherty TJ. Invited review: aging and sarcopenia. J Appl Physiol. 2003;95(4):1717–27.
14. Kanekar N, Aruin AS. The effect of aging on anticipatory postural control. Exp Brain Res. 2014;232(4): 1127–36.
15. Swinkels A, Newman JH, Allain TJ. A prospective observational study of falling before and after knee replacement surgery. Age Ageing. 2009;38(2):175–81.
16. Simmons S, Lephart S, Rubash H, Pifer GW, Barrack R. Proprioception after unicondylar knee arthroplasty

versus total knee arthroplasty. Clin Orthop Relat Res. 1996;331:179–84.

17. Knoop J, Steultjens MPM, Van der Leeden M, Van der Esch M, Thorstensson CA, Roorda LD, et al. Proprioception in knee osteoarthritis: a narrative review. Osteoarthritis Cartilage. 2011;19(4):381–8.

18. Rogers MW, Tamulevicius N, Coetsee MF, Curry BF, Semple SJ. Knee osteoarthritis and the efficacy of kinesthesia, balance & agility exercise training: a pilot study. Int J Exerc Sci. 2011;4(2):124.

19. Gstoettner M, Raschner C, Dirnberger E, Leimser H, Krismer M. Preoperative proprioceptive training in patients with total knee arthroplasty. Knee. 2011;18(4):265–70.

20. Pritchett JW. Bicruciate-retaining total knee replacement provides satisfactory function and implant survivorship at 23 years. Clin Orthop Relat Res. 2015;473(7):2327–33.

21. Relph N, Herrington L, Tyson S. The effects of ACL injury on knee proprioception: a meta-analysis. Physiotherapy. 2014;100(3):187–95.

22. Barrett DS, Cobb AG, Bentley G. Joint proprioception in normal, osteoarthritic and replaced knees. J Bone Joint Surg Br. 1991;73(1):53–6.

23. Warren PJ, Olanlokun TK, Cobb AG, Bentley G. Proprioception after knee arthroplasty. The influence of prosthetic design. Clin Orthop Relat Res. 1993;297:182–7.

24. Cash RM, Gonzalez MH, Garst J, Barmada R, Stern SH. Proprioception after arthroplasty: role of the posterior cruciate ligament. Clin Orthop Relat Res. 1996;331:172–8.

25. Ishii Y, Terajima K, Terashima S, Bechtold JE, Laskin RS. Comparison of joint position sense after total knee arthroplasty. J Arthroplasty. 1997;12(5):541–5.

26. Fuchs S, Thorwesten L, Niewerth S. Proprioceptive function in knees with and without total knee arthroplasty. Am J Phys Med Rehabil. 1999;78(1):39–45.

27. Swanik CB, Lephart SM, Rubash HE. Proprioception, kinesthesia, and balance after total knee arthroplasty with cruciate-retaining and posterior stabilized prostheses. J Bone Joint Surg Am. 2004;86-A(2):328–34.

28. Bäthis H, Perlick L, Blum C, Lüring C, Perlick C, et al. Midvastus approach in total knee arthroplasty: a randomized, double-blinded study on early rehabilitation. Knee Surg Sports Traumatol Arthrosc. 2005;13(7):545–50.

29. Isaac SM, Barker KL, Danial IN, Beard DJ, Dodd CA. et al. Does arthroplasty type influence knee joint proprioception? A longitudinal prospective study comparing total and unicompartmental arthroplasty. Knee. 2007;14(3):212–7.

30. Gauchard GC, Vançon G, Meyer P, Mainard D, Perrin PP. On the role of knee joint in balance control and postural strategies: effects of total knee replacement in elderly subjects with knee osteoarthritis. Gait Posture. 2010;32(2):155–60.

31. Vandekerckhove PJ, Parys R, Tampere T, Linden P, Van den Daelen L, Verdonk PC. Does cruciate retention primary total knee arthroplasty affect proprioception, strength and clinical outcome? Knee Surg Sports Traumatol Arthrosc. 2015;23(6):1644–52.

32. Baumann F, Bahadin Ö, Krutsch W, Zellner J, Nerlich M, Angele P, Tibesku CO. Proprioception after bicruciate-retaining total knee arthroplasty is comparable to unicompartmental knee arthroplasty. Knee Surg Sports Traumatol Arthrosc. 2017;25(6):1697–704.

33. Ishii Y, Noguchi H, Takeda M, Sato J, Kishimoto Y, Toyabe S-I. Changes of body balance before and after total knee arthroplasty in patients who suffered from bilateral knee osteoarthritis. J Orthop Sci. 2013;18(5):727–32.

34. Thewlis D, Hillier S, Hobbs SJ, Richards J. Preoperative asymmetry in load distribution during quite stance persist following total knee arthroplasty. Knee Surg Sports Traumatol Arthrosc. 2014;22(3):609–14.

35. Grayson CW, Decker RC. Total joint arthroplasty for persons with osteoarthritis. PM R. 2012;4((5): S97–S103.

36. Moraes MRB, Cavalcante MLC, Leite JAD, Macedo JN, Sampaio MLB, Jamacaru VF, et al. The characteristics of the mechanoreceptors of the hip with arthrosis. J Orthop Surg Res. 2011;6(1):58.

37. Ishii Y, Tojo T, Terajima K, Terashima S, Bechtold JE. Intracapsular components do not change hip proprioception. J Bone Joint Surg. 1999;81(2):345–8.

38. Karanjia PN, Ferguson JH. Passive joint position sense after total hip replacement surgery. Ann Neurol. 1983;13(6):654–7.

39. Nallegowda M, Singh U, Bhan S, Wadhwa S, Handa G, Dwivedi SN. Balance and gait in total hip replacement: a pilot study. Am J Phys Med Rehabil. 2003;82(9):669–77.

40. Szymanski C, Thouvarecq R, Dujardin F, Migaud H, Maynou C, Girard J. Functional performance after hip resurfacing or total hip replacement: a comparative assessment with non-operated subjects. Orthop Traumatol Surg Res. 2012;98(1):1–7.

41. Zati A, Degli Esposti S, Spagnoletti C, Martucci E, Bilotta TW. Does total hip arthroplasty mean sensorial and proprioceptive lesion? A clinical study. Chir Organi Mov. 1996;82(3):239–47.

42. Easley ME, Adams SB, Hembree WC, DeOrio JK. Results of total ankle arthroplasty. J Bone Joint Surg Am. 2011;93(15):1455–68.

43. Conti SF, Dazen D, Stewart G, Green A, Martin R, Kuxhaus L, et al. Proprioception after total ankle arthroplasty. Foot Ankle Int. 2008;29(11):1069–73.

44. Lee KB, Park YH, Song EK, Yoon TR, Jung KI. Static and dynamic postural balance after successful mobile-bearing total ankle arthroplasty. Arch Phys Med Rehabil. 2010;91(4):519–22.

45. Butler RJ, Thiele RAR, Barnes CL, Bolognesi MP, Queen RM. Unipedal balance is affected by lower extremity joint arthroplasty procedure 1 year following surgery. J Arthroplasty. 2015;30(2):286–9.

46. Cuomo F, Birdzell MG, Zuckerman JD. The effect of degenerative arthritis and prosthetic arthroplasty on shoulder proprioception. J Shoulder Elbow Surg. 2005;14(4):345–8.

47. Kasten P, Maier M, Rettig O, Raiss P, Wolf S, Loew M. Proprioception in total, hemi-and reverse shoulder arthroplasty in 3D motion analyses: a prospective study. Int Orthop. 2009;33(6):1641.

48. Schneeberger AG, Meyer DC, Yian EH. Coonrad-Morrey total elbow replacement for primary and revision surgery: a 2-to 7.5-year follow-up study. J Shoulder Elbow Surg. 2007;16(3):S47–54.

49. Lubiatowski P, Olczak I, Lisiewicz E, Ogrodowicz P, Bręborowicz M, Romanowski L. Elbow joint position sense after total elbow arthroplasty. J Shoulder Elbow Surg. 2014;23(5):693–700.

50. Felicetti G, Chiappano G, Molino A, Brignoli E, Maestri R, Maini M. Preliminary study on the validity of an instrumental method of evaluating proprioception in patients undergoing total knee arthroplasty. Eura Medicophys. 2003;39(2):87–94.

51. Pohl T, Brauner T, Wearing S, Stamer K, Horstmann T. Effects of sensorimotor training volume on recovery of sensorimotor function in patients following lower limb arthroplasty. BMC Musculoskelet Disord. 2015;16(1):195.

52. Bhave A, Marker DR, Seyler TM, Ulrich SD, Plate JF, Mont MA. Functional problems and treatment solutions after total hip arthroplasty. J Arthroplasty. 2007;22(6):116–24.

53. Liao C-D, Liou T-H, Huang Y-Y, Huang Y-C. Effects of balance training on functional outcome after total knee replacement in patients with knee osteoarthritis: a randomized controlled trial. Clin Rehabil. 2013;27(8):697–709.

54. Almeida GJ, Schroeder CA, Gil AB, Fitzgerald GK, Piva SR. Interrater reliability and validity of the stair ascend/descend test in subjects with total knee arthroplasty. Arch Phys Med Rehabil. 2010;91(6):932–8.

55. Meier W, Mizner R, Marcus R, Dibble L, Peters C, Lastayo PC. Total knee arthroplasty: muscle impairments, functional limitations, and recommended rehabilitation approaches. J Orthop Sports Phys Therapy. 2008;38(5):246–56.

56. Benedetti MG, Catani F, Bilotta TW, Marcacci M, Mariani E, Giannini S. Muscle activation pattern and gait biomechanics after total knee replacement. Clin Biomech. 2003;18(9):871–6.

57. Borsa PA, Lephart SM, Kocher MS, Lephart SP. Functional assessment and rehabilitation of shoulder proprioception for glenohumeral instability. J Sport Rehabil. 1994;3(1):84–104.

58. Lobet S, Pendeville E, Dalzell R, Defalque A, Lambert C, Pothen D, et al. The role of physiotherapy after total knee arthroplasty in patients with haemophilia. Haemophilia. 2008;14(5):989–98.

59. Di Monaco M, Castiglioni C. Which type of exercise therapy is effective after hip arthroplasty? A systematic review of randomized controlled trials. Eur J Phys Rehabil Med. 2013;49(6):893–907.

60. Levinger P, Menz HB, Morrow AD, Wee E, Feller JA, Bartlett JR, et al. Lower limb proprioception deficits persist following knee replacement surgery despite improvements in knee extension strength. Knee Surg Sports Traumatol Arthrosc. 2012;20(6):1097–103.

61. Moutzouri M, Gleeson N, Billis E, Tsepis E, Panoutsopoulou I, Gliatis J. The effect of total knee arthroplasty on patients' balance and incidence of falls: a systematic review. Knee Surg Sports Traumatol Arthrosc. 2017;25:3439–51.

62. Quelard B, Rachet O. Rehabilitation protocol following total knee arthroplasty. In: Bonnin M, Amendola NA, Bellemans J, MacDonald SJ, Menetrey J, editors. The knee joint: surgical techniques and strategies. Paris: Springer; 2013. p. 823–38.

63. Fung V, Ho A, Shaffer J, Chung E, Gomez M. Use of Nintendo Wii Fit™ in the rehabilitation of outpatients following total knee replacement: a preliminary randomised controlled trial. Physiotherapy. 2012;98(3):183–8.

64. Tugay N, Tugay BU. Proprioception after arthroplasty. In: Kaya D, editor. Proprioception: the forgotten sixth sense. Foster City: OMICS Group eBooks; 2016, pp. 145–157.

Return to Sports and Proprioception

13

Hayri Baran Yosmaoglu and Emel Sonmezer

13.1 Introduction

The return to sport is one of the most important phase in the rehabilitation of sports injuries. Many protocols and guides have been published on when it should take place after the various sports injuries. When examining the return criteria to sports contained in these guides, it is seen that the return to sport is associated with many factors. The type of injury, injury severity, the level of sport, and the intrinsic and extrinsic risk factors that will cause reinjury are some of them [1]. Besides, psychological, ethical, social, and legal factors other than injury that may affect the return to sport may need to be considered. When all these factors are taken into account, the difficulty of establishing a standard model based on scientific evidence, covering all injuries and sports is obvious. Nevertheless, various models and algorithms have been defined that can guide the decision to return to sport based on evidence [1, 2].

"How much is the effect of the sense of proprioception on the decision to return to sport?" In order to be able to answer this question correctly, the components of the decision to return to sport must be well analyzed. In this section, the factors effecting to return to sport following sports injury and the place of proprioception in return to sport and its effect on reinjury were examined in detail.

13.2 Evidence-Based Decision of Return to Sport

The return to sport, which is one of the main parts of the rehabilitation program after sports injuries, is one of the most important phases in terms of restoration of sportive performance. This phase of rehabilitation consists mainly of a variety of exercises based on strength, endurance, flexibility, agility, and restoration of reaction time. However, the sport-specific requirements that need to be improved are different for every athlete and injury. Therefore, the rehabilitation program needs to be designed and implemented individually. Perhaps the most critical decision on the return to sport is the timing of the return after injury. Timing is crucial to the risk of reinjury; therefore, efforts have been made to establish standards based on evidence to help ensuring that the decision to return to sport is given correctly [2]. It is defined that there are three basic evidence-based steps of the decision of the return to sport. These are: *Evaluation of health status, participation risk, and decision modification* [2].

H.B. Yosmaoglu, Ph.D., M.Sc., P.T. (✉)
E. Sonmezer, Ph.D., M.Sc., P.T.
Department of Physical Therapy and Rehabilitation,
Faculty of Health Sciences, Baskent University,
Ankara, Turkey
e-mail: hayribaran@baskent.edu.tr; emelsonmezer@gmail.com

© Springer International Publishing AG, part of Springer Nature 2018
D. Kaya et al. (eds.), *Proprioception in Orthopaedics, Sports Medicine and Rehabilitation*,
https://doi.org/10.1007/978-3-319-66640-2_13

The first step, *evaluation of health status*, is to assess whether the patient's general health status has reached the normal state before injury. Undoubtedly, the key factor that affects the decision in this step is tissue damage and the correct assessment of how well the injured tissue healed. However, it is of utmost importance that what extent the improvement in the measured tissue damage in this period or the decrease of symptoms affect the athlete's functional ability. Therefore, evaluation of improvement performed at this stage contains the subjective outcome measures and functional tests to be performed in clinics or field. The second step is the *evaluation of participation risk*. What should be assessed at this stage is to analyze how much the specific requirements of the sport are met by the athlete. For example, the sport-specific requirements and sport-related expectations of a football player and swimmer with an anterior cruciate ligament injury are different. This difference can even be observed in players playing in different positions in the same sport. For example, the risk of participating in a sport following upper extremity injury may be different for a goalkeeper and midfielder. Similar differences are also affected by factors such as competition level and effectiveness of the use of protective equipment [2]. Therefore, it is a very important advantage that the clinician has a good understanding of the athlete's special position for that sport and knowledge of the sport features. The third stage that affects the decision to return to sports is *decision modifiers*. These are external factors that are usually independent of the medical condition of the athlete resulting from injury. The situations such as the condition of the contract of the athlete, expectation from his career, the occurrence timing of the injury (inside or outside the season), and pressure of a coach or manager are the basic examples for the factors that modifies decision for the return to sport. Sometimes these factors can be much more effective than it is predicted. For example, an athlete who has come to the end of his/her career and is perhaps on the brink of losing his/her biggest contract can take considerably bigger risk.

13.3 The Role of Proprioception in the Return to Sport

The requirements for high level sportive activity are defined as strength, power, endurance, flexibility, balance, proprioception, speed, and agility [3]. As it is seen, proprioception is defined as a requirement for top-class sporting performance. However, although proprioception is the primary criteria for the decision to return to sport, it is not usually tested as isolated in practical applications. There are two reasons for this: First, there is no gold standard in the tests used to measure proprioceptive performance. It is not possible to suggest that the joint position sense and kinesthesia tests frequently used in scientific studies are isolated and precise measurement of the proprioceptive sensation [4]. Furthermore, even conflicting results have been reported in joint position sensation and kinesthesia tests performed after injuries leading to loss of proprioceptors, such as tearing anterior cruciate ligament [5]. The second possible reason is that these tests require specific clinical or laboratory conditions and equipment that the environmental conditions are well controlled. This makes proprioceptive tests difficult to use widely in clinical decision to the return of sport.

Instead, the tests conducted at the first step of the decision to return to the sport usually consist of performance tests that measure basic functions [4]. For example, one of the most frequent functional tests following knee injury is the functional hop test. It was shown that the painless score of this test was one of the lower extremity performance indicators and especially correlated with the quadriceps muscle strength [6]. Similarly, functional performance tests based on muscular, endurance, flexibility, and agility are frequently applied when a decision to return to sport is given but proprioception is not measured isolated during this period. However, what should not be overlooked at this point is that not performing proprioception tests in the decision of return to sport does not mean proprioceptive sense is completely ignored.

Stability and balance-related tests that can be applied when a decision to return to sport is given has proprioceptive components as well [7]. Because, proprioception is one of the important factors required for successful ensuring of postural stabilization, neuromuscular control, and functional movement [8]. Long-term analyses of active athletes show that the application of exercise programs with integrated proprioceptive approaches to the training program has improved sportive performance parameters and reduced the incidence of injuries by up to 400% [9].

13.4 Proprioceptive Tests and Exercises in Return to Sport

The disturbances in kinematic components of the functional movements can be seen after lower extremity ligament injuries. These disorders also increase the risk of reinjury during sports and limit the achievement of optimal performance [10–14]. Testing all of the factors while deciding to return to sport following the lower extremity ligament injuries is the most important step that can be taken to reduce the risk of reinjury. It has been reported that testing of the joint position sense or kinesthesia would be beneficial in reducing the risk of injury [4, 15]. Although there is no consensus on a reliable method to objectively determine the proprioception [4], direct proprioceptive tests can be used to measure proprioceptive deficits resulting from injury during the return to sport. *Active reproduction* and *threshold to detection of passive movement* are the tests directly used for the proprioception and is most commonly used to determine joint position sense after injury. Electrogoniometers or isokinetic measuring devices are used for these tests to be valid and reliable [16, 17]. The impairments of the kinesthesia and active reproduction test scores are expected after various ligament injuries. Studies have revealed that knee joint position sense is not restored after ACL injuries [18, 19] and reconstruction [20–23].

Similarly, study conducted with meniscus abnormality has shown that knee angle reproduction capability significantly reduces in subjects with medial meniscus injury compared to healthy controls [24]. Therefore, although joint position tests are not included in the standard criteria of the return to sport, they may be useful for the decision to return to sport safely after ligament injuries and surgery [25].

Another evaluation method that can be used in relation to proprioceptive sense in the return to sport is postural stability tests. Since the proprioception is closely related to postural control, functional stability and balance tests may be used as a predictor of return to sport safely. Modified Star Excursion Balance Test (SEBT), one of the most frequently used tests, measures not only the dynamic stability and neuromuscular control [26–28] but also lower limb strength, coordination, balance, and flexibility [29–32]. Modified SEBT has high test-retest reliability [33–35] as well as it has been shown that it is able to distinguish dynamic balance and proprioceptive control strategies between the extremities following unilateral lower extremity injury [36]. It was reported that the athlete after ACL surgery showed poorer and worse performance in both injured and uninjured extremities compared to uninjured athletes [37]. Therefore, this test can also be preferred in the decision to return to the sport phase to determine the functional stability status after lower extremity injuries.

Another method that can be used to measure postural stability in connection with proprioception in the return to sport is to detect postural sway. Postural sway can be recorded during the test on the computerized balance board called stabilometer [4, 38]. It has been widely used in athletes with lower extremity ligament injuries and defects in the performance of the injured side have been showed [38–40]. However, the disadvantage of these tests compared to the isolated proprioceptive tests is that it is not possible to attribute the result completely to the proprioception due to the balance can be affected by various parameters such as strength and flexibility as well as proprioceptive sense.

Although a valid and reliable proprioceptive test method is not described in the literature as a gold standard for the return to sport, it has been shown in studies that athlete should be tested proprioceptively before the return to sport. According to these test results, neuromuscular rehabilitation should be applied with proprioceptive education. These programs include training that allows the best postural response to sudden changes given in the sport, thus reducing the risk of reinjury [41]. The difficulty of exercise should be adjusted to the level of the athlete's neuromuscular control. It advances from low-density movements, usually concentrated on a single plane, to multi-planar high-density movements. Drills regarding to reflex activities that require rapid stabilization of the joints are used instead of planned and voluntary muscle activities [4, 42, 43].

It is the balance exercises that ignite the proprioceptive receptors. The most commonly used in clinics after lower extremity injuries is perturbation training on one foot in softer grounds with varying degrees of difficulty (Figs. 13.1 and 13.2).

In addition, leg press, squat, single leg hop, side and figure eight running, and crossover walking on unstable grounds will help improve joint neuromuscular control in more dynamic conditions. The most important point to be noticed during the vertical hop is to teach the right landing strategies. Exercises are often given as closed kinetic chain activity. This is due to the fact that limbs are used as a part of closed kinetic chains during sports and activities of daily living. Another reason is that mechanoreceptors can be stimulated more effectively during closed kinetic chains exercises [43]. In addition to these general stability exercises, sport-specific drills should be included. Such exercises help to reinforce the proprioceptive pathways that are specific to activities that the athletes may encounter in the return to sport [36]. At the same time, it provides application of sport-specific drills bearing the risk of reinjury in controlled conditions and will facilitate proprioceptive adaptation of the athlete to these conditions [4].

As a result, the decision to return to the sport is based on not only performance tests, but also social and psychological factors. Although proprioception is among performance-based multi-

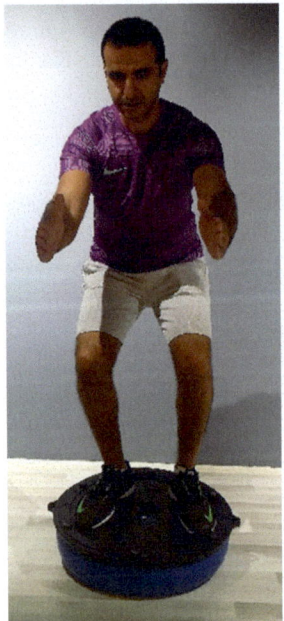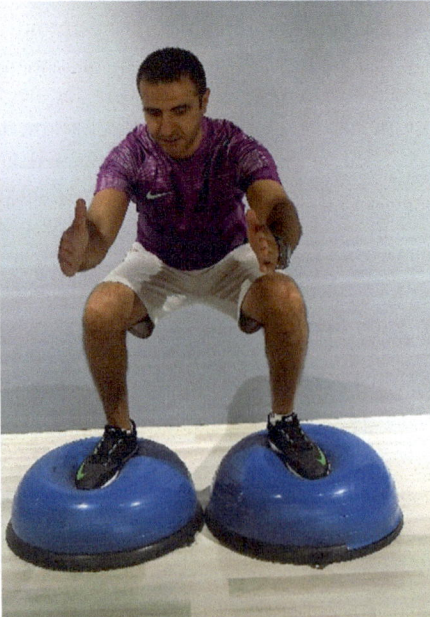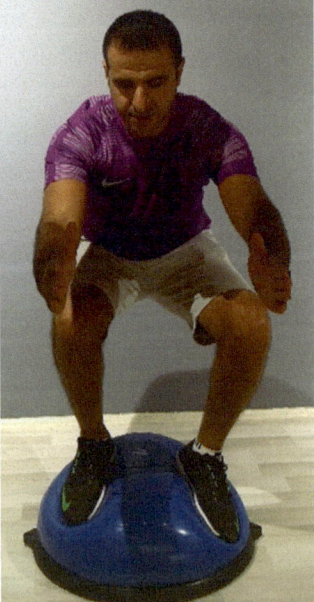

Fig. 13.1 Basic balance exercises for lower extremity

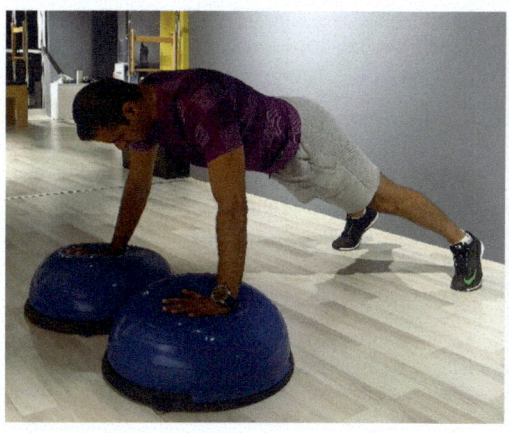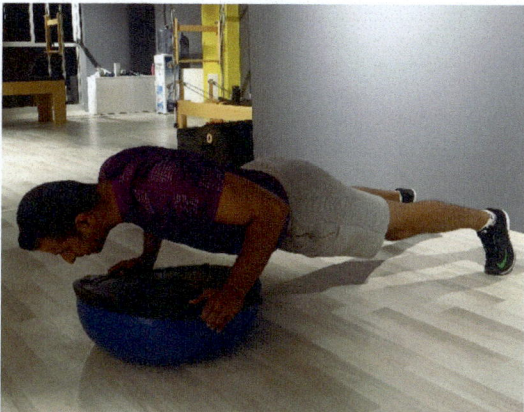

Fig. 13.2 Postural stability exercises for upper extremity and trunk

factorial factors, studies show conflicting results on a reliable method to objectively determine the proprioception. Athletes can show significant proprioceptive deficit following sports injuries but there is no consensus how to use proprioceptive test during return to sports. Establishing evidence-based standards for the use of proprioceptive tests in the decision to return to the sport may contribute to reduce reinjury risk.

References

1. Thomeé R, Suzanne W. Return to sport. Knee Surg Sports Traumatol Arthrosc. 2011;19:1795–7.
2. Creighton DW, Shrier I, Shultz R, Meeuwisse WH, Matheson GO. Return-to-play in sport: a decision-based model. Clin J Sport Med. 2010;20(5):379–85.
3. Reiman MP, Manske RC. Functional testing in human performance. Champaign, IL: Human Kinetics; 2009.
4. Hewett TE, Paterno MV, Myer GD. Strategies for enhancing proprioception and neuromuscular control of the knee. Clin Orthop Relat Res. 2002;402:76–94.
5. Gokeler A, Benjaminse A, Hewett TE, Lephart SM, Engebretsen L, Ageberg E, et al. Proprioceptive deficits after ACL injury: are they clinically relevant? Br J Sports Med. 2012;46(3):180–92.
6. Petschnig R, Baron R, Albrecht M. The relationship between isokinetic quadriceps strength test and hop tests for distance and one-legged vertical jump test following anterior cruciate ligament reconstruction. J Orthop Sports Phys Ther. 1998;28(1):23–31.
7. Lephart SM, Pincivero DM, Giraido JL, Fu FH. The role of proprioception in the management and rehabilitation of athletic injuries. Am J Sports Med. 1997;25(1):130–7.

8. Hassan BS, Mockett S, Doherty M. Static postural sway, proprioception, and maximal voluntary quadriceps contraction in patients with knee osteoarthritis and normal control subjects. Ann Rheum Dis. 2001;60(6):612–8.
9. Knobloch K, Martin-Schmitt S, Gösling T, Jagodzinski M, Zeichen J, Krettek C. Prospective proprioceptive and coordinative training for injury reduction in elite female soccer. Sportverletz Sportschaden. 2005;19(3):123–9.
10. Ageberg E, Zatterstrom R, Moritz U, Friden T. Influence of supervised and nonsupervised training on postural controlafter an acute anterior cruciate ligament rupture: a three year longitudinal prospective study. J Orthop Sports Phys Ther. 2001;31:632–44.
11. Decker MJ, Torry MR, Noonan TJ, Riviere A, Sterett WI. Landing adaptations after ACL reconstruction. Med Sci Sports Exerc. 2002;34:1408–13.
12. Keays SL, Bullock-Saxton J, Keays AC. Strength and function before and after anterior cruciate ligament reconstruction. Clin Orthop Relat Res. 2000; 373:174–83.
13. Neitzel JA, Kernozek TW, Davies GJ. Loading response following anterior cruciate ligament reconstruction during the parallel squat exercise. Clin Biomech (Bristol, Avon). 2002;17:551–4.
14. Paterno MV, Ford KR, Myer GD, Heyl R, Hewett TE. Biomechanical limb asymmetries in female athletes 2 years following ACL reconstruction. J Orthop Sports Phys Ther. 2005;35:A75.
15. Clanton TO, Matheny LM, Jarvis HC, Jeronimus AB. Return to play in athletes following ankle injuries. Sports Health. 2012;4(6):471–4.
16. Reider B, Arcand MA, Diehl LH, Mroczek K, Abulencia A, Stroud C, et al. Proprioception of the knee before and after anterior cruciate ligament reconstruction. Arthroscopy. 2003;19(1):2–12.
17. Daneshjoo A, Mokhtar AH, Rahnama N, Yusof A. The effects of comprehensive warm-up programs

on proprioception, static and dynamic balance on male soccer players. PLoS One. 2012;7(12):e51568.

18. Arockiaraj J, Korula RJ, Oommen AT, et al. Proprioceptive changes in the contralateral knee joint following anterior cruciate injury. Bone Joint J. 2013;95(2):188–91.

19. MacDonald PB, Hedden D, Pacin O, Sutherland K. Proprioception in anterior cruciate ligament-deficient and reconstructed knees. Am J Sports Med. 1996;24(6):774–8.

20. Angoules AG, Mavrogenis AF, Dimitriou R, et al. Knee proprioception following ACL reconstruction; a prospective trial comparing hamstrings with bone-patellar tendon-bone autograft. Knee. 2011;18(2):76–82.

21. Yosmaoglu HB, Baltacı G, Kaya D, ÖZER H, Atay A. Comparison of functional outcomes of two anterior cruciate ligament reconstruction methods with hamstring tendon graft. Acta Orthop Traumatol Turc. 2001;45(4):240–7.

22. Yosmaoglu HB, Baltacı G, Kaya D, Özer H. Tracking ability, motor coordination, and functional determinants after anterior cruciate ligament reconstruction. J Sport Rehabil. 2011;20(2):207–18.

23. Yosmaoglu HB, Baltacı G, Kaya D, Özer H, Atay A. Effects of additional gracilis tendon harvest on muscle torque, motor coordination, and knee laxity in ACL reconstruction. Knee Surg Sports Traumatol Arthrosc. 2011;19(8):1287–92.

24. Jerosch J, Prymka M, Castro WH. Proprioception of knee joints with a lesion of the medial meniscus. Acta Orthop Belg. 1996;62(1):41–5.

25. Zazulak BT, Hewett TE, Reeves NP, Goldberg B, Cholewicki J. The effects of core proprioception on knee injury. Am J Sports Med. 2007;35(3):368–73.

26. Aminaka N, Gribble PA. Patellar taping, patello femoral pain syndrome, lower extremity kinematics, and dynamic postural control. J Athl Train. 2008;43:21–8.

27. Earl JE, Hertel J. Lower-extremity muscle activation during the Star Excursion Balance Tests. J Sport Rehabil. 2001;10:93–104.

28. Hale SA, Hertel J, Olmsted-Kramer LC. The effect of a 4-week comprehensive rehabilitation program on postural control and lower extremity function in individuals with chronic ankle instability. J Orthop Sports Phys Ther. 2007;37:303–11.

29. Fitzgerald D, Trakarnratanakul N, Smyth B, Caulfield B. Effects of a wobble board-based therapeutic exergaming system for balance training on dynamic postural stability and intrinsic motivation levels. J Orthop Sports Phys Ther. 2010;40:11–9.

30. Leavey VJ, Sandrey MA, Dahmer G. Comparative effects of 6-week balance, gluteus medius strength,

and combined programs on dynamic postural control. J Sport Rehabil. 2010;19:268–87.

31. McLeod TC, Armstrong T, Miller M, Sauers JL. Balanceimprovements in female high school basketball players after a 6-week neuromuscular-training program. J Sport Rehabil. 2009;18:465–81.

32. Wojtys EM, Huston LJ. Longitudinal effects of anterior cruciate ligament injury and patellar tendon auto graft reconstruction on neuromuscular performance. Am J Sports Med. 2000;28:336–44.

33. Hertel J, Miller SJ, Denegar CR. Intratester and intertester reliability during the star excursion balance tests. J Sport Rehabil. 2000;9:104–16.

34. Kinzey SJ, Armstrong CW. The reliability of the star-excursion test in assessing dynamic balance. J Orthop Sports Phys Ther. 1998;27:356–60.

35. Plisky PJ, Rauh MJ, Kaminski TW, Underwood FB. Star Excursion Balance Test as a predictor of lower extremity injury in high school basketball players. J Orthop Sports Phys Ther. 2006;36:911–9.

36. Herrington L, Hatcher J, Hatcher A, McNicholas M. A comparison of Star Excursion Balance Test reach distances between ACL deficientpatientsandasymptomaticcontrols. Knee. 2009;16:149–52.

37. Clagg S, Paterno MV, Hewett TE, Schmitt LC. Performance on the modified star excursion balance test at the time of return to sport following anterior cruciate ligament reconstruction. J Orthop Sports Phys Ther. 2015;45(6):444–52.

38. Mizuta H, Shiraishi M, Kubota K, Kai K, Takagi K. A stabilometric technique forevaluation of functional instability in anterior cruciate ligament-deficient knee. Clin J Sports Med. 1992;2:235–9.

39. Harrison EL, Duenkel N, Dunlop R, Russell G. Evaluation of single-legstandingfollowinganterior cruciateligamentsurgeryandrehabilitation. Phys Ther. 1994;74:245–52.

40. Zatterstrom R, Friden T, Lindstrand A, Moritz U. The effect of physiotherapy on standing balance in chronic anterior cruciate ligament insufficiency. Am J Sports Med. 1994;22:531–6.

41. Griffin LY, Agel J, Albohm MJ, Arendt EA, Dick RW, Garrett WE, Johnson RJ. Noncontact anterior cruciate ligament injuries: risk factors and prevention strategies. J Am Acad Orthop Surg. 2000;8(3):141–50.

42. Brand RA. Knee ligaments: a new view. J Biomech Eng. 1986;108:106–10.

43. Laskowski ER, Newcomer-Aney K, Smith J. Refining rehabilitation with proprioceptive training: expediting return to play. Phys Sports Med. 1997;25:89–102.

Proprioception After Soft Tissue Regenerative Treatment

14

Barış Gülenç, Ersin Kuyucu, and Mehmet Erdil

14.1 Introduction

Proprioception is a word of Latin origin which is formed by the combination of the words "proprius" (person-specific) and "-ception" (perception, intuition) and first coined in 1932 by Charles Scott Sherrington, a Nobel laureate in psychology. It is defined as the perception of joints and extremities provided by the neural inputs through receptors found in joints and surrounding tissues. It can be simply described as "awareness of the location of one's body parts in 3-dimensional space." Sharma defined proprioception in its most comprehensive form as "gathering of inputs from somatosensorial, vestibular, and visual systems by central nervous system to regulate periarticular muscle activity that provides joint stabilization" [1, 2].

Proprioceptiom is achieved by afferent stimuli which comes from reseptors found in joint capsule, muscles, tendons,ligaments, other intraarticular structures (e.g., meniscus), and skin. These receptors are composed of mechanoreceptors that are responsible for the sensations of

position and movement, and nociceptors that are responsible for pain transmission.

Mechanoreceptors are composed of three different structures (Fig. 14.1).

Pacini bodies are found in deep capsular layers, anterior cruciate ligament, meniscofemoral and collateral ligaments, intra- and extra-articular fat pads, and inner meniscus. They are especially sensitive to acceleration and deceleration. They are not stimulated in static conditions and when joints move at a constant pace, and they react to rapid changes of movement.

Ruffini bodies are especially abundant in superficial layers and joint capsule, and also in cruciate ligaments, meniscofemoral and collateral ligaments, and menisci. Ruffini receptors have a high sensitivity for mechanical stress and have a slow adaptation. They can detect intra-articular pressure, joint rotations, static joint position, and joint width and speed.

Golgi tendon organ receptors are found in menisci, cruciate ligaments, and collateral ligaments. They show a slow adaptation; they have a higher sensitivity for mechanical stimuli; and they are completely inactive in stationary joints. As Golgi tendon receptors have a high threshold, they are considered to measure the threshold points of the normal movement series of a joint (Fig. 14.1).

Nociceptors are abundant in joint capsule, cruciate ligaments, and in menisci, with their number in the latter being greater than other receptors. These endings are myelinated or

B. Gülenç, M.D, (✉) • E. Kuyucu, M.D. • M. Erdil, M.D.
Department of Orthopedics and Traumatology,
Faculty of Medicine, Istanbul Medipol University,
Istanbul, Turkey
e-mail: barisgulenc@yahoo.com;
ersinkuyucu@yahoo.com.tr;
drmehmeterdil@gmail.com

© Springer International Publishing AG, part of Springer Nature 2018
D. Kaya et al. (eds.), *Proprioception in Orthopaedics, Sports Medicine and Rehabilitation*,
https://doi.org/10.1007/978-3-319-66640-2_14

Fig. 14.1 Neuromuscular control pathway (by Lephart and Henry) [9]

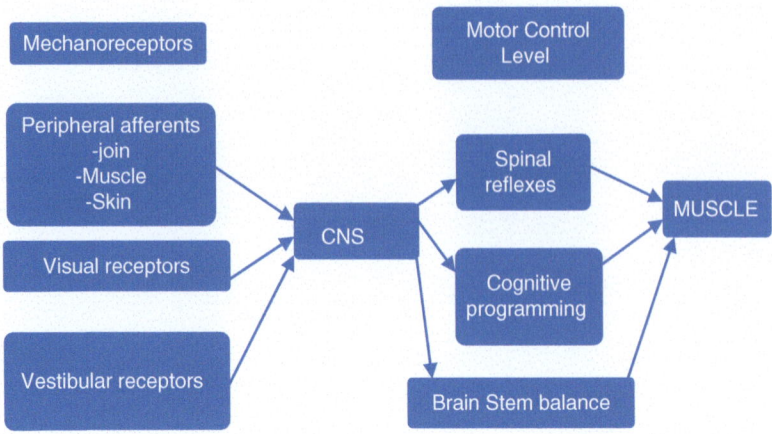

unmyelinated axons with a diameter ranging between 0.5 and 5 mm. Most nerve endings remain silent under normal conditions; they are activated when a joint is subjected to mechanical force or certain agents.

All these receptors may be injured when the hosting tissue is injured, operated, or reconstructed. Loss of proprioception causes an increased rate of recurrent injuries so proprioceptive rehabilitation aims both reduce the risk of injury and affects positively outcomes of surgical therapy. Studies on athletes have shown that this type of rehabilitation may increase performance not only in those who sustain injuries, but also in healthy athletes [3, 4].

Treatment of soft tissue injuries should be dealt with care by orthopedic surgeons and physical therapy specialists. An important aspect of recovery and post-recovery rehabilitation process is the replacement of the injured tissue's sensation of proprioception [5, 6].

Joint motion (kinesthesia) and joint position are the two important elements of proprioception measurement. Kinesia forms the dynamic part of proprioception and is thus regulated by the Pacini bodies that react to rapid changes. On the other hand, joint position is responsible for the static part of proprioception and is basically regulated by the Ruffini bodies and Golgi tendon organ [7, 8].

Although recent studies on athletes have indicated beneficial effects of elastic bandages,

splints, bandaging, and surgical treatment on proprioception, no standard treatment exists for proprioceptive rehabilitation and studies are ongoing. In this chapter, we aimed to discuss data on the change of proprioception following regenerative treatments applied mainly after articular, muscular, and other soft tissue injuries.

14.2 Evaluation of the Change in Proprioception After Knee Injuries

In the knee joint proprioceptive data and neuromuscular feedback mechanisms coming from joint and muscle receptors play an important role for muscle tonus, coordination, and control of contraction, i.e., establishing and maintenance of joint stability. A properly coordinated muscle co-activation protects normal joint cartilage from overload. The protective muscle activity pattern occurs when ligaments are subjected to stress [10]. The relationship between sensory input and motor response has been stressed in many studies where the correlation between the sensation of proprioception and motor function has been evaluated. In the knee joint, especially the cruciate ligaments are rich in proprioceptive receptors. It has been shown that the injury or surgical repair or reconstruction of these structures adversely affects proprioception [10, 11].

14.3 Anterior Cruciate Ligament (ACL)

ACL is one of the most important ligaments limiting knee translation and rotation. Prospective studies that have been done following its injury have shown that 40–90% of the affected persons develop radiological osteoarthritis 7–12 years after the event [12, 13].

Pacini, Ruffini, and Golgi tendon organ are found at femoral and tibial attachment sites. ACL tears cause a reduction of afferent inputs sent from these receptors, lowering the number of receptors. Hence, ACL tears not only lead to mechanical knee instability, but also markedly reduced proprioception, with resulting impairment of balance, strength, and activity level of the quadriceps muscle, putting persons at risk of recurrent injuries.

There is no standard method for evaluating proprioception after ACL injury. Joint position sensory test and TTDPM (threshold to detect passive motion) are the most commonly employed tests for measuring proprioception after ACL injuries. TTDPM is sensitive to changes in Pacini bodies stimulated by rapid changes in knee joint. On the other hand, JPS primarily evaluates changes in receptors that respond to slower changes such as Golgi tendon organ and Ruffini bodies. The tests are used to assess the difference between injured knee and normal knee, or between post-injury and post-treatment states [11, 14].

Kim et al., in a metaanalysis of studies on proprioception after ACL tears, reported that the JPS scores were greater in the normal knee compared to the injured knee [15]. Similar results were provided by studies comparing patients with ACL injury and an external control group, with the latter having a better JPS score. The same study revealed no significant difference between the TTDPM scores compared to the contralateral knee. Comparisons using control groups indicated that the scores were better in control groups, as is the case for JPS [16].

Studies evaluating treatment outcomes have shown that both TTDPM and JPS dramatically improved following treatment. Outcomes following this improvement are superior to both the external control group and the contralateral knee. When both tests are compared, although the opposite has been suggested, since metaanalyses revealed that JPS scores yield more consistent results after ACL injuries, it has been recommended to use them as the evaluation test. TDDPM and JPS scores below 5 are not considered significant in clinical practice [17–24].

The lack of change in proprioception with ACL tears can be explained by the abovementioned fact stating that these tests are sensitive to stimuli coming from different receptors. Additionally, ACL contain 1% of all mechanoreceptors of knee, and the remaining ones are localized in joint capsule and adjacent muscles. Golgi tendon organ, which is more abundant in muscles and tendons, can be a reason why severe loss of proprioception does not occur after ACL injury [18, 20].

It has been shown that proprioceptive sense in reconstructed ligaments does not recover for about 6 months after ACL injury. Post-reconstruction rehabilitation program should aim at increasing the number and activity of mechanoreceptors found in joint capsule and muscles. The number and activity of the receptors at this anatomic site may explain why some patients with ACL deficit are more resistant than others against recurrent injuries [21, 23].

Among studies comparing single bundle augmentation (SBA), double bundle (DB) and single bundle (SB) reconstruction with one another, the one by Ma et al. where balance ability and proprioception were evaluated, joint stability, balance ability, and proprioception were better among patients undergoing DB and SBA at 6th and 12th months. Gains in joint stability and proprioception occurred more rapidly in patients undergoing DB than those undergoing other two methods. On the other hand, muscle strength was similar in the three groups [25].

14.4 Menisci

In daily life meniscal injuries occur with axial overload and knee rotation. Patients present to clinicians with mechanical knee symptoms (locking, sound). In symptomatic tears the treatment of choice is arthroscopic surgery. Depending on the site, time, and type of the tear, as well as patient age and activity level, repair or debridement of tear is performed. Repair is preferentially selected in central tears, young patients, and acute tears.

Menisci are innervated by the posterior articular branch of the tibial nerve. The majority of innervation is at the anterior and posterior horns and the greatest in the peripheral two-third of the meniscus. Exactly like the ACL, there also exist free nerve endings (nociceptors) and mechanoreceptors within the menisci. While free nerve endings are responsible for pain sensation, Pacini bodies sense joint acceleration and deceleration, while Ruffini bodies send information about a joint's static position to the central nervous system. The physical stimuli sent with these receptors' afferent inputs mediate reflex protective responses against joint changes [26].

There is a paucity of information regarding the change in proprioception after meniscal tears and their treatment. The basic reason of this is the heterogeneity of meniscal tears and technical difficulty of measuring proprioception. Dynamic postural stability measurement with stabilometry is one of the available methods used for the measurement of proprioception after meniscal tears. In this method, dynamic postural stability on a single leg is assessed to evaluate proprioception. It allows the evaluation of both afferent and efferent reflex pathways. Additionally, TTDPM and JPS can also be used for post-meniscal evaluation [27].

A prospective study followed 50 patients who underwent partial meniscectomy for symptomatic meniscal tear for a mean of 63 weeks and showed that proprioception was markedly reduced after meniscal tear compared to the contralateral side, but despite a statistically significant improvement in clinical scores the patients did not show significant improvement of stabilometry results after surgery [28].

Palm et al. reported that there was no significant difference between postural stability among knees with and without tear after surgical treatment of meniscal tear. However, the limitation of that study was that none of the patients was compared with the external control group [29].

In another study where pre- and postsurgical meniscal tear was compared with a control group, there occurred a significant reduction in proprioception than the control group after meniscal tear, which was not improved with external bandaging. When postoperative outcomes were analyzed, on the other hand, a significant increase in proprioception was noted compared to the peroperative values although no significant difference was evident compared with the control group [30].

Whereas total meniscectomy was once a commonly preferred surgical method, it is now abandoned. Thijs et al. prospectively evaluated 14 patients undergoing total meniscectomy with the JPS testing at 30–70°. They found a significant proprioception deficit in the meniscectomy group, which partially recovered 6 months after fresh frozen meniscus transplantation [31]. In another study where a change in quadriceps muscle strength was evaluated, both EMG activity and muscle strength were significantly improved at 6th month although there was no discernible change in muscle diameter after meniscus surgery; this result was attributed to a postsurgical decrease in neural activity [32].

There is a paucity of information about the state of proprioception after meniscal repair and further studies are warranted.

14.5 Posterior Cruciate Ligament (PCL)

In just the same way as ACL, PCL consists of two branches and its injury may lead to knee atrophy and instability relatively rapidly. Unlike ACL, it is more likely to recover after injury because of a large synovial sheath found around it and its proximity to middle geniculate artery. Therefore, its isolated injuries have been mostly treated conservatively in the past, but the tendency to use surgery has been increasing due to recent advancements in surgical technique, and also due to reports indicating a tibiofemoral and patello-femoral arthrosis risk in the long term. Single branch PCL reconstruction preserving PCL residue is one of the most preferred techniques because of both graft revascularization and preserved proprioception. PCL contains Golgi body, Pacini and Ruffini bodies in its structure and its defects have been associated with loss of proprioception [33–36]. Adachi et al. reported that JPS was rapidly reduced at early postoperative period after PCL reconstruction and could reach the same level as the contralateral knee by only 24 months. TTDPM tests evaluated by different authors at different angles showed that the values in knees with PCL tear were lower than the intact side [37]. Lee et al. retrospectively studied TTDPM and RPP (reproduction of patient positioning) values in knees undergoing PCL reconstruction and found no difference from the contralateral side at 61 months [38]. Li et al. studied the effect of three different PCL reconstruction techniques on proprioception. They used autograft in one group, hybrid graft in the other, and reconstruction with PCL treated with gamma radiation in another. The authors found no significant difference between the three groups with respect to proprioception and functional outcomes at the end of a 5.5-month follow-up period [39].

14.6   Evaluation of a Change in Proprioception After Soft Tissue in the Ankle Injuries

As the knee region, ankle region is rich in proprioceptive receptors. Freeman et al. were the first to report that afferent nerve endings were reduced in number, leading to recurrent ankle sprain following chronic ankle instability. The time and ability of standing on a single foot after ankle sprain was reported to be reduced compared to those on the intact side [40].

Kinesthesia, sensation of joint position, and RPP (reproduction of proprioception) values are also reportedly decreased after ankle sprain. A significant reduction in peroneal reaction time

was also reported after rapid inversion following these injuries [41].

The main problem mentioned in a number of papers is the association of reduced number of mechanoreceptors with chronic instability and postural disorder. Postural control is the main factor for maintaining balance, and its loss results in falls and injuries. The risk of recurrent ankle sprain is increased in these patients [42, 43].

Li et al. reported that postural control significantly increased at postoperative period compared to the preoperative period after ATFL reconstruction (modified Bröstrom). It has also been reported that postural sway at anteroposterior plane was also significantly lowered following surgery [44, 45].

Several studies have examined ankle proprioception after achilles tendon injuries. Bressel et al. studied the changes in ankle proprioception after achilles tendon injuries and found that ankle proprioception was significantly reduced at both sides compared to the control group after a mean of 5.8 years after primary achilles tendon repair [46].

Kaya et al. studied 19 patients after percutaneous achilles tendon repair and found no difference between the intact side and the repaired side with respect to muscle strength and sensation of joint position at 10° dorsiflexion whereas there was a significant difference between both groups' sensation of joint position at 15° plantar flexion. Although they detected a significant reduction at the affected side compared to the control group, no significant difference was detected between the intact side and the control group [47].

14.7   Evaluation of a Change in Proprioception After Soft Tissue Injuries Involving Shoulder Region

Shoulder joint is a spheroid joint that can move at each of the three anatomic axes. Only a third of humeral head is covered by glenoid. Capsulolabral structures around the joint increase the depth of the glenoid and contribute to joint stability. External injury to these structures may result in instability. The recommended treatment after a first dislocation episode is conservative follow-up with the arm resting in a sling; the rate of recurrent episodes of dislocation has been reported to be 60% especially in the second decade. Surgical labrum repair is the standard surgical modality for recurrent dislocations. Among the surgical techniques, the most commonly preferred ones are arthroscopic or open capsulorrhaphy, labrum repair, and glenoid reconstruction [48–50].

In a histological study by Vangness et al., Both pacini bodies and ruffini receptors were shown in glenohumeral ligamentous complex. However, there are no mechanoreceptors and only nociceptors exist in labrum and subacromial bursa. Proprioception is one of the involuntary dynamic stabilizers of the shoulder joint; it regulates joint movements and prepares the shoulder for the stages of the preparation and response to stress reaction. The sensation of joint position is necessary for the maintenance of harmony between joint surfaces during shoulder movement arch. Stretching of intra-articular and periarticular structures during shoulder elevation promotes the sensation of proprioception. It is thought that by this way joint harmony is maintained properly at the extremes of joint motion arch [51–53].

14.8 Instability Surgery

Shoulder instability is the basic subject of studies investigating proprioception and shoulder. As mentioned above, there is a plethora of studies examining how the sensation of joint position, which is considered among dynamic stabilizers, is affected in case of instability, and to which degree it contributes to instability.

Lephart et al., in a study where they measured and compared kinesthesia and sensation of joint position among healthy, unstable patients undergoing instability surgery, demonstrated that the values were worse in the instability group compared to the healthy subjects, and that their values approximated to those of healthy subjects following surgery. Edmunds et al. examined proprioception after immobilization with conservative sling immobilization and primer arthroscopic

surgery and found no difference between the groups [54, 55]. Fremery et al. compared EMG and proprioception of shoulder muscles after open instability surgery (capsulolabral repair) with those of the control group. They reported that while there was no significant difference between both groups' shoulder proprioception, deltoid muscle activity level at EMG examination at 90° abduction and throwing positions was significantly lower at the operation side compared to the control group. According to the authors, the use of an open dissection was the reason of a lower deltoid activity in the operated patients. They reported that in 6 to 33 months proprioception returned to the same level as the contralateral shoulder [56].

In another study where open surgery and arthroscopic surgery was compared, the arthroscopy and control groups showed no significant difference from arthroscopic surgery in terms of acceleration/movement time ratio and peak/mean velocity ratio, and the values were lower with open surgery compared to the other two groups [57].

Sullivan et al. compared proprioception after different capsulorrhaphy types and found no significant differences between the thermal, open, and arthroscopic capsulorrhaphy groups with respect to the sensation of joint position for external rotation movement. Another study examining proprioception and muscle strength after open inferior capsular shift and anterior capsulolabral reconstruction indicated that, although proprioception and muscle strength returned to normal 1 year after operation in both groups, that improvement was achieved later in patients who underwent inferior capsular shift with detachment of subcapsularis than the reconstruction group, but both muscle strength and proprioception returned to normal 6 months after operation in the reconstruction group [58].

Today, arthroscopic capsulolabral interventions are considered ideal for preserving sensation of joint position because they minimize tissue injury and associated loss of deep sensation after open surgery.

Multidirectional shoulder instability is a condition characterized by subluxation or dialocation of shoulder joint in multiple directions. It is characterized by recurrent pain and subluxation sensation. Its pathogenesis involves loosening due to disrupted shoulder joint capsule attachment. Studies involving these patients have found a markedly reduced sensation of dynamic upper extremity proprioception [59].

Anderson et al. compared patients with chronic rotator cuff pain syndrome with a control group and the contralateral shoulder, and found that the sensation of joint position was lower in the injured side than both groups [60].

14.9 Evaluation of Change of Proprioception After Soft Tissue Injuries Involving Hand–Wrist Region

Impairment of proprioception is among important parameters after hand and wrist injuries. The wrist is innervated by median, ulnar, radial nerves, and the articular branches of the musculocutaneous nerve. There are mechanoreceptors in the extensor and flexor musculotendineous junction providing the sensation of position of the wrist. Ruffini bodies are the dominant mechanoreceptor type in the hand; they are activated by low amplitude motion and they respond to loading and stretching. Mechanoreceptors found in the skin are an important part of hand proprioception and aid in the coding and regulation of the sensation of position. The degree of innervation shows difference among the structures of wrist and it is greater in distal radiocarpal and distal intercarpal ligaments [61, 62].

An in vivo proprioception and EMG study on the scafolunate ligament (SLL) by Hagert et al. showed that proprioception and EMG conduction velocities were different in SLL injuries from those of normal subjects. In that study, it was shown that antagonist muscles were activated by this reflex pathway as a result of injury to the ligaments. It was reported that SL ligament reflexively performed volar flexion motion when stimulated with the wrist in flexion position. It was noted that when the area of SL ligament was desensitized, the protective reflexes were eliminated [63].

In cases of wrist hypermobility and palmar midcarpal instability, the use of orthesis and extensor carpi ulnaris strengthening exercise program to preserve afferent sensory conduction has been reported in the literature [64, 65].

In patients for whom conservative treatment would not suffice and surgical therapy is required, a careful dissection and care taken not to severe nervous structures are important in order to prevent deep sensory loss. Instability surgery can currently be applied with the arthroscopic method. Arthroscopic electrothermal shrinkage has been reported to enable to shrink and tighten failing ligaments by applying thermal stimulus, and to provide favorable outcomes. Hagert et al. stated that the outcome may be limited due to injured receptors after this surgery [65–67].

References

1. Sharma L. Proprioceptive impariment in knee osteoarthtitis. Rheum Dis Clin North. 1999;25:299–314.
2. Sherrington CS. The integrative action of the nervous system. New Haven, CT: Yale University Press; 1906.
3. Akseki D, Erduran M, Kaya D. Sports injuries and proprioception: current trends and new horizons. In: Sports injuries. Berlin Heidelberg: Springer; 2012. p. 67–71.
4. Zimmy ML. Mechanoreseptors in articular tissues. Am J Anat. 1988;182:16–32.
5. Kaminski TW, Buckley BD, Powers ME, Hubbard TJ, Ortiz C. Effect of strength and proprioception training on eversion to inversion strength ratios in subjects with unilateral functional ankle instability. Br J Sports Med. 2003;37:410–5.
6. Verhagen E, Beek A, Twisk J, Bouter L, Bahr R, Mechelen W. The effect of a proprioceptive balance board training program for the prevention of ankle sprains: a prospective controlled trial. Am J Sports Med. 2004;32:1385–93.
7. Xu D, Hong Y, Li J, Chan K. Effect of tai chi exercise on proprioception of ankle and knee joints in old people. Br J Sports Med. 2004;38:50–4.
8. Robbins S, Waked E, Rappel R. Ankle taping improves proprioception before and after exercise in young men. Br J Sports Med. 1995;29:242–7.
9. Lephart SM, Henry TJ. The physiological basis for open and closed kinetic chain rehabilitation for the upper extremity. J Sport Rehabil. 1996;5:71–87.
10. Lee HM, Cheng CK, Liau JJ. Correlation between proprioception, muscle strength, knee laxity, and dynamic standing balance in patients with chronic anterior cruciate ligament deficiency. Knee. 2009;16:387–91.

11. Corrigan JP, Cashman WF, Brady MP. Proprioception in the cruciate deficient knee. J Bone Joint Surg. 1992;74(2):247–50.

12. O'Connor BL, Brant KD. Neurogenic factors in the etiopathogenesis of osteoarthritis. Rheum Dis Clin N Am. 1993;19:581–605.

13. Pai YC, Rymer WZ, Chang RW, Sharma L. Effect of age and osteoarthritis on knee proprioception. Arthritis Rheum. 1997;40:2260–5.

14. Barrack RL, Skinner HB, Buckley SL. Proprioception in the anterior cruciate deficient knee. Am J Sports Med. 1989;17(1):1–6.

15. Kim HJ, Lee JH, Lee DH. Proprioception in patients with anterior cruciate ligament tears. Am J Sports Med. 2017;45:2916–22. https://doi.org/10.1177/0363546516682231.

16. Fischer-Rasmussen T, Jensen PE. Proprioceptive sensitivity and performance in anterior cruciate ligament-deficient knee joints. Scand J Med Sci Sports. 2000;10:85–9.

17. Fremerey RW, Lobenhoffer P, Zeichen J, et al. Proprioception after rehabilitation and reconstruction in knees with deficiency of the anterior cruciate ligament: a prospective, longitudinal study. J Bone Joint Surg Br. 2000;82:801–6.

18. Ozenci AM, Inanmaz E, Ozcanli H, et al. Proprioceptive comparison of allograft and autograft anterior cruciate ligament reconstructions. Knee Surg Sports Traumatol Arthrosc. 2007;15:1432–7.

19. Mir SM, Hadian MR, Talebian S, et al. Functional assessment of knee joint position sense following anterior cruciate ligament reconstruction. Br J Sports Med. 2008;42:300–3.

20. Anguoles AG, Mavrogenis AF, Dimitriou R, Karzis K, Drakoulakis E, Michos J, et al. Knee proprioception following ACL reconstruction; a prospective trial comparing hamstring with bone-patellar tendon-bone autograft. Knee. 2011;18:76–82.

21. Relph N, Herrington L, Tyson S. The effects of ACL injury on knee proprioception: a meta-analysis. Physiotherapy. 2014;100:187–95.

22. Barrack RL, Munn BG. Effects of knee ligament injury and reconstruction on proprioception. In: Lephart SM, Fu FH, editors. Proprioception and neuromuscular control in joint stability. Champaign: Human Kinetics; 2000.

23. Pinczewski LA, Lyman J, Salmon LJ, Russell VJ, Roe J, Linklater J. A 10-year comparison of anterior cruciate ligament reconstructions with hamstring tendon and patellar tendon autograft: a controlled, prospective trial. Am J Sports Med. 2007;35:564–74.

24. Reider B, Arcand M, Diehl HL, Mroczek K, Abulencia A, Stroud CC, Palm M, Gilbertson J, Staszak P. Proprioception of the knee before and after anterior cruciate ligament reconstruction. Arthroscopy. 2003;19:2–12.

25. Ma Y, Deie M, Iwaki D, Asaeda M, Fujita N, Adachi N, Ochi M. Balance ability and proprioception after single-bundle, single-bundle augmentation, and double-bundle ACL reconstruction. Sci World J. 2014;2014:342012.

26. Hewett TE, Paterno MV, Myer GD. Strategies for enhancing proprioception and neuromuscular control of the knee. Clin Orthop Relat Res. 2002;402:76–94.

27. Lephart SM, Pincivero DM, Rozzi SL. Proprioception of the ankle and knee. Sports Med. 1998;25:149–55.

28. Al-Dadah O, Shepstone L, Donell ST. Proprioception following partial meniscectomy in stable knees. Knee Surg Sports Traumatol Arthrosc. 2011;19:207–13.

29. Palm HG, Laufer C, von Lubken F, Achatz G, Friemert B. Do meniscus injuries affect postural stability? Orthopade. 2010;39:486–94.

30. Jerosch J, Prymka M, Castro WH. Proprioception of knee joints with a lesion of the medial meniscus. Acta Orthop Belg. 1996;62:41–5.

31. Thijs Y, Witvrouw E, Evens B, et al. A prospective study on knee proprioception after meniscal allograft transplantation. Scand J Med Sci Sports. 2007;17:223–9.

32. Glatthorn JF, Berendts AM, Bizzini M, Munzinger U, Maffiuletti NA. Neuromuscular function after arthroscopic partial meniscectomy. Clin Orthop Relat Res. 2010;468:1336–43.

33. Bray RC, Leonard CA, Salo PT. Vascular physiology and long-term healing of partial ligament tears. J Orthop Res. 2002;20:984–9.

34. Petersen W, Tillmann B. Blood and lymph supply of the posterior cruciate ligament: a cadaver study. Knee Surg Sports Traumatol Arthrosc. 1999;7:42–50.

35. Clark P, MacDonald PB, Sutherland K. Analysis of proprioception in the posterior cruciate ligament-deficient knee. Knee Surg Sports Traumatol Arthrosc. 1996;4:225–7.

36. Safran MR, Allen AA, Lephart SM, Borsa PA, Fu FH, Harner CD. Proprioception in the posterior cruciate ligament deficient knee. Knee Surg Sports Traumatol Arthrosc. 1999;7:310–7.

37. Adachi N, Ochi M, Uchio Y, Iwasa J, Ishikawa M, Shinomiya R. Temporal change of joint position sense after posterior cruciate ligament reconstruction using multi-stranded hamstring tendons. Knee Surg Sports Traumatol Arthrosc. 2007;15:2–8.

38. Lee CD, Shon JO, Kwack HB, Lee JS. Proprioception and clinical results of anterolateral single-bundle posterior cruciate ligament reconstruction with remnant preservation. Knee Surg Relat Res. 2013;25:126–32.

39. Li J, Kong F, Gao X, Shen Y, Gao S. Prospective randomized comparison of knee stability and proprioception for posterior cruciate ligament reconstruction with autograft, hybrid graft, and γ-irradiated allograft. Arthroscopy. 2016;32:2548–55.

40. Freeman MAR, Wyke B. The innervation of the knee joint. An anatomical and histological study in the cat. J Anat. 1964;101:505–32.

41. Garn SN, Newton RA. Kinesthetic awareness in subjects with multiple ankle sprains. Phys Ther. 1988;68:1667–71.

42. Glencross D, Thorton E. Position sense following joint injury. J Sports Med Phys Fitness. 1982;21:23–7.

43. Konradson L, Ravn JB. Ankle instability caused by prolonged peroneal reaction time. Acta Orthop Scand. 1990;61:388–90.

44. Li HY, Zheng JJ, Zhang J, Cai YH, Hua YH, Chen SY. The improvement of postural control in patients with mechanical ankle instability after lateral ankle ligaments reconstruction. Knee Surg Sports Traumatol Arthrosc. 2016;24:1081–5.
45. McKeon PO, Hertel J. Systematic review of postural control and lateral ankle instability, part I: can deficits be detected with instrumented testing? J Athl Train. 2008;43:293–304.
46. Bressel E, Larsen BT, McNair PJ, Cronin J. Ankle joint proprioception and passive mechanical properties of calf muscles after an Achilles tendon rupture: a comparison with matched controls. Clin Biomech. 2004;19:284–91.
47. Kaya D, Doral MN, Nyland J, Toprak U, Turhan E, Donmez G, Citaker S, Atay OA, Callaghan MJ. Proprioception level after endoscopically guided percutaneous Achilles tendon. Knee Surg Sports Traumatol Arthrosc. 2013;21:1238–44.
48. Hawkins RB. Arthroscopic stapling repair for shoulder instability: a retrospective study of 50 cases. Arthroscopy. 1989;5:122–8.
49. Matthews LS, Vetter WL, Oweida SJ, Spearman J, Helfet D. Arthroscopic staple capsulorrhaphy for recurrent anterior shoulder instability. Arthroscopy. 1988;4:106–11.
50. Morgan CD, Bodenstab AB. Arthroscopic Bankart suture repair: technique and early results. Arthroscopy. 1987;3:111–22.
51. Vangsness CT Jr, Ennis M, Taylor JG, Atkinson B. Neural anatomy of the glenohumeral ligaments, labrum, and subacromial bursa. Arthroscopy. 1995;11:180–4.
52. Jerosch J, Steinbeck J, Schroder M, Westhues M. Intraoperative EMG recording in stimulation of the glenohumeral joint capsule. Unfallchirurg. 1995;98:580–5.
53. Myers JB, Lephart SM. The role of the sensorimotor system in the athletic shoulder. J Athl Train. 2000;35:351–63.
54. Janwantanakul P, Magarey ME, Jones MA, Dansie BR. Variation in shoulder position sense at mid and extreme range of motion. Arch Phys Med Rehabil. 2001;82:840–4.
55. Lephart SM, Warner JJ, Borsa PA, Fu FH. Proprioception of the shoulder joint in healthy, unstable, and surgically repaired shoulders. J Shoulder Elb Surg. 1994;3:371–80.
56. Fremerey R, Bosch U, Freitag N, Lobenhoffer P, Wippermann B. Proprioception and EMG pattern after capsulolabral reconstruction in shoulder instability: a clinical and experimental study. Knee Surg Sports Traumatol Arthrosc. 2006;14:1315–20.
57. Uri O, Pritsch M, Oran A, Liebermann DG. Upperlimb kinematics after arthroscopic and open shoulder stabilization. J Shoulder Elb Surg. 2015;24:399–406.
58. Sullivan JA, Hoffman MA, Harter RA. Shoulder joint position sense after thermal, open, and arthroscopic capsulorrhaphy for recurrent anterior instability. J Shoulder Elb Surg. 2008;17:389–94.
59. An YH, Friedman RJ. Multidirectional instability of the glenohumeral joint. Orthop Clin North Am. 2000;31:275–85.
60. Anderson VB, Wee E. Impaired joint proprioception at higher shoulder elevations in chronic rotator cuff pathology. Arch Phys Med Rehabil. 2011;92:1146–51.
61. Hagert E, Garcia-Elias M, Forsgren S, Ljung BO. Immunohistochemical analysis of wrist ligament innervation in relation to their structural composition. J Hand Surg Am. 2007;32:30–6.
62. Mataliotakis G, Doukas M, Kostas I, Lykissas M, Batistatou A, Beris A. Sensory innervation of the subregions of the scapholunate interosseous ligament in relation to their structural composition. J Hand Surg Am. 2009;34:1413–21.
63. Hagert E, Persson JK. Desensitizing the posterior interosseous nerve alters wrist proprioceptive reflexes. J Hand Surg Am. 2010;35:1059–66.
64. Lluch Bergada A, Leon Lopez MM, Llusa Perez M, Garcia-Elias M. Neuromuscular control of the carpus in simulated palmar midcarpal instability. Thesis in progress, Institut Kaplan, Barcelona University, Spain; 2015.
65. Smith TO, Bacon H, Jerman E, et al. Physiotherapy and occupational therapy interventions for people with benign joint hypermobility syndrome: a systematic review of clinical trials. Disabil Rehabil. 2014;36:797–803.
66. Hargreaves DG. Arthroscopic thermal capsular shrinkage for palmar midcarpal instability. J Wrist. 2014;3:162–5.
67. Hagert E, Lluch A, Rein S. The role of proprioception and neuromuscular stability in carpal instabilities. J Hand Surg Eur Vol. 2016;4:94–101.

Osteoarthritis and Proprioception 15

Cetin Sayaca, Yavuz Kocabey,
and Engin Ilker Cicek

15.1 Overview of Osteoarthritis

Osteoarthritis (OA) is the most common joint arthritis in the world [1–3]. It is seen in older people who are 65 years of age with clinical symptoms and radiographic changes [4]. Other names of osteoarthritis are **osteoarthrosis**, **degenerative joint disease**, **degenerative arthritis**, **decaying cartilage**, and **degenerative changes** [3].

OA is a chronic disease that develops slowly in a while [3]. OA is defined as degeneration of cartilage and hypertrophy of subchondral bone. Especially it often affects hands and weight-bearing joints of the body like knee, hip, cervical-lumbosacral spine, and first metatarsal phalangeal joint [3–7]. OA affects cartilage and tissues around the joint, that is, subchondral bone, ligaments, muscle, and synovium [3]. Classification of OA is given in Table 15.1 according to American College of Rheumatology [8].

15.2 Pathology of OA

The main special features of OA are progressive degeneration of cartilage, subarticular sclerosis, osteophyte formation, synovial irritation, and fibrosis of joint capsule. The changes of cartilage are seen very early [9] and the first change of OA is fibrillation that decreases the cartilage [10]. The cartilage is smooth, strong, white, and elastic in healthy people. The aim of cartilage is to help articular face of bones to move painlessly and smoothly. In mild OA, the cartilage is less smooth, insufficient, and thinner so that joint space becomes narrow. As a result movement becomes hard, and pressure of soft tissue around the joint is increased. After degenerated cartilage and imbalance of pressure, little bony spurs that entitle osteophytes thrive. Finally, the cartilage is very thin, osteophytes are bigger than in the beginning, and subchondral bone is thickened in severe osteoarthritis [3]. Cysts improve where pressure is high and trabecula around cysts becomes sclerosed. After that, intraosseous pressure increases. During that time, osteophytes are formed in cartilage that has no stress or pressure.

C. Sayaca, P.T., Ph.D. (✉)
Department of Physiotherapy and Rehabilitation,
Faculty of Health Sciences, Uskudar University,
İstanbul, Turkey
e-mail: cetin.sayaca@uskudar.edu.tr

Y. Kocabey, M.D.
Health Services Vocational School, Acibadem
University, İstanbul, Turkey

Orthopedy and Traumatology Department, Golcuk
Necati Celik State Hospital, Turkish Republic Health
Ministry, Izmıt, Turkey
e-mail: drkocabey@yahoo.com

E.I. Cicek, M.D.
Orthopedy and Traumatology Department, Golcuk
Necati Celik State Hospital, Turkish Republic
Health Ministry, Izmıt, Turkey
e-mail: drenginilkercicek@yahoo.com

© Springer International Publishing AG, part of Springer Nature 2018
D. Kaya et al. (eds.), *Proprioception in Orthopaedics, Sports Medicine and Rehabilitation*,
https://doi.org/10.1007/978-3-319-66640-2_15

Table 15.1 American College of Rheumatology criteria for classification of osteoarthritis

I. Idiopathic

A. Localized

1. **Hands** (e.g., Heberden's and Bouchard's nodes [nodal], erosive interphalangeal arthritis [nonnodal]): scaphometacarpal, scaphotrapezial

2. **Foot** (e.g., hallux valgus, hallux rigidus, contracted toes [hammer/cock-up toes]): talonavicular

3. **Knee**

   (a) Medial compartment

   (b) Lateral compartment

   (c) Patellofemoral compartment (e.g., chondromalacia)

4. **Hip**

   (a) Eccentric (superior)

   (b) Concentric (axial, medial)

   (c) Diffuse (coxae senilis)

5. **Spine** (particularly cervical and lumbar)

   (a) Apophyseal

   (b) Intervertebral (disk)

   (c) Spondylosis (osteophytes)

   (d) Ligamentous (hyperostosis [Forestier disease or diffuse idiopathic skeletal hyperostosis])

6. **Other single sites** (e.g., shoulder, temporomandibular, sacroiliac, ankle, wrist, acromioclavicular)

B. Generalized: includes three or more areas listed above (Kellgren-Moore)

1. Small (peripheral) and spine

2. Large (central) and spine

3. Mixed (peripheral and central) and spine

II. Secondary

A. Posttraumatic

B. Congenital or developmental diseases

1. **Localized**

   (a) **Hip diseases** (e.g., Legg-Calvé-Perthes, congenital hip dislocation, slipped capital femoral epiphysis, shallow acetabulum)

   (b) **Mechanical and local factors** (e.g., obesity, unequal lower extremity length, extreme valgus/varus deformity, hypermobility syndromes, scoliosis)

2. **Generalized**

   (a) **Bone dysplasias** (e.g., epiphyseal dysplasia, spondyloapophyseal dysplasia)

   (b) **Metabolic diseases** (e.g., hemochromatosis, ochronosis, Gaucher disease, hemoglobinopathy, Ehlers-Danlos syndrome)

Table 15.1 (continued)

C. Calcium deposition disease

1. **Calcium pyrophosphate deposition disease**

2. **Apatite arthropathy**

3. **Destructive arthropathy** (shoulder, knee)

D. Other bone and joint disorders (e.g., avascular necrosis, rheumatoid arthritis, gouty arthritis, septic arthritis, Paget's disease, osteopetrosis, osteochondritis)

E. Other diseases

1. **Endocrine diseases** (e.g., diabetes mellitus, acromegaly, hypothyroidism, hyperparathyroidism)

2. **Neuropathic arthropathy** (Charcot joints)

3. **Miscellaneous** (e.g., frostbite, Kashin-Beck disease, caisson disease)

From Altman R, Asch E, Bloch D, et al. (1986) Development of criteria for the classification and reporting of osteoarthritis. Classification of osteoarthritis of the knee. Diagnostic and Therapeutic Criteria Committee of the American Rheumatism Association. Arthritis Rheu 29:1039–49

As a result, all of these activities which are construction and demolition are seen in OA together [9]. Enzymes secreted as a result of damage to the circumference of the joint degenerate the cells and synovitis develops. In the late stage, fibrosis develops around the articulation capsule and then it may cause stiffness of joint [9]. Normally cartilage and synovium don't have nerves [3, 9] but the chances in subchondral and capsular area cause pain, because of nerves in that area [9]. Therefore OA progresses silently. When patients are aware, it may be too late.

15.3 Risk Factors for OA

A lot of risk factors are defined for OA and a single factor is not responsible for its occurrence [3]. Epidemiological studies refer to a lot of risk factors but especially six main factors are important for OA. These are age, obesity, trauma, abnormal biomechanics, genetic, and change of joint shape [11, 12]. Mechanical and genetic factors are important for OA, but age is the most important factor than others [13].

Symptoms increase with age and sex. OA is seen in radiologic imaging in 90% of all people by age 40 [6]. Especially it is seen in a lot of people in 65 years and 80% of over age 75 [2]. Sex is an important risk factor because of most frequent occurrence in women than in men [6, 14]. But OA is seen more frequently in men before 50 years of age. After 50 years of age, frequent increase in women [15, 16]. Another important risk factor is obesity that affects the knee, hand, and probably hip joints [6]. This factor increases the load to joint surface and soft tissue around joint. So the cartilage is exposed with extreme stress for a long time. In terms of ethnicity, knee OA has higher rates in African-American women but not men. African-American people have a higher risk of OA than white people but there is a little difference for hand OA [17]. Otherwise, according to Anderson and Felson and Jordan et al., there are no differences in the prevalence of OA ethnically [18, 19] and hip OA [20]. Most of the genes are responsible and affect the prevalence of OA [21], for example the vitamin D receptor gene, insulin-like growth factor I genes, and cartilage oligomeric protein genes [22]. Biomechanical changes affect healthy and pathological joint directly [23]. Abnormalities of biomechanics increase degenerative force on the cartilage of joint. Malalignment of knee is a risk factor for knee OA [24] and hip joint geometry alter the distribution of loading forces across the hip joint [25]. Geometry of hip can distribute the stress that comes on the hip joint. If there is a wrong position of the geometry of hip, the stress increases on some area and OA develops. Trauma, like a fracture of articular surface, menisci, or ligament tears, is a reason for joint instability. The risk of posttraumatic OA increases with obesity [26, 27]. Bone and cartilage pathologies are related with OA [28]. For example, upper femoral epiphyseal shift or congenital acetabular dysplasia is associated with greater risk for OA, as it causes alterations in the joint surface [9].

Out of these risk factors, sports/physical activity, muscle weakness, and occupation are also risk factors for OA. During sports or physical activity, ligament or meniscal injury damages joint and increases the risk of OA. Repeated movements in daily activities increase the risk of OA. However, muscle weakness is another important risk factor. Muscle weakness around the joint breaks down the stability and increases loading on joint [29]. Some risk factors are not changed from person to person. It is important that people manage their risk factors that are changeable for decreasing the incidence of OA. For example, exercise and decreasing of weight are important for protecting joints from osteoarthritis [23]. In addition, biological, quality of life, and socioeconomic factors may affect the prevalence of OA.

15.4   Diagnosis of OA

There are two groups of arthritis. The first group is atrophic that is characterized by synovial inflammation and decreasing of cartilage and bone like a rheumatoid arthritis or septic arthritis. The other group is hypertrophic that is called osteoarthritis [2]. To explain the joint pattern is important for diagnosis of arthritis. It is explained to answer these questions: Is there inflammation, and how many and which joints are affected? Within 30 min will morning stiffness, swelling, and inflammation of joint clear? Characteristic joint patterns of OA are monoarticular, minimal inflammation, and distal interphalangeal joint involvement. All of these signs are important to distinguish OA from another form of arthritis [6]:

* No systemic symptoms
* Degeneration and minimal inflammation of joint
* In rest pain decreases
* The morning stiffness for a short time
* General features in the radiographic review: decreased joint space, osteophyte formation, bony cysts, high mineral density of subchondral bone in X-ray [2]

15.5   Clinical Signs of OA

The symptoms of OA are frequent pain and stiffness and decrease in pain in a few minutes after movement but occurrence of pain at rest in chronic stage. Normally, inflammation and swelling are very mild in OA [6]. But, in serious pathology, inflammation and its symptoms like swelling and heat may be seen [3]:

- Joint stiffness
- Pain increases with motion and weight-bearing activity
- Pain reduces with rest
- DIP and PIP nodes are remarkable
- Limitation of range of motion in affected joint
- Crepitus
- Mild inflammation and swelling
- Any systemic signs
- No rise in erythrocyte sedimentation rate and other laboratory signs of inflammation
- Osteophyte, bone cysts, decreasing joint area, and intensive subchondral bone in radiograph

15.6   Radiographic Definitions of OA

Radiography is the gold standard for definition of OA [17]. The Kellgren-Lawrence radiographic grading scale divided OA into five levels [30]. In "Grade 0" there are no changes and in "Grade 4" there is a lot of degeneration in joint (Table 15.2). To use this classification of OA with the Kellgren-Lawrence radiographic grading scale, there must be osteophytes in joint. This has been criticized by another researcher [31]. But it is often used by clinicians.

Table 15.2 Kellgren-Lawrence radiographic grading system for osteoarthritis

Grade	Classification	Description
0	Normal	No characteristic finding about OA
1	Doubtful	İnsignificant osteophytes
2	Minimal	Certain osteophytes but intact joint space
3	Moderate	Moderate reducing of joint space
4	Severe	Severe reducing of joint space and sclerosis of subchondral bone

Adapted from Kellgren JH, Lawrence JS, editors. The epidemiology of chronic rheumatism, atlas of standard radiographs. Oxford: Blackwell Scientific; 1963

15.7   Proprioception in OA

Awareness and definition of movement in space called proprioception are important. There are three important specialties of proprioception that limits excessive movement, stabilizes joint position, and coordinates during movement [32]. Proprioception could be identified as awareness of velocity, force, and position of extremity in space [33] and it originates from mechanoreceptors that are in muscles, joint capsule tendons, ligaments, and skin [34]. Intact innervation of joint is important for proprioception. Damage of mechanoreceptors that are around the joint affects neuromuscular control and as a result non-coordinated motion appears [35].

Proprioception is important for the strength of muscle which prevents loading excessive stress on joint during walking [35]. Joint receptors provide information input for the central nervous system about joint position and movements. In OA, primarily the joint receptors change, while muscle receptors change over time [32]. So the proprioceptive input decreases and impairs. Proprioceptive input is important and essential for homeostasis [36, 37]. Proprioceptive deficits may result in functional instability leading to future microtrauma and reinjury [38]. Decreasing of proprioception affects the pathophysiology of knee OA [39, 40]. But it doesn't affect another joint proprioception like knee or wrist in patient with knee OA [41]. However, there are relationships between strength, proprioception, and loading in the lower extremity with affected hip OA. Especially, there are deficits of proprioception and muscle strength in OA [42]. In addition, proprioception decreases with age and it is a risk for knee OA. As a result, poor proprioception continues with functional disability in knee OA [40].

There are two types of proprioceptive receptors classified as slow and fast. Fast receptors, like Pacinian corpuscles, react quickly to external stimuli and issue nerve impulses. The main function of Pacinian corpuscles is to detect movement which is acceleration or deceleration and beginning or completion. Slow receptors, like Ruffini corpuscles, free nerve endings, Golgi tendon organ, and muscle spindles, proceed to sense stimuli over time whose main role is to sense change of position and accurate positioning of joints [43].

Proprioceptors may be classified into three main parts in terms of their localization such as cutaneous, joint, and muscle receptors, respectively. Joint receptors are free nerve endings, Pacinian corpuscle, Ruffini's nerve endings, Golgi ligament endings, and Golgi Mazzoni corpuscles [44, 45]. Muscle receptors are Golgi tendon organs and muscle spindle [46]. Information gained from these receptors are processed in the somatosensorial cortical areas and resulted with the perception of the joint kinematics.

1. **Joint Receptors**: Joint receptors (JR) are located in the joint structures. JR are sensitive to the changes in the joint structures like stretch and relaxation. The information of joint position and movement are transmitted to the upper cortical systems. Joint receptors are generally defined in terms of their response to the stimuli and characteristics as the joint state, intensity of the stimuli (low threshold/high threshold), and adaptation to the stimuli (slow adapting/rapid adapting) [47].
   - **Free nerve ending (FNE)**: FNEs are bare dendrites found in every body structure. FNEs are especially intense in epithelial and connective tissue. FNEs are tiny sensorial fibers capable for detecting pressure, pain, and temperature and act as pain receptor/nociceptive system in the synovial joints. Typically, joint capsule, periosteum beneath the joint, and intra-articular fat pad have numerous FNEs. Inactivate FNEs are activated with the stimuli (mechanical and chemical stimulations) including inflammatory fluids and inflammatory agents (bradykinin, histamine, etc.), pain, pressure, and temperature alterations.
   - **Pacinian corpuscle (PC)**: PCs are conical and extended corpuscles, capable of sensing initial pressure and vibrations. These featured receptors are located in the connective tissue capsules. PCs are found much in deeper layers of fibrous joint capsule; therefore these are sensitive to initial

deep pressure. PCs are often lined up along with articular vessel. PCs are inactive in resting joint and active during joint compression and perturbations for short-term duration of 1 s and less [48]. PCs have low activation threshold and they adapt rapidly to the persistent stimuli [47].
   - **Ruffini's nerve ending (RNE)**: RNEs are thin capsulated globular/ovoid corpuscles generally located in the superficial layer of joint capsules. Meniscofemoral, collateral, and anterior cruciate ligaments have also RNE. These receptors are low-threshold and slowly adapting mechanoreceptors. RNEs are sensitive to joint position, intra-articular pressure, amplitude, and velocity of movement and they are always active either in static or dynamic position [47].
   - **Golgi ligament endings (GLEs)**: GLEs are located in ligaments and menisci. GLEs have sensitivity for tension or stretching forces on ligaments and are active in case of joint dynamic with high activation threshold. Their response to the persistent stimuli is slow adaptation. When GLE detects the stretching of tendon, they trigger the reflex pathways in order to inhibit the muscle contraction to protect the tendon or muscle from injury.
   - **Golgi Mazzoni corpuscles (GMCs)**: GMCs are located in joint capsule for detecting the joint compression. Weight-bearing activities stimulate these mechanoreceptors.

2. **Muscle Receptors**: There are two types of muscle receptors: Golgi tendon organ (GTO) and muscle spindle [46]. These receptors inform the muscle length and tension.
   - **Golgi tendon organ (GTO)**: GTOs are located in the tendons that attach muscles to the bones. GTO gives information about muscle tension and is very sensitive to the changes under force because each organ is connected to the small muscle fibers. These receptors can be able to give response to the forces even less than 0.1 g [49].
   - **Muscle spindles (MSs)**: MSs are encapsulated structures that lie parallel to the muscle fibers. MSs are sensitive to muscle

length and velocity [46]. MSs play a role in the control of the posture. These structures also detect sudden motion and stretch of the muscle.

Mechanoreceptors provide proprioceptive sensation which is essential for normal activities and also stimulating the protective reflex arcs in physically challenging tasks. Degenerative pathologies affecting the tissues where these receptors are located also cause proprioceptive deficits. The integrity and control of sensorimotor systems are essential for balanced and stable normal gait [50]. Specific range of motion of the knee joint has different extent of the role of proprioception [51]. All receptors are activated to prevent injuries at the last angles of motion range. Muscle spindle receptors take the sense of changing position of the knee joint in the middle angles of motion range.

Joint cartilage damage could stimulate joint mechanoreceptors and this process evokes abnormal sensory information to the central nervous system that decelerates voluntary activation [52]. Afferent fibers originating from joint mechanoreceptors transduce stimuli onto alpha motoneurons located in spinal cord that activates muscle fibers extra-fusally [53, 54]. Articular degenerative damages result in abnormal signalization, following which alpha motoneuron excitation is decelerated that results in decreased voluntary activation of quadriceps [53, 54]. Joint mechanoreceptors' afferent pathway has also projection onto gamma motoneurons in the spinal cord. Intra-fusal muscle fibers are activated by gamma motoneurons and comprised muscle spindles. The regulation of muscle spindle sensitivity is provided by gamma motoneuron excitability. The sensitivity of muscle spindle decreases, and therefore perception sensitivity of the joint decreases [55, 56]. Barrett et al. claimed that laxity of joint capsule and ligaments was due to loss of cartilage and bone height, and lytic enzymes may damage the receptors [55].

15.8 Proprioception After Knee Replacement Surgery

Knee arthroplasty was first introduced in the 1950s. Ligaments were replaced with the hinged design of the prosthesis. In early designs, stability had been the major issue for the replacement. Approaches aiming normal knee kinematics have been the major expectation in the designs in course of time. With the clinical usage of methyl methacrylate cement there has been improved fixation of the prosthesis. This integration of components with the bone surface allowed surface design modifications for the normal articular motion kinematics. Despite scarification of menisci, anterior cruciate ligament and posterior cruciate ligament are not denied that significant influence on the knee proprioception impairment during the knee replacement surgery, and proprioceptive receptors are also located in the joint, ligaments, capsule, skin, surrounding muscles, synovium, and subcutaneous tissue. From another point of view, the knee proprioception will continue with the help of these structures. Proper ligament balance may partly contribute to better proprioception after total knee arthroplasty. The designers believed that posterior cruciate ligament preservation resulted in more balanced and anatomic replaced knee joint. The PCL preservation in total knee arthroplasty also increased the proprioceptive sensation [55, 57, 58].

It should be kept in mind that even though these receptors are preserved during knee arthroplasty, these receptors are worn out in the gonarthrosis pathophysiological process and therefore an effective proprioceptive sensation will not occur, despite the benefit of all these receptors. Knee replacement surgery with the new designs has benefits for pain relief and function; candidates have to improve the strength of the surrounding structures especially muscle and ligaments and neuromuscular control by means of proprioception. This aim can be achieved with the preoperative and postoperative well-programmed exercises

[59]. These exercise protocols enhanced proprioceptive sensation and also stability of the prosthetic motion, resulting with the increase in durability of prosthesis.

Wada et al. evaluated the effects of total knee arthroplasty on joint proprioception and the absolute angular error of the knee in patients with knee osteoarthritis before and after total knee arthroplasty [60]. Angular error of knee was found to be much more seen in the knees which had anterior cruciate ligament deficiency than normal-appearing ACL before surgery and they concluded that deficiency of the anterior cruciate ligament may not adversely affect proprioception in severe knee osteoarthritis [60].

Moutzouri and colleagues reviewed systematically 13 studies in order to identify the extent of the effects of total knee arthroplasty on balance and incidence of falls. These studies interpreted balance and incidence of falls without physiotherapeutic intervention after total knee arthroplasty. The results showed that single-limb standing balance and dynamic balance were improved in 1-year period following surgery [61]. Also, fear of falling and incidence of falls decreased after TKA. They claimed that knee extension strength, proprioception, and symmetrization of postural strategies are not exactly amended after TKA and addressed that these deficits have to be solved with physiotherapy before surgical intervention [61].

Ries evaluated the effect of anterior cruciate ligament on knee kinematics after total knee arthroplasty [62]. He claimed that posterior cruciate-retaining total knee arthroplasties are resulted with paradoxical motion since the tibia is subluxed anteriorly during knee extension movement and the femur translates anteriorly during knee flexion movement. The author concluded that preserving the anterior cruciate ligament (ACL) resulted in better knee kinematics and function with unicompartmental and patellofemoral arthroplasties, when compared with conventional knee arthroplasty [63].

Expectations for normal knee kinematics improve prosthesis technologic development for new designs. Bicruciate-retaining models have been developed for this purpose. Bauman et al. commented on the balance ability in order to measure proprioception sensation in patients with a bicruciate-retaining total knee arthroplasty [63]. They found better static balance ability after preservation of both cruciate ligaments in arthroplasty of the knee and also this study indicated better proprioceptive function when compared with the control group of patients after unicondylar knee arthroplasty and posterior stabilized total knee arthroplasty. They conclude that kinematics and long-term survivorship of bicruciate-retaining implants had to be investigated with the prospective and randomized studies [63].

15.9 Proprioceptive Rehabilitation Approaches for OA

In OA, there is a degeneration of cartilage and other tissues around joint, like ligaments and muscle. So this degeneration of all tissues can affect proprioceptor in these tissues, in OA. There is no consensus about exercise effects, type, time, duration, etc. on OA. The aim of rehabilitation in OA is to increase quality of life with improving range of motion, increase strength, and decrease pain. Therapeutic approaches are shown to have evident improvements on proprioception. In addition, rehabilitation is different in every joint. But their aims are similar. Physical work capacity is important to protect joint cartilage from losing [64].

15.10 Exercise Therapy

Exercises are the most effective intervention and important part of rehabilitation in OA and included aerobic, strengthening, range-of-motion [65], stretching, and flexibility exercises [66]. It can be used for restoration pain and function and its clinical result is meaningful [67]. Exercise therapy of OA is to increase muscle strength, improve balance and coordination of movements, and improve joint mobility [68] and muscle strength is associated with functional level in OA [69]. Muscle weakness is a mechanical risk factor for OA around the joint [70]. When muscles around the joint are strong, joint can be protected from progression of OA.

Cartilage develops during activity that is known, but during overexercise cartilage might progress in both directions [70]. Eckstein et al. did not find any difference significantly in the in vivo deformational behavior of cartilage between non-athletes and athletes (weight lifters, sprinter, etc.). But in animal study, weight-bearing exercises protect joint from OA during physical activity. On the contrary, there are conflicting results in human study about physical activity affecting cartilage thickness [71]. Articular cartilage is changeable with mechanical stimulation and it is adaptive to new conditions so it can change morphology and composition [72] although some studies didn't offer exercise for OA [73, 74]. But if people don't move enough, it affects cartilage negatively. In a study, rate of cartilage was worse in spinal cord injury than OA due to nonuse [75]. True exercise is important to keep cartilage healthy.

Joint loading in the weight-bearing exercises stimulates Ruffini's endings due to increase in joint articular pressure, by the way proprioceptive accuracy is advanced [76]. Some exercises can be harmful in the long term like running and step aerobics. They may not be chosen for OA by physiotherapist or patients [70].

15.10.1 Exercise Therapy in Hand OA

Exercise and education of joint protection are used in hand OA. Especially stretching and strengthening exercises are used commonly [77]. Also there is lack of evidence about exercise's effect on hand OA [78]; strengthening and range-of-motion exercise is often used [79] for decreasing pain and improving range of motion and strength in hand OA [80].

15.10.2 Exercise Therapy in Hip OA

Exercise treatment is recommended mostly in hip OA. Strength, stretching, and flexibility exercises are recommended [66]. Improving joint stability of hip might be done by strengthening exercise for stabilizer muscles of hip [81]. In idiopathic OA, if there is degeneration in one hip, it effects OA in another hip [82]. Therefore, bilateral exercises may start to protect. If needed, lumbo-pelvic stabilization exercise is added by physical therapist [83]. Aerobic, strengthening, and range-of-motion exercise could be used to decrease pain [66, 84] and aerobic exercises are very cheap like walking, swimming, and cycling that patient enjoys [83]. There are positive effects of strength exercises on pain, range of motion, stiffness, disability, and physical function in a short time [66]. Otherwise, neuromuscular exercise education is beneficial for hip OA even in the last stage [85]. Svege et al. reported that exercise might delay replacement of hip joint by 44%. Despite everything, there are limited number of studies about the effects of exercise on pain, function, and quality of life in hip OA [86, 87]. Even so, exercise is an important part of rehabilitation and this condition continues for a long time.

15.10.3 Exercise Therapy in Knee OA

Exercise therapy is an important branch of physical therapy for improving proprioceptive accuracy including knee position and motion sense. Two main branches of exercise protocol are aforementioned. These are proprioceptive exercises and muscle-strengthening exercises. Proprioceptive exercises are performed as non-weight-bearing and weight-bearing exercises. Muscle-strengthening exercises are also divided in terms of loading perspective of the joint (weight-bearing and non-weight-bearing muscle-strengthening exercises). There is no consensus on which exercise protocol corrects proprioceptive accuracy more than the other. Quadriceps weakness is an important risk factor of knee OA. Especially, increasing instability of knee decreases shock absorption behavior of muscle by weakness of quadriceps [88, 89]. However, strengthening the hamstrings with quadriceps is useful for attenuated symptoms in knee OA [90].

15.10.4 Intensity and Duration of Proprioceptive Exercises

Strengthening exercise program may be started with isometric, but it is improved to isotonic as long as it is tolerated [70]. Multitype exercise programs were not effective than single-type exercise programs [91]. However, it should be noted that the exercise program must be designed specifically for the patients each time. In literature, there are no significant differences within high- versus low-intensity exercise about pain, function, and quality of life in patients with hip or knee OA [92] or intensity and duration of the sessions [91].

Exercises are continued 3–6 months after therapy for reduction in pain and improvement in physical function [93]. Strength exercises must be done minimum 8–24 weeks for effects to be seen [66]. Exercise program must be continued three times in a week and the effect of exercises increases with the number of sessions [91].

15.11 Aquatherapy

There are a lot of different names of aquatic exercise, like pool therapy, hydrotherapy, or balneotherapy. The basic aim of it is that people do their exercise in water. The water's heat is generally 32–36 °C. Aquatic exercises are used to relieve pain and improve function and usually chosen for knee or hip, or both in OA [94]. Exercises that are done in the water are more effective in hip OA [65].

Aquatic exercises may be more expensive than exercise therapy and is difficult to provide hygiene. But it might have advantages as relieving pain, decreasing stiffness, or relaxing muscle [95]. Therefore, aquatic exercises might be preferred in session initially if there is a stiffness or a lot of pain in extremity.

15.12 Specialized Proprioceptive Techniques

Proprioceptive exercises are important to restore neuromuscular control, regain dynamic and static stability of joint, and improve functional status of people. With the damage of mechanoreceptors around the joint, neuromuscular control is lost, and as a result smooth, coordinated movement cannot be seen [35], so it affects function [38, 96, 97], because stability of joint depends on afferent impulses from nerve endings [98]. Exercises are important to restore proprioception and equilibrium, like walking, retrowalking, closed kinetic chain, kinesthetic, balance, aerobic dancing, Tai Chi, and aquatic exercises [99, 100, 101]. Direction, velocity, load, surface, and unexpected impulse can be changed or added to increase the difficulty level of proprioception in exercise therapy. The common point of exercises may be to give a mechanical stimulation for mechanoreceptors during weight bearing, range-of-motion exercises, or progressive resistive exercises, but doing exercises in weight-bearing position are effective than these exercises [102]. For example, closed kinetic chain exercises may be better than open kinetic chain exercises, because they affect a few joints during the exercise, so a lot of impulses from mechanoreceptors stimulate cortex [103, 104]. In addition, giving sensory input may increase proprioception [38]. If proprioception is increasing, it can improve knee muscle strength too [43]. Proprioceptive exercises improve the joint position sense in OA [105].

15.13 Manuel Therapy Approaches

Manual therapy includes high-velocity manipulations, stretching, traction, massage, and myofascial trigger point release. Joint-based manual therapy techniques relieve pain with activating inhibitory system of pain from cortical area [106]. In one study, manual therapy caused hypoalgesia immediately in knee OA [107]. It is applied in a lot of sessions but there is no consensus about the total number of sessions using it. Manual therapy may be used between 2 and 8 weeks in the treatment [108–111]. In addition, there are a lot of parameters that may affect therapy result like force, speed, amplitude, rate, repetition, and duration. As a result, manual therapy may be used to decrease pain and improve function for short-term benefits. But there isn't enough evidence about the benefit on pain and function for knee and hip OA [112].

15.14 Therapeutic Ultrasound

Therapeutic ultrasound (TUS) is used very often than other physiotherapy modalities in rehabilitation of OA. TUS includes high-frequency vibrations [113] and consists of pulsed or continuous mode. Pulsed mode affects tissue with nonthermal properties and continuous mode affects tissue with thermal properties [114]. It can be used to decrease pain and increase function in knee OA, despite the quality of evidence being limited. So it can affect proprioception positively. In addition, there was no knowledge about safety of ultrasound and effects on hip OA in literature [115].

15.15 Thermotherapy

In OA, sometimes inflammation can be increased by edema. Thermotherapy can be used for decreasing edema, relieving pain, and increasing movement and function. In physiotherapy, heat and cryotherapy are used very often for pain with combining other physiotherapy interventions. When cold is applied longer than 20 min, "hunting reaction" may occur and as a result pain may recur or increase [116]. Ice massaging that may be used for 20 min per session, 5 sessions per week, for 2 weeks improves quadriceps strength, range of motion, and functional status significantly in knee OA. But there are no important changes that are measured by knee circumference [117]. But another study showed that using cold pack reduces knee edema after ten sessions. In addition, there was no change in knee edema when using hot packs in this study [118].

15.16 Acupuncture

Acupuncture is very popular for reducing musculoskeletal pain [119, 120]. It can be used with or without mechanical or electrical stimulation [87]. But there is no evidence for using acupuncture in OA [121]. Effects of acupuncture are little on pain in knee OA.

References

1. Lawrence RC, Hochberg MC, Kelsey JL, et al. Estimates of the prevalence of selected arthritic and musculoskeletal diseases in the United States. J Rheumatol. 1989;16:427–41.
2. Arden N, Cooper C. Osteoarthritis handbook. Arden N, Cooper C, editors. London: Taylor and Francis Group; 2006. p. 1–2.
3. Prieto-Alhambra D, Arden N, Hunter DJ The facts osteoarthritis. 2nd ed. Oxford: Oxford University Press; 2014. p. 3–12.
4. Goldring SR, Goldring MB. Clinical aspects, pathology and pathophysiology of osteoarthritis. J Musculoskelet Neuronal Interact. 2006;6(4):376–8.
5. Wood PHN, Badley EM. Epidemiology of individual rheumatic disorders. In: Scott JT, editor. Copeman's textbook of the rheumatic disases. 6th ed. Edinburgh and London: Churchill Livingstone; 1986. p. 59–142.
6. Hellmann DB, İmboden JB. Rheumatologic, ımmunologic and allergic disorder. In: Papadakis MA, Mcphee SJ, editors. Current medical dignosis and treatment. 55th ed. New York: McGraw-Hill Education; 2016. p. 812–5. ISBN 978-0-07-184509-0.
7. Kasper DL, Fauci AS, Hauser SL, Longo DL, Jameson JL, Loscalzo J. Harrison's principles of internal medicine. 19th ed. New York: ABD; 2016. p. 2226–30. ISBN 978-0-07-180215-4.
8. Altman R, Asch E, Bloch D, et al. Development of criteria for the classification and reporting of osteoarthritis. Classification of osteoarthritis of the knee. Diagnostic and Therapeutic Criteria Committee of the American Rheumatism Association. Arthritis Rheum. 1986;29:1039–49.
9. Solomon L, Warwick D, Nayagam S. Apley and Solomon's concise system of orthopaedics and trauma. 4th ed. London: Taylor & Francis Group; 2014. p. 46–8.
10. Huber M, Trattnig S, Lintner F. Anatomy, biochemistry and physiology of articular cartilage. Investig Radiol. 2000;35:573–80.
11. Felson DT. Epidemiology of hip and knee osteoarthritis. Epidemiol Rev. 1988;10:1–28.
12. Scott JC, Hochberg MC. Osteoarthritis: 1. Epidemiology. Md State Med J. 1984;33:712–6.

13. Felson DT, Zhang Y. An update on the epidemiology of knee and hip osteoarthritis with a view to prevention. Arthritis Rheum. 1998;41:1343–55.
14. Felson DT, Naimark A, Anderson J, Kazis L, Castelli W, Meenan RF. The prevalence of knee osteoarthritis in the elderly. The Framingham Osteoarthritis Study. Arthritis Rheum. 1987;30:914–8.
15. van Saase JL, van Romunde LK, Cats A, Vandenbroucke JP, Valkenburg HA. Epidemiology of osteoarthritis: Zoetermeer survey. Comparison of radiological osteoarthritis in a Dutch population with that in 10 other populations. Ann Rheum Dis. 1989;48:271–80.
16. Lawrence JS, Sebo M. The geography of osteoarthritis. In: Nuki G, editor. The aetiopathogenesis of osteoarthritis. Kent: Pitman Medical; 1980. p. 155–83.
17. Nelson AE, Jordan JM. Rheumatology. In: Hochberg MC, et al., editors. 6th edn. Philadelphia: Elsevier Mosby; 2015. p. 1433–40.
18. Anderson JJ, Felson DT. Factors associated with osteoarthritis of the knee in the first national Health and Nutrition Examination Survey (HANES I). Evidence for an association with overweight, race, and physical demands of work. Am J Epidemiol. 1988;128:179–89.
19. Jordan JM, Linder GF, Renner JB, Fryer JG. The impact of arthritis in rural populations. Arthritis Care Res. 1995;8:242–50.
20. Tepper S, Hochberg MC. Factors associated with hip osteoarthritis: data from the first National Health and Nutrition Examination Survey (NHANES-I). Am J Epidemiol. 1993;37:1081–8.
21. Clark AG, Jordan JM, Vilim VV, Renner JB, Dragomir AD, Luta G, et al. Serum cartilage oligomeric matrix protein reflects osteoarthritis presence and severity: the Johnston County Osteoarthritis Project. Arthritis Rheum. 1999;42:2356–64.
22. Wright GD, Hughes AE, Regan M, Doherty M. Association of two loci on chromosome 2q with nodal osteoarthritis. Ann Rheum Dis. 1996;55:317–9.
23. Guilak F. Biomechanical factors in osteoarthritis. Best Pract Res Clin Rheumatol. 2011;25:815–23.
24. Moyer RF, Birmingham TB, Chesworth BM, Kean CO, Giffin JR. Alignment, body mass and their interaction on dynamic knee joint load in patients with knee osteoarthritis. Osteoarthr Cartil. 2010;18:888–93.
25. Lenaerts G, Bartels W, Gelaude F, Mulier M, Spaepen A, Van der Perre G, et al. Subject-specific hip geometry and hip joint centre location affects calculated contact forces at the hip during gait. J Biomech. 2009;42:1246–51.
26. Buckwalter JA, Lane LE. Athletics and osteoarthritis. Am J Sports Med. 1997;25:873–81.
27. Honkonen SE. Degenerative arthritis after tibial plateau fractures. J Orthop Trauma. 1995;9:273–7.
28. Julie C, LePain B, Lane NE. Role of bone architecture and anatomy in osteoarthritis. Bone. 2012;51:197–203.
29. Garstang SV, Stitik TP. Osteoarthritis: epidemiology, risk factors, and pathophysiology. Am J Phys Med Rehabil. 2006;85:2–11.
30. Kellgren JH, Lawrence JS. Radiological assessment of osteo-arthrosis. Ann Rheum Dis. 1957;16:494–502.
31. Schiphof D, Boers M, Bierma-Zeinstra SM. Differences in descriptions of Kellgren and Lawrence grades of knee osteoarthritis. Ann Rheum Dis. 2008;67:1034–6.
32. Knoop J, Steultjens MPM, van der Leeden M, van der Esch M, Thorstensson CA, Roorda LD, et al. Proprioception in knee osteoarthritis: a narrative review. Osteoarthr Cartil. 2011;19(4):381–8.
33. Stillman BC. Making sense of proprioception. The meaning of proprioception, kinaesthesia and related terms. Physiotherapy. 2002;88:667–76.
34. Olsson L, Lund H, Henriksen M, Rogind H, Bliddal H, et al. Test-retest reliability of a knee joint position sense measurement method in sitting and prone position. Adv Physiother. 2004;6:37–47.
35. Lephart SM, Fu FH. Proprioception and neuromuscular control in joint stability. Champaign, IL: Human Kinetics; 2000.
36. Sjölander P, Johansson H, Djupsjöbacka M. Spinal and supraspinal affects of activity in ligament afferents. J Electromyogr Kinesiol. 2002;12:167–76.
37. Diederichsen LP, Nørregaard J, Krogsgaard M, Fischer-Rasmussen T, Dyhre-Poulsen P. Reflexes in the shoulder muscles elicited from the human coracoacromial ligament. J Orthop Res. 2004;22:976–83.
38. Lephart SM, Pincivero DM, Giraldo JL, Fu FH. The role of proprioception in the management and rehabilitation of athletic injuries. Am J Sports Med. 1997;25:130–7.
39. Lund H, Juul-Kristensen B, Hansen K, Christensen R, Christensen H, Danneskiold-Samsoe B, Bliddal H. Movement detection impaired in patients with knee osteoarthritis compared to healthy controls: a cross-sectional case–control study. J Musculoskelet Neuronal Interact. 2008;8:391–400.
40. Pai YC, Rymer WZ, Chang RW, Sharma L. Affect of age and osteoarthritis on knee proprioception. Arthritis Rheum. 1997;40:2260–5.
41. Shanahan CJ, Wrigley TV, Michael J, Shanahan CJF, Wrigley TV, Farrell MJ, Bennell KL, Hodges PW. Poprioceptive impairments associated with knee osteoarthritis are not generalized to the ankle and elbow joints. Hum Mov Sci. 2015;41:103–13.
42. Shakoor N, Foucher KC, Wimmer MA, Mikolaitis-Preuss RA, Fogg LF, Block JA. Asymmetries and relationships between dynamic loading, muscle strength, and proprioceptive acuity at the knees in symptomatic unilateral hip osteoarthritis. Arthritis Res Ther. 2014;16:455. https://doi.org/10.1186/s13075-014-0455-7.
43. Hewett TE, Paterno MV, Myer GD. Strategies for enhancing proprioception and neuromuscular control of the knee. Clin Orthop Relat Res. 2002;402:76–94.

44. Grigg P. Peripheral neural mechanisms in proprioception. Sport Rehabil. 1994;3:1–17.

45. Haus J, Halata Z. Innervation of the anterior cruciate ligament. Int Orthop. 1990;14:293–6.

46. Gordon J, Ghez C. Muscle receptors and spinal reflexes: the stretch reflex. In: Kandel E, Schwartz J, Jessell T, editors. Principles of neural science. 3rd ed. New York, NY: Elsevier Science Publishing Co.; 1991. p. 564–80.

47. Williams GN, Chmielewski T, Rudolph K, Buchanan TS, Snyder-Mackler L. Dynamic knee stability: current theory and implications for clinicians and scientists. J Orthop Sports Phys Ther. 2001;31(10):546–66.

48. Moraes MR, Cavalcante ML, Leite JA, Ferreira FV, Castro AJ, Santana MG. Histomorphometric evaluation of mechanoreceptors and free nerve endings in human lateral ankle ligaments. Foot Ankle Int. 2008;29(1):87–90.

49. Houk J, Henneman E. Responses of Golgi tendon organs to active contractions of the soleus muscle of the cat. Neurophysiology. 1967;30:466–81.

50. Fitzpatrick R, McCloskey D. Proprioceptive, visual and vestibular thresholds for the perception of sway during standing in humans. J Physiol. 1994;478(1):173–86.

51. Angoules AG, Mavrogenis AF, Dimitriou R, et al. Knee proprioception following ACL reconstruction; a prospective trial comparing hamstrings with bone patellar tendon-bone autograft. Knee. 2011;18:76–82.

52. Hurley MV, Newham DJ. The influence of arthrogenous muscle inhibition on quadriceps rehabilitation of patients with early, unilateral osteoarthritic knees. Br J Rheumatol. 1993;32:127–31.

53. Baldissera F, Hultborn H, Illert M. Integration in spinal neurone systems. In: Brooks V, editor. Handbook of physiology. Bethesda, MD: American Physiological Society; 1981. p. 509–97.

54. McCrea DA. Can sense be made of spinal interneuron circuits? Behav Brain Sci. 1992;15:633–9.

55. Barrett DS, Cobb AG, Bentley G. Joint proprioception in normal, osteoarthritic and replaced knees. J Bone Joint Surg Br. 1991;73(1):53–6.

56. Ferrell W, Crighton A, Sturrock R. Position sense at the proximal interphalangeal joint is distorted in patients with rheumatoid arthritis of finger joints. Exp Physiol. 1992;77:678–80.

57. Andriacchi TP, Galante JO. Retention of the posterior cruciate in total knee arthroplasty. J Arthroplast. 1988;3(1):13–9.

58. Dorr LD, Ochsner JL, Gronley J, Perry J. Functional comparison of posterior cruciate-retained versus cruciate-sacrificed total knee arthroplasty. Clin Orthop Relat Res. 1988;236:36–43.

59. Gstoettner M, Raschner C, Dirnberger E, Leimser H, Krismer M. Preoperative proprioceptive training in patients with total knee arthroplasty. Knee. 2011;18(4):265–70.

60. Wada M, Kawahara H, Shimada S, Miyazaki T, Baba H. Joint proprioception before and after total knee arthroplasty. Clin Orthop Relat Res. 2002;403:161–7.

61. Moutzouri M, Gleeson N, Billis E, Tsepis E, Panoutsopoulou I, Gliatis J. The effect of total knee arthroplasty on patient's balance and incidence of falls: a systematic review. Knee Surg Sports Traumatol Arthrosc. 2017;25(11):3439–51.

62. Ries M. Effect of ACL sacrifice, retention, or substitution on kinematics after TKA. Orthopedics. 2007;30(8):74–6.

63. Baumann F, Bahadin Ö, Krutsch W, Zellner J, Nerlich M, Angele P, Tibesku CO. Proprioception after bicruciate-retaining total knee arthroplasty is comparable to unicompartmental knee arthroplasty. Knee Surg Sports Traumatol Arthrosc. 2017;25(6):1697–704.

64. Foley S, Ding C, Cicuttini F, et al. Physical activity and knee structural change: a longitudinal study using MRI. Med Sci Sports Exerc. 2007;39:426–34.

65. Zhang W, Moskowitz RW, Nuki G, Abramson S, Altman RD, Arden N, et al. OARSI recommendations for the management of hip and knee osteoarthritis. Part II: OARSI evidence-based expert consensus guidelines. Osteoarthritis Cartilage. 2008;16:137–62.

66. Brosseau L, Wells GA, Pugh AG, Smith CA, Rahman P, Alvarez Gallardo IC, et al. Ottawa panel evidence-based clinical practice guidelines for therapeutic exercise in the management of hip osteoarthritis. Clin Rehabil. 2015 [Epub ahead of print. PMID: 26400851 (pii: 0269215515606198)].

67. Walsh NE, Pearson J, Healey EL. Physiotherapy management of lower limb osteoarthritis. Br Med Bull. 2017:1–11. https://doi.org/10.1093/bmb/ldx01.

68. Ageberg E, Roos EM. Neuromuscular exercise as treatment of degenerative knee disease. Exerc Sport Sci Rev. 2015;43(1):14–22.

69. Gur H, Cakin N, Akova B, Okay E, Küçükoğlu S. Concentric versus combined concentric-eccentric isokinetic training: effects on functional capacity and symptoms in patients with osteoarthrosis of the knee. Arch Phys Med Rehabil. 2002;83(3):308–16.

70. Hunter DJ, Eckstein F. Exercise and osteoarthritis. J Anat. 2009;214:197–207.

71. Otterness IG, Eskra JD, Bliven ML, et al. Exercise protects against articular cartilage degeneration in the hamster. Arthritis Rheum. 1998;41:2068–76.

72. Carter DR, Beaupre GS, Wong M, Smith RL, Andriacchi TP, Schurman DJ. The mechanobiology of articular cartilage development and degeneration. Clin Orthop Relat Res. 2004;427(Suppl):69–77.

73. Kujala UM, Kettunen J, Paananen H, et al. Knee osteoarthritis in former runners, soccer players, weight lifters, and shooters. Arthritis Rheum. 1995;38:539–46.

74. Spector TD, Harris PA, Hart DJ, et al. Risk of osteo-arthritis associated with long-term weight-bearing sports: a radiologic survey of the hips and knees in female ex-athletes and population controls. Arthritis Rheum. 1996;39:988–95.
75. Vanwanseele B, Eckstein F, Knecht H, et al. Longitudinal analysis of cartilage atrophy in the knees of patients with spinal cord injury. Arthritis Rheum. 2003;48:3377–81.
76. Jan MH, Lin CH, Lin YF, Lin JJ, Lin DH. Effects of weight-bearing versus nonweight-bearing exercise on function, walking speed, and position sense in participants with knee osteoarthritis: a random-ized controlled trial. Arch Phys Med Rehabil. 2009;90(6):897–904.
77. Dziedzic K, Nicholls E, Hill S, Hammond A, Handy J, Thomas E, et al. Self-management approaches for osteoarthritis in the hand: a 2_2 factorial randomised trial. Ann Rheum Dis. 2015;74:108–18.
78. Osteras N, Hagen KB, Grotle M, Sand-Svartrud AL, Mowinckel P, Kjeken I. Limited effects of exer-cises in people with hand osteoarthritis: results from a randomized controlled trial. Osteoarthr Cartil. 2014;22:1224–33.
79. Zhang W, Doherty M, Leeb BF, Alekseeva L, Arden NK, Bijlsma JW, et al. EULAR evidence based rec-ommendations for the management of hand osteo-arthritis: report of a Task Force of the EULAR Standing Committee for International Clinical Studies Including Therapeutics (ESCISIT). Ann Rheum Dis. 2007;66:377–88.
80. Kjeken I, Grotle M, Hagen KB, Osteras N. Development of an evidence-based exercise pro-gramme for people with hand osteoarthritis. Scand J Occup Ther. 2015;22:103–16.
81. Nguyen C, et al. Rehabilitation (exercise and strength training) and osteoarthritis: a critical narra-tive review. Ann Phys Rehabil Med. 2016;59:190–5.
82. Philippon MJ. The role of arthroscopic ther-mal capsulorrhaphy in the hip. Clin Sports Med. 2001;20:817–29.
83. Rannou F, Poiraudeau S. Non-pharmacological approaches for the treatment of osteoarthritis. Best Pract Res Clin Rheumatol. 2010;24:93–106.
84. Fernandes L, Hagen KB, Bijlsma JW, Andreassen O, Christensen P, Conaghan PG, et al. EULAR recom-mendations for the non-pharmacological core man-agement of hip and knee osteoarthritis. Ann Rheum Dis. 2013;72:1125–35.
85. Villadsen A, Overgaard S, Holsgaard-Larsen A, Christensen R, Roos EM. Immediate efficacy of neuromuscular exercise in patients with severe osteoarthritis of the hip or knee: a secondary analy-sis from a randomized controlled trial. J Rheumatol. 2014;41:1385–94.
86. Hernandez-Molina G, Reichenbach S, Zhang B, Lavalley M, Felson DT. Effect of therapeutic exer-cise for hip osteoarthritis pain: results of a meta-analysis. Arthritis Rheum. 2008;59:1221–8.
87. Bennell KL, Hall M, Hinman RS. Osteoarthritis year in review 2015: rehabilitation and outcomes. Osteoarthr Cartil. 2016;24:58–70.
88. Slemenda C, Heilman DK, Brandt KD, et al. Reduced quadriceps strength relative to body weight: a risk factor for knee osteoarthritis in women? Arthritis Rheum. 1998;41:1951–9.
89. Hurley MV. The role of muscle weakness in the pathogenesis of osteoarthritis. Rheum Dis Clin N Am. 1999;25:283–98.
90. Al-Johani AH, Kachanathu SJ, Ramadan Hafez A, Al-Ahaideb A, Algarni AD, Meshari Alroumi A, et al. Comparative study of hamstring and quadriceps strengthening treatments in the management of knee osteoarthritis. J Phys Ther Sci. 2014;26:817–20.
91. Juhl C, Christensen R, Roos EM, et al. Impact of exercise type and dose on pain and disability in knee osteoarthritis: a systematic review and meta-regression analysis of randomized controlled trials. Arthritis Rheumatol. 2014;66:622–36.
92. Regnaux JP, Lefèvre-Colau MM, Trinquart L, Nguyen C, Boutron I, Brosseau L, et al. High-intensity versus low-intensity physical activity or exercise in people with hip or knee osteoarthritis. Cochrane Database Syst Rev. 2015;(10):CD010203.
93. Bartels EM, Juhl CB, Christensen R, Hagen KB, Danneskiold-Samsøe B, Dagfinrud H, Lund H. Aquatic exercise for the treatment of knee and hip osteoarthritis. Cochrane Database Syst Rev. 2016;(3):CD005523. doi: https://doi.org/10.1002/14651858. CD005523. pub3.
94. Fransen M, McConnell S, Hernandez-Molina G, et al. Exercise for osteoarthritis of the hip. Cochrane Database Syst Rev. 2014:CD007912. doi:https://doi.org/10.1002/14651858. CD007912.pub2.
95. Elkayam O, Wigler I, Tishler M, Rosenblum I, Caspi D, Segal R, et al. Effect of spa therapy in Tiberias on patients with rheumatoid arthritis and osteoarthritis. J Rheumatol. 1991;18(12):1799–803.
96. Sharma L. Proprioceptive impairment in knee osteo-arthritis. Rheum Dis Clin N Am. 1999;25:299–314.
97. Hurley MV, Scott DL. Improvement in quad-riceps sensorimotor function and disability of patients with knee osteoarthritis following a clini-cally practicable exercise regime. Br J Rheumatol. 1998;37:1181–7.
98. Hagert E, Lee J, Ladd AL. Innervation patterns of thumb trapeziometacarpal joint ligaments. J Hand Surg Am. 2012;37:706–14.
99. Ledin T, Kronhed AC, Möller C, Möller M, Odkvist LM, et al. Effects of balance training in elderly eval-uated by clinical tests and dynamic posturography. J Vestib Res. 1990;1:129–38.
100. Hain TC, Fuller L, Weil L, Kotsias J. Effects of T'ai Chi on balance. Arch Otolaryngol Head Neck Surg. 1999;125:1191–5.
101. Messier SP, Royer TD, Craven TE, O'Toole ML, Burns R, et al. Long-term exercise and its effect on balance in older, osteoarthritic adults: results from

the Fitness, Arthritis, and Seniors Trial (FAST). J Am Geriatr Soc. 2000;48:131–8.

102. Walla DJ, et al. Hamstring control and their unstable anterior cruciate ligament- deficient knee. Am J Sports Med. 1985;13:34.

103. Fitzgerald GK. Open versus closed kinetic chain exercise: issues in rehabilitation after anterior cruciate ligament reconstructive surgery. Phys Ther. 1997;77:1747–54.

104. Beard DJ, Dodd CA, Trundle HR, Simpson AH. Proprioception enhancement for anterior cruciate ligament deficiency. A prospective randomised trial of two physiotherapy regimes. J Bone Joint Surg Br. 1994;76:654–9.

105. Metgud S, Putti BB. Effect of proprioceptive exercises in osteoarthritic and replaced knees. Int J Physiother Res. 2015;3(6):1294–300.

106. Skyba DA, Radhakrishnan R, Rohlwing JJ, Wright A, Sluka KA. Joint manipulation reduces hyperalgesia by activation of monoamine receptors but not opioid or GABA receptors in the spinal cord. Pain. 2003;106(1–2):159–68.

107. Moss P, Sluka K, Wright A. The initial effects of knee joint mobilization on osteoarthritic hyperalgesia. Man Ther. 2006;12(2):109–18.

108. Pollard H, Ward G, Hoskins W, Hardy K. The effect of a manual therapy knee protocol on osteoarthritic knee pain: a randomised controlled trial. J Can Chiropr Assoc. 2008;52(4):229–42.

109. Tucker M, Brantingham JW, Myburg C. Relative effectiveness of a non-steroidal antiinflammatory medication (Meloxicam) versus manipulation in the treatment of osteo-arthritis of the knee. Eur J Chiropractic. 2003;50(3):163–83.

110. Hoeksma HL, Dekker J, Ronday HK, Heering A, van der Lubbe N, Vel C, et al. Comparison of manual therapy and exercise therapy in osteoarthritis of the hip: a randomized clinical trial. Arthritis Care Res. 2004;51(5):722–9.

111. Perlman AI, Sabina A, Williams AL, Njike VY, Katz DL. Massage therapy for osteoarthritis of the knee: a randomized controlled trial. Arch Intern Med. 2006;166(22):2533–8.

112. French HP, Brennan A, White B, Cusack T. Manual therapy for osteoarthritis of the hip or knee e a systematic review. Man Ther. 2011;16:109–17.

113. Nelson RM, Hayes KW, Currier DP. Clinical electrotherapy. 3rd ed. Stamford, CT, Appleton & Lange; 1999.

114. Rand SE, Goerlich C, Marchand K, Jablecki N. The physical therapy prescription. Am Fam Physician. 2007;76(11):1661–6.

115. Rutjes AW, Nüesch E, Sterchi R, et al. Therapeutic ultrasound for osteoarthritis of the knee or hip. Cochrane Database Syst Rev. 2010:CD003132. doi:10.1002/14651858. CD003132.pub2.

116. Knight KL. Cryotherapy for sports injuries management. Windsor: Human Kinetics; 1995.

117. Yurtkuran M, Kocagil T. TENS, electroacupuncture and ice massage: comparison of treatment for osteoarthritis of the knee. Am J Acupunct. 1999;27:133–40.

118. Hecht PJ, Backmann S, Booth RE, Rothman RH. Effects of thermal therapy on rehabilitation after total knee arthroplasty: a prospective randomized study. Clin Orthop Relat Res. 1983;178:198–201.

119. Barnes PM, Bloom B, Nahrin NL. Complementary and alternative medicine use among adults and children: United States, 2007. Natl Health Stat Rep. 2008;12:1–23.

120. Jong MC, van de Vijver L, Busch M, Fritsma J, Seldenrijk R. Integration of complementary and alternative medicine in primary care: what do patients want? Patient Educ Couns. 2012;89:417–22.

121. Nelson AE, Allen KD, Golightly YM, Goode AP, Jordan JM. A systematic review of recommendations and guidelines for the management of osteoarthritis: the chronic osteoarthritis management initiative of the U.S. bone and joint initiative. Semin Arthritis Rheum. 2014;43:701–12.

The manufacturer's authorised representative in the EU is Springer
Nature Customer Service Centre GmbH, Europaplatz 3, 69115 Heidelberg,
Germany. If you have any concerns regarding our products, please
contact ProductSafety@springernature.com

Printed and bound by CPI Group (UK) Ltd, Croydon, CR0 4YY
29/04/2026
02099516-0003